T0257963

Advances in Calcific Aortic Valve Disease Research

Advances in Calcific Aortic Valve Disease Research

Edited by **Samuel Ostroff**

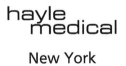

New York

Published by Hayle Medical,
30 West, 37th Street, Suite 612,
New York, NY 10018, USA
www.haylemedical.com

Advances in Calcific Aortic Valve Disease Research
Edited by Samuel Ostroff

© 2015 Hayle Medical

International Standard Book Number: 978-1-63241-025-2 (Hardback)

Contents

Preface

Calcific aortic valve disease (CAVD) is one of the most common forms of valve disease. It has become the most widespread cardiac valve disease in the economically advanced nations. Population ageing is one of the major reasons for this increasing rate. There is no definite treatment which may slow down the disease progression; valve replacement is the only adequate treatment. This book provides comprehensive information on bicuspid aortic valve (BAV) disease and discusses various therapeutic measures. This book will facilitate people to know about CAVD and other aspects concerning valve biology. It also emphasizes on the prospective chances of curbing the disease from rising in future.

All of the data presented henceforth, was collaborated in the wake of recent advancements in the field. The aim of this book is to present the diversified developments from across the globe in a comprehensible manner. The opinions expressed in each chapter belong solely to the contributing authors. Their interpretations of the topics are the integral part of this book, which I have carefully compiled for a better understanding of the readers.

At the end, I would like to thank all those who dedicated their time and efforts for the successful completion of this book. I also wish to convey my gratitude towards my friends and family who supported me at every step.

Editor

Bicuspid Aortic Valve

The Bicuspid Aortic Valve

Mehmet Demir

Additional information is available at the end of the chapter

1. Introduction

Bicuspid aortic valve (BAV) represents the most common cardiac congenital malformation in the adult age, with strong male predominance. It may occur in isolation, or in association with other congenital heart diseases. The BAV is seen in 1% to 2% of the population and may be complicated by aortic stenosis or aortic insufficiency and infective endocarditis. It may be associated with abnormalities of the aortic wall such as coarctation of the aorta, aortic dissection, and aortic aneurysm. Most patients with a BAV develop some complications during life [1,2].

Congenital coronary anomalies, coronary atherosclerosis, and calcification have been described in association with BAV[3].

BAV has been identified at a prevalence of 4.6 cas-es per 1000 live births. The prevalence of BAV according to sex has been found to be 7.1 cases per 1000 among male neonates, and 1.9 per 1000 among female neonates.

The congenitally BAV may function normally throughout life, may develop progressive calcification and stenosis or may develop regurgitation with or without infection. Aortic root dilatation is common in BAV, even when the valve is haemodynamically normal, and consequently aortic dissection usually occurs in previously asymptomatic patients [4,5].

Aortic stenosis and regurgitation, infective endocarditis and aortic dissection are the most common complications. Left coronary artery dominance is more common in patients with a BAV (29-56.8%) and in 90% of cases, the left main coronary artery is less than 5 mm in length [6-8]. The ignorance of these associations may cause an inadequate myocardial preservation and an increased risk of myocardial infarction[9,10].

Accordingly, associated congenital cardiovascular anomalies have been reported in as many as 25% of patients. Patent ductus arteriosus and ventricular septal defect are the most frequent heart defects associated with BAVdisease [11].

1.1. Embryology and pathogenesis

The definitive fetal cardiac structure is evident from the second week of gestation, whereas separation of the heart into four chambers is completed during the sixth and seventh weeks of gestation resulting in separated systemic and pulmonary circulation[12]. The process of aortic valve morphogenesis begins from the cardiac cushions located in the ventricular outflow tract of the primary heart tube. In the outflow tract, the truncal cushion swellings contribute to form three leaflet valves of the aorta and pulmonary artery.The initial endocardial cushions, which will contribute to all four cardiac valves, are formed by the thickening of the extracellular matrix in the region of the atrioventricular and outflow tract.This process is initiated by the secretion of extracellular matrix proteins such as fibronectin and transferrin across the cardiac jelly to the adjacent endocardium. The endocardium then secretes transforming growth factor beta family members, which act synergistically with bone morphogenetic protein-2 secreted by the myocardium, to increase mesenchyme formation and proliferation, which results in the growth of the endothelial cushions. The myocardial cells then invade the margins of the cellular endothelial cushions [13].

The semilunar valves form the division of the truncus arteriosus into two separate channels which form the aortic and pulmonary trunks..The channels are created by the fusion of two truncal ridges across the lumen. In each channel a third swelling occurs opposite the first two which will form the 3rd leaflet. In the normal aortic valve the left and right leaflets of the adult valve are formed from the respective swellings while the posterior leaflet is formed from a swelling in the aortic trunk.

The pathogenesis of BAV is not yet fully understood. There is certainly a genetic component, especially given the association of BAV with other congenital abnormalities. However, fusion of the right and left valve cushions at the beginning ofvalvulogenesis appears to be a key factor in BAV formation [14].

A previous study suggested that BAV is a consequence of the anomalous behavior of cells derived from the neural crest because BAV often is associated with congenital aortic arch malformations and other neural crest-derived systems [15]. Other studies suggest that extracellular matrix proteins may affect the initiation of cell differentiation during valvulogenesis, while a molecular abnormality in this process may lead to the formation of abnormal cusps [16,17]. Some researchers suggest that a molecular abnormality in the extracellular matrix may lead to abnormal valvulogenesis, becouse matrix proteins help direct cell differentiation and cusp formation during valvulogenesis [16-18]. This could also explain why BAVis often linked to other cardiovascular anomalies.

These abnormalities cause the fusion of two cusps and lead to one larger cusp; therefore, the BAV usually includes two unequally sized cusps, the presence of a central raphe, and smooth cusp margin. A previous studies showed that raphal position was between the right and left cusp in 86% of cases [19]. An anomalous origin of coronary arteries depends on the spatial orientation of the two cusps. When the orientation of the cusps is anteroposterior, the coronary arteries originate from the anterior sinus or if cusps laterlateral oriented the right coronary artery originate from the common trunk and right Valsava's sinus [20].

A recent study has demonstrated that BAVs with fused right and noncoronary leaflets and those with fused right and left leaflets are different etiological entities. BAVs with fused right and noncoronary leaflets result from a morphogenetic defect that occurs before cardiac outflow tract septation on the basis of an exacerbated nitric oxide-dependent epithelialto-mesenchymal transformation. On the other hand, BAVs with fused right and left leaflets result from anomalous septation of the proximal portion of the cardiac outflow tract, caused by dysfunctional neural crest cells [21].

The pulmonary valve can also be bicuspid, although this is much rarer and is most commonly associated with congenital heart disease such as Tetralogy of Fallot. There have been less than 10 cases reported in the literature of an isolated bicuspid pulmonary valve [22].

Deficient fibrillin-1 content in the vasculature of BAV patients may trigger matrix metalloproteinase production, thereby leading to matrix disruption and dilation. It has been noted that the fibrillin-1 content was remarkably reduced in the aorta of BAV patients, compared with that of patients with a tricuspid aortic valve. Aortic elasticity measurements of BAV patients suggest that diminished aortic elasticity is at least part of its causation [23-25].

1.2. Anatomy

The bicuspid valve is composed of two leaflets, of which one is usually larger (due to fusion of two cusps leading to one larger cusp), and unequal cusp size the presence of a central raphe (usually in the center of the larger of the two cusps). The raphe or fibrous ridge is the site of congenital fusion of the two components of the conjoined cusps and does not contain valve tissue (Figure 1) Three morphologies are identified: type 1, fusion of right coronary cusp and left coronary cusp; type 2, fusion of right coronary cusp and noncoronary cusp; and type 3, fusion of left coronary cusp and noncoronary cusp. The most common is type 1 (70% to 85%), followed by type 2 (10% to 30%) and most rare type 3 (1%) [13,19,26] (Figure 2).

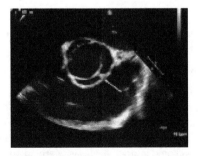

Figure 1. Transesophageal short-axis view of a BAV. There is fusion of the right and left cusps. The arrow points to the raphe.

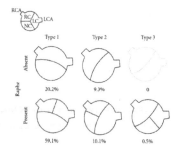

Figure 2. The classification and incidence of BAVs.

The site of cusp fusion can have e • ects on the prognosis of BAV [27], with the suggestion that type 1 BAVs are more likely to stenose as adults while type 2 valves will have complications at a younger age. The fused valve leaflet in BAV is actually smaller in area. Valvular incompetence is usually caused by the redundancy of one cusp, since the two cusps usually have different dimensions [28]

The coronary anatomy can be abnormal. Most patients with BAV disease have a left dominant coronary circulation [29]. This left coronary can arise from the pulmonary artery. The left main can also be up to 50% shorter than in normal in up to 90% of cases. This is an important consideration for any aortic valve surgery. The commonest abnormality associated with BAV is dilatation of the thoracic aorta, also known as aortopathy. This is thought not only to be due to the altered flow in the aorta, but also due to cellular structural abnormalities including decreased fibrillin, causing smooth muscle cell detachment, and cell death [30].

The other abnormality found in conjunction with BAV disease is coarctation of the aorta. [22,31]. The presence of coarctation and a poor result from repair can lead to more rapid failure of the valve or aortic dissection.

1.3. Genetics

BAV is an inheritable disorder, with a family recurrence rate of approximately 35% [33]. Recent clinical studies have reported a 9% prevalence of BAV in first-degree relatives of patients with BAV which was the estimated population prevalance of 1-2% [33-35].

BAV is likely due to mutations in different genes with dissimilar patterns of inheritance [33].

The first genetic cause of BAV is Anderson syndrome, which is reported to be a result of mutations in the potassium channel gene KCNJ2 (chromosome 17q24.3)], whereas it clinically presents as ventricular arrhythmias, periodic paralysis, and scoliosis [36]. Another mutations in a gene called NOTCH1(gene map locus 9q34.3), a transmembrane receptor that has a role in determining cell outcome in organogenesis, were noted in two families with BAV [37]. Regions 18q, 5q, and 13q are reported to contain genes responsible for BAV and/or associated cardiovascular malformations [38,39]. The region 10q contains the ACTA2 gene, which encodes for smooth muscle alpha-actin (ACTA2), and mutation in this gene can result in thoracic aneurysm and, in some instances, BAV [40]. Also the ubiquitin fusion degradation 1–like gene UFD1L (chromosome 22q11.2) expressed in the outflow tract during embryogenesis is down-regulated in BAV tissue when compared with trileaflet valve tissue [41]. The UFD1L gene encodesa component of a multi-enzyme complex involved in the degradation of ubiquitin fusion proteins, and is highly expressed during embryogenesis in certain tissues. It seems to play a key role in the development of ectoderm-derived structures, including neural crest cells.downregulation of the UFD1L gene, hypothetically resulting from an anomalous behavior of neural crest cells, may lead to reduced degradation activities, and may finally lead to fusion of valve cushions, a key factor in the development of congenital BAV[42]. Recent American College of Cardiology (ACC)/American Heart Association (AHA) adult congenital heart disease guidelines suggest echocardiographic screening for BAV and aortopathy in first-degree relatives of patients with BAV [43,44].

Although these valves are more common in males than females by a factor of 2:1 in the general population, the prevalance was equal in males and females in families having more than one affected individual [45,46].

2. Diagnosis

Clinical findings are usually limited to auscultation with most patients having an ejection systolic murmur heard loudest at the apex [47]. The S1 usually is normal but sometimes may be associated with ejection click. The S2 is soft, and when aortic stenosis is present, S2 occurs simultaneously with P2. In aortic stenosis, an ejection systolic murmur is heard in the left second intercostal space but may also be transmitted to the carotid arteries. If aortic incompetence is present, a diastolic murmur of aortic regurgitation may be heard.

The electrocardiogram is usually normal; and ECG changes are not specific in patients with BAV: left ventricular hypertrophy, atrial enlargement, and arrhythmias may be present.

The mainstay of diagnosis is echocardiography (transthoracic or transoesophageal) which can provide a definitive diagnosis in the majority of patients [92% sensitivity and 96% specificity) [48,49]. Transesophageal echocardiography (TEE) is also very important for evaluating the aortic valve and thoracic aorta, whereas the sensitivity and specifity of multiplane technique for assessing aortic valve morphology is high [13].

The parasternal short axis view allows for direct visualization of the valve cusps. In this view the normal triangular opening shape is lost, becoming more "fish mouth-"like in appearance, more similar to the mitral valve. This is especially pronounced in systole, as in diastole the raphe can appear similar to a commissure of the third cusp. Differentiating severe bicuspid aortic stenosis from severe other aortic stenosis can also be difficult. In order to establish the diagnosis, the valve must be visualized in systole in the short-axis view. In the long-axis view, the valve often has an eccentric closure line and there is doming of the leaflets. If there is uncertainty in diagnosis, a TEE can improve visualization of the leaflets [50].

For BAV associated with stenosis, mean gradient and maximal flow velocity should be measured, but when regurgitation is present, the effective regurgitant area and Doppler jet size should be evaluated. For asymptomatic patients with aortic stenosis, echocardiography is recommended for evaluating disease progression. In asymptomatic patients, TTE recommended: every year for severe aortic stenosis, ever 1-2 years for moderate aortic stenosis and every 3-5 years for mild aortic stenosis [51].

In patients with poor acustic window, cardiac magnetic resonance (MRI) and multidetector computed tomography are useful for measuring the aortic valve area and is an alternative method to echocardiography in selected cases. MRI especially will enable views of the valve to be obtained without interference from calcification. It also allows for excellent assessment of the aorta. A recent study of 123 patients with confirmed BAV found that 10% of the patients were misidentified as having a tricuspid valve using transthoracic echo and 28% had a nondiagnostic study, in comparison to 4% being misidentified as having a tricuspid valve by MRI and 2% having a non-diagnostic study [52].

The current guidelines suggest that cardiac magnetic resonance imaging or cardiac computed tomography is reasonable in patients with BAVs when aortic root dilatation is detected by echocardiography to further quantify severity of dilatation and involvement of theascending aorta (Clas IIa; Level of Evidence: B)[53].

3. Clinic

The clinical presentation of patients with BAV can vary from severe valve disease in infancy to asymptomatic valve disease in old age. It may be associated with abnormalities of the aortic wall such as coarctation of the aorta, aortic dissection, and aortic aneurysm. Most patients with a BAV develop some complications during life [1,2].

Congenital coronary anomalies, coronary atherosclerosis, and calcification have been described in association with BAV[3].

The congenitally BAV may function normally throughout life, may develop progressive calcification and stenosis or may develop regurgitation with or without infection. Aortic root dilatation is common in BAV, even when the valve is haemodynamically normal, and consequently aortic dissection usually occurs in previously asymptomatic patients [4,5].

Sudden death may occur as a result of obstruction of the left ventricular outflow tract by a congenital BAV [54]. BAV are in most cases remain undetected until infection or calcification supervenes [55].

Aortic stenosis and regurgitation, infective endocarditis and aortic dissection are the most common complications. Left coronary artery dominance is more common in patients with a BAV (29-56.8%) and in 90% of cases, the left main coronary artery is less than 5 mm in length [7,8]. The ignorance of these associations may cause an inadequate myocardial preservation and an increased risk of myocardial infarction[9,10].

Symptoms associated with aortic stenosis are angina pectoris, syncope, and congestive heart failure. The most common complication of aortic stenosis is congestive heart failure symptomatically presented with dyspnea, which is a result of combined diastolic and systolic dysfunction [56]. Angina pectoris occurs in patients with severe aortic stenosis and in those who do not have coronary artery disease; it may be a result of ventricular hypertrophy.

Syncope is another common symptom in patients with BAV. Syncope reflects the cerebral hypoperfusion caused by the inability to increase stroke volume during physical activity.

The clinical presentation in patients with BAV and presence of other cardiac congenital defects depends from structural complexity of the heart. In patients with interventricular septal defects, the clinical presentation depends on the size of the defect area and the grade of aortic stenosis. If the interventricular defect is small, the patient may be asymptomatic, but when the interventricular defect is large, cardiac output will decrease and Eisenmenger syndrome will develop.

Two large recent series reported that clinical course of unoperated patients with BAV depends on age, stenosis, and aortic incompetence. The severe aortic stenosis, and severe aortic incompetence in older patients increases the risk of primary cardiac events including cardiac death. Both these studies suggest that intervention on the basis of early symptoms or incipient cardiac dysfunction may decreases the mortality of patients with BAV [57,58].

The natural history of BAV has been evaluated several cohort studies. It is known to be variable and of course somewhat dependent on associated abnormalities. It can range from severe aortic stenosis in childhood to asymptomatic disease until old age. There have indeed been incidental findings of a minimally calcified BAV in patients in their 70s.More commonly however [in around 75% of patients] there is progressive fibrocalcific stenosis of the valve eventually requiring surgery. This usually leads to presentation in middle age only around 2% of children have clinically significant BAV disease [59].

The prevalence of fibrosis, cystic medial necrosis, elastic fragmentation, and inflammation has been shown to be significantly higher in patients with fusion of the left coronary and right coronary cusps. fusion of the left coronary and right coronary cusps was associated with a larger aortic root diameter and a smaller aortic arch,than was fusion of the right coronary and non-coronary cusps. Another study demonstraed that fusion of the right coronary and non-coronary cusps correlated with the more rapid growth of ascending aortic diameter in the pediatric population [60-63].

There have been a couple of studies looking at long-term followup of patients with unoperated BAV. A cohort of 212 asymptomatic patients with BAV were found to have the same 20-year survival rate as the normal population but an increased frequency of cardiac events including aortic valve surgery, ascending aorta surgery and any other cardiovascular surgery. Predictive factors for cardiovascular events were found to be age ≥50 years and valve degeneration at diagnosis while baseline ascending aorta ≥40 mm independently predicted surgery for aorta dilatation. Another study [64] 642 patients were followed up for a mean of 9 years, again with a 10-year survival rate similar to the normal population [96%]. One or more primary cardiac events occurred in 25% including cardiac death in 3, intervention on aortic valve or ascending aorta in 22%, aortic dissection or aneurysm in 2%, and congestive heart failure requiring hospital admission in 2%. Independent predictors of primary cardiac events were age older than 30 years, moderate or severe aortic stenosis, and moderate or severe aortic regurgitation [50].

In the another study [61].the incidence of aortic dissection was found to be 1.5% in all patients regardless of the progression of BAV; however this increased markedly in patients aged 50 or older at baseline to 17.4% and even more in those found to have aneurysm formation at baseline to [44.9%]. 25-year rate for aortic surgery was 25% and there was a significant burden of progression of disease to cause aortic dissection with 49 of the 384 patients without baseline aneurysms developing them during followup [22].

Although the clinical presentation of patients with BAV can vary from severe valve disease in infancy to asymptomatic valve or thoracic aortic disease in old age, symptomstypically develop in adulthood. The clinical manifestations relate to the function of the aortic valve,the aortopathy/dissection, and acquired complications such as endocarditis. However in childhood, BAV disease is commonly asymptomatic [61]

Estimates of late cardiac events were approximately 25% at a mean age of 44 years in the study from Toronto and 40% at a mean age of 52 years in the Olmsted County study [62,63]. In the Olmsted County series, 27% of adults with BAV and no significant valve disease at baseline required cardiovascular surgery within 20 years of follow-up. Twenty-two percent of the patients in the Toronto cohort required intervention within 9 years of follow-up. In both studies, age was an important determinant of outcomes supporting the notion held by many that eventually most patients with BAV would require some form of intervention.

3.1. Aortic stenosis

A common complication of BAV disease is aortic stenosis. BAV is recognized as a frequent cause of aortic stenosis in adults. Aortic stenosis has been found in 72% of adults with BAV. In 388 patients with severe aortic valve disease alone, BAVs were found in 45% of the patients with aortic stenosis and 24% of the patients with aortic regurgitation. In 110 patients with severe combined aortic and mitral valve disease, BAVs were found in only 12% [64].

Among the 600 patients analyzed, 213 (36%) had pure aortic stenosis, 265 (44%) had pure aortic regurgitation and 122 (20%) had combined stenosis and regurgitation. BAVs represented 18%, as the third most important cause of aortic disorder following degenerative and rheumatic changes, followed by infective endocarditis (5%) [65].

The main symptoms are exertional dyspnea, syncope, and chest pain. These patients should be evaluated and managed similarly to patients with tricuspid aortic valve stenosis.

In the Joint Study of the Natural History of Congenital Heart Defects, one-third of the children in the cohort had increases in catheterization gradients during the 4- to 8-year follow-up period. In the follow-up study, children with baseline peak left ventricular to aortic gradients >50 mm Hg were at risk for serious cardiac events at a rate of 1.2% per year. In theUnited Kingdom cohort.20% of children with mild aortic stenosis at baselinehad mild disease after 30 years of follow-up. Age was the primary determinant of valvular disease progression [50,66].

In adults, with BAV, stenosis occurs by similar methods to the process in patients with tricuspid aortic valves. It is felt to be due to calcification, endothelial dysfunction, inflammation, lipoprotein deposition, and ossification of the aortic side of the valve leaflets. There has been a suggestion that leaflet orientation may be a predictive factor in the rate of valve stenosis. The folding and creasing of the valves and the turbulent flow are felt to contribute to development of fibrosis and calcification [59].more rapid progression in aortic valve gradients occurred in patients with anteroposteriorly located cusps[60]. However, not all studies have found this association, and the 2 large studies in adults have not identified leaflet orientation as a risk factor for late adverse events. Olmsted County study identified a composite index of valve degeneration, which incorporated valve thickening, calcification, and mobility, that was an independent predictor of long-term cardiac events in a population of adults with no baseline valve dysfunction. The predictive role of both morphology and function in adults with BAV parallels that observed in series examining older adults with aortic stenosis mostly of acquired basis [50,62,63].

3.2. Aortic incompetence

Primary aortic regurgitation without infective endocarditis was uncommon, and 32% had an apparently normally functioning aortic valve [67].

One cohort of 118 BAV patients found that of 70 patients without aortic stenosis, 28 (40% had moderate to severe aortic regurgitation. The mechanisms of aortic incompetence in children are usually due to prolapsing cusps, myxoid degeneration, postvalve surgery and after balloon valvuloplasty or endocarditis, while as the patients age dilatation of the ascending aorta can lead to a functionally regurgitant valve[68,69]. With age, aortic incompetence may also develop secondary to dilation of the ascending aorta. In the Olmstead study of asymptomatic adults, 47% had some degree of aortic incompetence at baseline; however, interventions for severe aortic incompetence were relatively uncommon, occurring in only 3% of the cohort during follow-up. In the Toronto study 21% of the population had moderate or severe aortic incompetence at baseline; however, only 6% had an intervention for symptomatic aortic incompetence or progressive left ventricular dysfunction [62,63].

3.3. Aortopathy/aortic dissection

BAV patients tend to develop vascular abnormalities of the aorta, such as dilation, coarctation and dissection. Aortic dilation in BAV patients is thought to be caused by intrinsic aortic disease that is characterized by cystic medial necrosis and disruption of the extracellular matrix due to fibrillin deficiency. BAV is often associated with dilatation of the aortic root and the ascending aorta. This is otherwise known as aortopathy. This can lead to aneurysm and dissection. The dilatation has been reported during childhood, and it has also been suggested that increased aortic size at baseline is predictive for earlier dilatation and worse outcomes. Aortic size is larger generally in patients with BAV compared to those with normal valves. The most likely risk factor for progression is felt to be age. Aortic root size itself is related to valve morphology and the presence of significant disease [22,6]; however, a recent study did suggest that while most patients with BAV and ascending aortic aneurysm had severe valve dysfunction, there was a small proportion of patients (5%) who did have aneurysm formation without any aortic valve dysfunction [50].

In the ascending aorta as well as the pulmonary trunk, the severity of cystic medial necrosis, elastic fragmentation and changes in the smooth muscle cell orientation have been found to be significantly more severe in patients with bicuspid valves than in those with tricuspid valves.

Factors leading to aortic dissection four years after the Bentall operation have been considered to be an impact of congenital BAV or proximal anastomosis of venous grafts, or both [70].

Studies have suggested that patients with BAV have an intrinsic defect in the aortic wall that results in aortic disease, regardless of aortic valve function. BAV was associated with significantly less intimal change, and less fragmentation and loss of elastic tissue, compared with patients with a tricuspid aortic valve. Type I and III collagens were significantly decreased in dilated aortas of BAV patients, compared with controls, particularly at the convexity. Expression of messenger RNA [ribonucleic acid] for collagens was lower than normal only in the regurgitant subgroup. Fewer smooth muscle cells and greater severity of elastic fiber fragmentation were observed at the convexity than at the concavity [71-73].

Among 119 cases of fatal dissecting aneurysm of the aorta, 11 cases of congenital BAV (9%) were observed. Among the latter, three had coarctation of the aorta and one had Turner's syndrome without coarctation. In each case, cystic medial necrosis of the aorta was present. Hypertension was either established or inferred from cardiac weight in 73% of the cases. The high incidence among subjects with dissecting aneurysm suggested a causative relationship between BAV and aortic dissecting aneurysm [74].

Many theories have been postulated for the mechanism of BAV aortopathy. For a long time there has been felt to be a genetic component; however there is increasing evidence for a haemodynamic mechanism. It is felt that it is due to defects in the aortic media, such as elastin fragmentation, loss of smooth muscle cells, and an increase in collagen [6,22]. Systemic features have also been noted in BAV patients which may predispose to aneurysm formation including systemic endothelial dysfunction and higher plasma levels of matrix metalloproteinases [75].

Pathological examination of surgical specimens from the aortic wall of patients with aortic dissection associated with BAV showed cystic medial necrosis or mucoid degeneration [76].

Matrix metalloproteinases (endogenous enzymes that degrade matrix components) have been implicated in atherosclerotic aortic aneurysm formation and appear to be elevated in the aorta of patients with BAVs [77].

The histological findings of BAV are nonspecific, and had been described by several authors in patients with Marfan syndrome [78-80]. The histopathological appearance of thoracic aortic aneurysm in Marfan and BAV is similar, and includes evidence of vascular smooth muscle cell (VSMC) apoptosis and extracellular matrix degeneration in the absence of a significant inflammatory response [81].

Abnormalities in the ascending aorta of the patients with BAV, specifically premature medial layer VSMC apoptosis, have been described, explaining the higherthan-expected prevalance of aortic dissection in these patients [82].

Also recently studies show less elastic tissue in the aortas of BAV patients [83,84].

In patient with BAV there are fibrillin, fibronectin, and tenascin abnormality. Additionally Bonderman et al suggested that a primary role for VMSC apoptosis in the development of aneurysm these patients [85].

The FBN1 gene encodes fibrillin-1, a large glycoprotein that is secreted from cells and deposited in the extracellular matrix in structures called microfibrils. Microfibrils are found at the periphery of elastic fibers, including the elastic fibers in the medial layer of the ascending aorta, and in tissues not associated with elastic fibers.

The histopathological appearance of thoracic aortic aneurysm in Marfan and BAV is similar, and includes evidence of VSMC apoptosis and extracellular matrix degeneration in the absence of a significant inflammatory response. Abnormalities in the ascending aorta of the patients with BAV, specifically premature medial layer smooth muscle cell apoptosis, have been described, explaining the higherthan-expected prevalance of aortic dissection in these patients [82,83].

Aortic root dilation has been documented in childhood, suggesting that this process begins early in life. Furthermore, children with BAV have greater increases in aortic dimensions than do children with trileaflet valves. In both children and adults, progressive dilation of the aorta is more common in patients with larger aortas at baseline. In BAV disease, the aortic annulus, sinus, and proximal ascending aorta are larger than those found in adults with trileaflet valves [50].

In the Olmsted County study, the prevalence of ascending aorta dilation (>40 mm) was 15% and in the subset of patients with repeat measurements, the prevalence increased to 39% at study completion. Dilation of the ascending aorta was an independent risk factor for ascending aorta surgery. Although there are a number of risk factors associated with dilation of the ascending aorta including increased systolic blood pressure, male sex, and significant valve disease, the most important variable is likely age [50,63,64]. Aortic root size is shown to be related to valve morphology and the presence of significant valve disease. In the Toronto series, the prevalence of dissection was 0.1% per patient-year of follow-up, and in the Olmsted County study, there were no cases of dissection. Despite the low rates of dissection, the increasedprevalence of BAV disease relative to Marfan syndrome make dissections due to BAV equal to or more common than dissections due to Marfan syndrome [86]. Dissection in BAV, when it occurs, typically involves the ascending aorta, but involvement of the descending aorta has been reported in older patients. Although dissection is more common in patients with dilated aortas, there are reports of dissection in normal-sized aortic roots and after valve replacement. Risk factors for dissection have included aortic size, aortic stiffness, male sex, family history, and the presence of other lesions such as coarctation of the aorta or Turner syndrome [50].

3.4. Endocarditis

Endocarditis is more common in BAV. The estimated incidence is 0.16% per year in unoperated children and adolescents [87]. In adults the case series by Michelena give an incidence of 2% per year [56].

Outcomes in BAV patients with infective endocarditis tend to be worse than in those with normal valves. A recent study of 310 patients with infective endocarditis found that the 50 patients with BAV were younger at presentation and had a higher incidence of aortic perivalvular abscess. In-hospital mortality and 5-year survival were also comparable to patients with normal valves [22].

Most patients are unaware of their condition until the onset of infective endocarditis

Patients with BAV endocarditis are young, and there is strong male predominance. Staphylococci and viridans streptococci account for nearly three-quarters of the cases affecting BAVs. Endocarditis can lead to severe acute aortic incompetence, heart failure and it is poorly tolerated [88].

Endocarditis risk was estimated to range between 2% or 0.3%/year. Because the risk of endocarditis is felt to be low, the ACC/AHA practice guidelines no longer suggest bacterial endocarditis prophylaxis in patients with straightforward BAV disease, except in patients with a prior history ofendocarditis [50,89].

3.5. Coronary artery disorders

Some reports have also suggested that the involvement of coronary arteries, including congenital coronary artery anomalies, coronary artery fistulas, spontaneous coronary artery dissection, immediate bifurcation and a shorter length of the left main coronary artery [6,13]. The incidence of left dominance in BAVs has been found to be unusually high (24.4-56.8%), compared with the incidence in tricuspid valves [9.5%]. Patients with BAVs have higher incidence of immediate bifurcation of the left main coronary artery, and higher incidence of left main coronary length less than 10 mm. The mean length of the left main coronary artery is significantly shorter in BAV patients [90].

Anomalous origins of the right 20,21 and left 22 coronary arteries, association with annuloaortic ectasia, and anomalous origins of the left circumflex coronary artery 23 and single left coronary artery,24 have been noted in patients with BAVs. Spontaneous coronary artery dissection may occur in BAV patients [91]

There have also been some case reports describing patients with BAVdisease associated with coronary heart disease [92] and even with acute myocardial infarction[10].

Also Recently studies[93]Yuan et al. suggested that the prevalence rate of angiographic coronary heart disease was higher among the patients with BAVdisease.

3.6. Congenital heart defects

Patent ductus arteriosus and ventricular septal defect are the most frequent congenital heart defects associated with BAV. Patent ductus arteriosus is usually present in pediatric patients with BAV and may be associated with hand anomalies. BAV is reported to be present in up to 30 % of adult patients with small ventricular septal defects. However, BAV may also be associated with large ventricular septal defects and poor clinical outcome. There is significantly higher incidence of aortic arch obstruction (51.1%). The frequency of BAV in specimens with complete transposition of great arteries has been found to be 1% [13,50].

Hypoplastic left heart syndrome, complete atrioventricular canal defect, Ebstein's anomaly, partial or total anomalous pulmonary venous return, tetralogy of Fallot, double-outlet right ventricle, septal left ventricular diverticulum,Williams syndrome,Down syndrome and annuloaortic ectasia are occasionally associated with BAV. Shone's complex, which is defined by four cardiovascular defects including supravalvular mitral membrane, valvular mitral stenosis with a parachute mitral valve, subaortic stenosis and aortic coarctation, is a rare entity and forms another association in BAV cases [94].

It has been reported that BAV is presented in > 50 % of patients with coarctation of the aorta [COA]. Patients with COA and BAV are reported to have more severe disease associated with aortic stenosis, aortic regurgitation, and aortic aneurysm. The risk of dissection of the aorta and death is greater when COA and BAV are comorbid.

Turner syndrome characterized by a defect in or the absence of one X chromosome. Except for gonadal dysgenesis, cardiovascular defects are commonly present in this group of patients. Clinical research on patients with Turner Syndrome reports that BAV is present in 30% of cases, that over 95% of BAV s result from fusion of the right and left coronary leaflets, and that aortic ascending diameters are significantly greater in this group of patients [13].

3.7. Thromboembolism

Thrombus formation in a native BAV is a rare complicaton. Pathological studies have indicated that post-inflammatory changes ocur in the resected BAV, which is prone to develop thrombosis on the valve surface or in the calcification area [95].

Microthrombus formation and valve thickening with incompetence could result in embolization, and subsequent cerebrovascular events [96].

Embolization from calcific BAVs may lead to stroke and myocardial infarction. Conservative management with anticoagulation, to treat associated post-stagnation thrombosis, or aortic valve replacement as the treatment, is debatable [97].

4. Management

4.1. Medical

Medical therapies are to try and alleviate symptoms and slow progression. It is generally felt that blood pressure should be aggressively controlled to try and slow the progression of aortopathy [51].

High blood pressure should be aggressively treated in patients with BAV disease. In Marfan-associated aortopathy, treatment with beta-blockers to slow the rate of progression is the standard of care at many centers, although debate exists about their effectiveness [50,101]. The ACC/AHA guidelines for the management of adult congenital heart disease and guidelines for the management of patients with valvular heart disease suggest that it is reasonable to use beta-blockers in this population [Class IIa recommendation] [53]. There are emerging data in animal models and in 1 small study in humans supporting the use of angiotensin II receptor blockers to decreased aortic root dilation in Marfan syndrome [50]. Whether these agents will have a role in BAV aortopathy has not yet been demonstrated. Also long-term vasodilator therapy in BAV disease with aortic regurgitation is only recommended if there is concomitant systemic hypertension [47]. The relationship between risk factors for atherosclerosis and the development and progression of degenerative aortic valve disease has been well studied [99]. However, the role of treatment with cholesterol-lowering agents is unresolved. The use of lipid lowering agents specifically in young patients with BAV has not been studied, and the current ACC/AHA guidelines for the management of patients with valvular heart disease do not endorse the use of statins to slow the degenerative process in this population [51]. Concomitant conditions and risk factors should be treated as in the normal population.

4.2. Surgical

Indications for valve surgery in patients with BAV are similar to those with tricuspid aortic valve disease or degenerative aortic valve disease [100].

The 2006 AHA/ACC guidelines also suggest concomitant replacement of the ascending aorta if it is greater than 45 mm in diameter [51]. Estimated 15-year freedom from complications was 86% in patients with an aortic diameter less than 40 mm, dropping down to 81% in those with diameter 40–44 and 43% in patients with a diameter 45 mm or greater.

When rheumatic disease is excluded, a significant portion of adults undergoing surgery for aortic valve disease will have a congenitally malformed valve. During childhood, insertion of a prosthetic valve is suboptimal because of the continuing growth of the child. Fortunately, at this stage, the aortic valve is usually not calcified and valvuloplasty can successfully disrupt the commissural fusion and relieve obstruction. Valvuloplasty is the interventional strategy of choice in children and in some young adults with BAV and aortic stenosis. Symptomatic aortic stenosis is an indication for intervention, similar to standard indications for trileaflet valve disease. However, in the pediatric setting, indications include children with peak-topeak gradients >50 mm Hg who develop symptom at rest or with exercise. An additional indication includes asymptomatic children with peak-to-peak gradients >60 mm Hg. In adulthood, aortic valve replacement is the most common intervention for either aortic valve stenosis or incompetence, and valvuloplasty is rarely performed [50,51,62].

BAV disease involves younger patients and involves both the valves and the ascendan aorta; therefore, surgical decision making is more complicated. Approximately 30% of adults undergoing aortic valve replacement will also need aortic root surgery[63]. The guideline suggest that a cutoff of 5.0 cm be used for intervention or 4.5 cm if the surgery is otherwise being performed for valve indications. In addition, suggest that changes in root size more than 0.5 cm/year are an indication for root replacement [53].

Recently published Guidelines [53] for the diagnosis and management of patients with thoracic aortic disease recommendations for BAV are summarized below:

CLASS I

1. First-degree relatives of patients with a BAV, premature onset of thoracic aortic disease with minimal risk factors, and/or a familial form of thoracic aortic aneurysm and dissection should be evaluated for the presence of a BAV and asymptomatic thoracic aortic disease. (Level of Evidence: C)

2. All patients with a BAV should have both the aortic root and ascending thoracic aorta evaluated for evidence of aortic dilatation (Level of Evidence: B)

3. Should undergo elective operation at smaller diameters (4.0 to 5.0 cm)to avoid acute dissection or rupture. ()Level of Evidence: C)

4. Patients with a growth rate of more than 0.5 cm/year in an aorta that is less than 5.5 cm in diameter should be considered for operation. (Level of Evidence: C)

5. Patients undergoing aortic valve repair or replacement and who have an ascending aorta or aortic root of greater than 4.5 cm should be considered for concomitant repair of the aortic root or replacement of the ascending aorta. (Level of Evidence: C)

6. Elective aortic replacement is reasonable for patients with BAV when the ratio of maximal ascending or aortic root area ($\pi r2$) in cm2 divided by the patient's height in meters exceeds 10 (CLASS IIa, Level of Evidence: C).

In regard to valve surgery, there is controversy regarding the use of the Ross procedure and the use of valve repairs in this population. Abnormalities of the media are seen in both the aorta and the pulmonary artery in BAV disease. Intrinsic abnormalities in the wall of the pulmonary artery [neoaorta] may contribute to progressive neoaortic root dilation and/or aortic regurgitation when the pulmonary root is placed in the systemic position [101].

When to surgically treat asymptomatic patients with BAV remains controversial. The risk of sudden death in asymptomatic adult patients with severe aortic stenosis is reported to be less than 1% per year, however, current practice guidelines recommended aortic valve replacement in patients with reduced left ventricular systolic function (EF< 50%) without other explanation even when they are asymptomatic [51].

For high-risk patients to undergo conventional novel methods including aortic balloon valvulotomy or transfemoral valve implantation may be helpful. A patient considered inoperable should be treated orally with angiotensin converting enzyme (ACE) inhibitors, diuretics, and digitalis. In patients with depressed LV associated with pulmonary congestion and atrial fibrillation, diuretics and digitalis may be used with the understanding that in some cases intensive hemodynamic monitoring is needed. Patients with aortic root dilatation > 4.0cm who are not candidate for surgical treatment should be given β-adrenergic blocking agents [51].

4.3. Pregnancy

During pregnancy there are changes in hemodynamics as well as changes in the aortic media, and therefore, women with BAV and significant aortic stenosis and/or dilated aortic roots are at risk for complications during pregnancy.

In rare instances, women will develop progressive symptoms during pregnancy and require either valvuloplasty or valve surgery. Both interventions can be performed during pregnancy, but are associated with both maternal and fetal risks and should be performed only when necessary.

Although pregnancy can be successfully completed in most instances, aortic surgery may be required early after pregnancy in some women with severe aortic stenosis. Pregnancy itself seems to accelerate the need for surgery postpartum in women with moderate or severe aortic stenosis, perhaps by affecting the ability of the left ventricle to adapt to the fixed outflow obstruction. It is therefore important that women be counseled about both the risk of pregnancy and the potential for late complications [102,103].

Additionally, guidelines suggest that women with BAV and significant aortopathy (ascending aorta diameter >4.5 cm)"should be counseled against the high risk of pregnancy" [43].

4.4. Exercise

There are little data available to support recommendations regarding exercise in subjects with BAV. In children with congenital severe aortic stenosis, for instance, sudden death can occur during exercise [121]. The Task Force on Exercise in Patients with Heart Disease recommends that athletes with severe aortic stenosis or severe aortic incompetence with left ventricular dilation [left ventricular dimensions >65 mm] should not participate in competitive athletics. Athletes with or without aortic valve disease who have dilated aortic roots (>45 mm) are advised to only participate in low-intensity competitive sports. No restrictions exist for those with BAV with no significant valve dysfunction or aortic root/ascending aorta dilation(>40 mm) [50,104,105].

5. Conclusions

Consequently aortic stenosis and regurgitation, infective endocarditis and aortic dissection are the most common complications of BAV additionaly this process continues after valve replacement. The person with BAV requires continuous surveillance to treat associated lesions and prevent complications. Arterial hypertension should be meticulously controlled. Smoking should be discouraged and control of hypercholesterolaemia considered, in view of the impact of these factors on the development of aortic stenosis. Aortic root dilatation is common in BAV, even when the valve is haemodynamically normal, and consequently aortic dissection usually occurs in previously asymptomatic patients. Beta-blockers and statins are the possibilities for medical treatment, and aortic valve repair/replacement and ascending aorta replacement are indicated for patients with a severely diseased aortic valve and aorta. All patients should therefore be regularly reviewed to identify progressive root dilatation [6,94].

Author details

Mehmet Demir

Bursa Yüksek İhtisas Education and Research Hospital, Cardiology Department, Bursa, Turkey

References

[1] Braverman AC, Güven H, Beardslee MA, et al.The bicuspid aortic valve. Curr Probl Cardiol 2005;30:470-522.

[2] Yener N, Oktar GL, Erer D, et al. Bicuspid aortic valve. Ann Thorac Cardiovasc Surg. 2002 Oct;8[5]:264-7.

[3] Ward C. Clinical significance of the bicuspid aortic valve. Heart 2000; 83: 81–5.

[4] Tadros TM, Klein MD, Shapira OM. Ascending aortic dilatation associated with bicuspid aortic valve: pathophysiology, molecular biology, and clinical implications Circulation. 2009 17;119[6]:880-90.

[5] Pachulski RT, Weinberg AL, Chan KL. Aortic aneurysm in patients with functionally normal or minimally stenotic bicuspid aortic valve. Am J Cardiol 1991; 67:781–2.

[6] Demir M. Current Approach to Bicuspid Aortic Valve: Review. Global Advanced Research Journal of Medicine and Medical Sciences. 2012: 1[5]; 105-107.

[7] Hutchins GM, Nazarian IH, Bulkley BH. Association of left dominant coronary arterial system with congenital bicuspid aortic valve. Am J Cardiol 1978; 42: 57–9.

[8] Higgins CB, Wexler L. Reversal of dominance of the coronary arterial system in isolated aortic stenosis and bicuspid aortic valve. Circulation 1975; 52: 292–6.

[9] Presbitero P, Demarie D, Villani M, et al. Long term results [15-30 years] of surgical repair of aortic coarctation. Br Heart J 1987; 57: 462–7.

[10] Demir M. Acute myocardial infarction in a young patient with bicuspid aortic valve. Turk Kardiyol Dern Ars. 2009 Oct;37[7]:490-2.

[11] Suzuki T, Nagai R, Kurihara H, et al. Stenotic BAVassociated with a ventricular septal defect in an adult presenting with congestive heart failure: a rare observation. European Heart Journal. 1994;15:402-403.

[12] Rabkin-Aikawa E, Farber M, Aikawa M,et al. Dynamic and reversible changes of interstitial cell phenotype during remodeling of cardiac valves. The Journal of heart valve disease 2004; 13:841-847.

[13] Blerim Berisha, Xhevdet Krasniqi,Dardan Kocinaj, Ejup Pllana and Masar Gashi Bicuspid Aortic Valve.In: Ying-Fu Chen and Chwan-Yau Luo. (ed) Aortic valve. Rijeka: InTech; 2011.

[14] Sans-Coma V, Fernández B, Durán AC, et al. Fusion of valve cushions as a key factor in the formation of congenital bicuspid aortic valves in Syrian hamsters. Anat Rec. 1996;244[4]:490-8.

[15] Kappetein AP, Gittenberger-de Groot AC, Zwinderman AH, et al. The neural crest as a possible pathogenetic factor incoarctation of the aorta and bicuspid aortic valve. The Journal of Thoracic and Cardiovascular Surgery 1991; 102[6]:830-836.

[16] Eisenberg LM, Markwald RR. Molecular regulation of atrioventricular valvuloseptal morphogenesis. Circulation Research, 1995; 77[1]: 1-6.

[17] Fedak PW, Verma S, DavidTE,et al. Clinical and pathophysiological implications of a bicuspid aortic valve. Circulation 2002;106:900-4.

[18] Hinton RB, Jr, Lincoln J, Deutsch GH, et al. Extracellular matrix remodeling and organization in developing and diseased aortic valves. Circulation Research 2006; 98[11]:1431-1438.

[19] Sabet HY, Edwards WD, Tazelaar HD, et al. Congenitally bicuspid aortic valves: a surgical pathology study of 542 cases [1991 through 1996] and a literatüre review of 2715 additional cases. Mayo Clinic Proceedings 1996;74[1]:14–26.

[20] Schang SJ, Pepine CJ, Bemiller CR, et al. Anomalous coronary artery origin and bicuspid aortic valve. Vasc Surg 1975; 9: 67–72.

[21] Fernández B, Durán AC, Fernández-Gallego T, et al. Bicuspid aortic valves with different spatial orientations of the leaflets are distinct etiological entities. J Am Coll Cardiol.2009;54[24]:2312-8.

[22] Ify Mordi, Nikolaos Tzemos. BAVDisease: A Comprehensive Review. Cardiology Research and Practice 2012];

[23] Leme MP, David TE, Butany J, et al. Molecular evaluation of the great vessels of patients with BAVdisease. Rev Bras Cir Cardiovasc. 2003;18[2]:148-56.

[24] Sá MPL, Bastos ES, Murad H. Valva aórtica bicúspide: fundamentos teóricos e clínicos para substituição simultânea da aorta ascendente [Bicuspid aortic valve: theoretical and clinical aspects of concomitant ascending aorta replacement]. Rev Bras Cir Cardiovasc.2009;24[2]:218-24.

[25] Yap SC, Nemes A, Meijboom FJ, et al. Abnormal aortic elastic properties in adults with congenital valvular aortic stenosis. Int J Cardiol. 2008;128:336–41.

[26] Fernandes SM, Sanders SP, Khairy P, et al. Morphology of BAVin children and adolescent. Journal of the American College of Cardiology 2004;44[8]:1648-1651.

[27] T. J. Calloway, L. J. Martin, X. Zhang, et al. "Risk factors for aortic valve disease inbicuspid aortic valve: a family-based study," American Journal of Medical Genetics 2011;155[5]:1015–1020.

[28] De Mozzi P, Longo UG, Galanti G, et al. Bicuspid aortic valve: a literature review and its impact on sport activity. British Medical Bulletin 2008;85:63-85.

[29] W. C. Roberts. The congenitally bicuspid aortic valve. A study of 85 autopsy cases. The American Journal of Cardiology 1970;26[1]:72–83.

[30] E. S. Murphy, J Rosch, S. H. Rahimtoola. Frequency and significance of coronary arterial dominance in isolated aortic stenosis. American Journal of Cardiology 1977;39[4]: 505–509.

[31] B. Stewart, R. Ahmed, C. M. Travill,et al. Coarctation of the aorta life and health 20–44 yers after surgery repair. British Heart Journal 1993;69[1]:65–70.

[32] Larson EW, Edwards WD. Risk factors for aortic dissection: a necropsy study of 161 cases. Am J Cardiol 1984;53:849-55.

[33] Cripe L, Andelfinger G, Martin J, Shooner K, Benson DW. BAVis heritable. J Am Coll Cardiol 2004;44:138-43.

[34] Huntington K, Hunter AG, Chan KL. A prospective study to assess the frequency of familial clustering of congenital bicuspid aortic valve. J Am Coll Cardiol 1997;30:1809-12.

[35] Glick BN, Roberts WC. Congenitally BAVin multiple family members. Am J Cardiol 1994;73:400–4.

[36] Andelfinger G, Tapper AR, Welch RC, et al. KCNJ2 mutation results in Andersen syndrome with sex-specific cardiac and skeletal muscle phenotypes. American Journal of Human Genetics 2002;71[3]:663-668.

[37] Garg V, Muth AN, Ransom JF, et al. Mutations in NOTCH1 cause aortic valve disease. Nature 2005;437:270–4.

[38] Mohamed SA, Aherrahrou Z, Liptau H, et al. Novel missense mutations [p.T596M and p.P1797H] in NOTCH1 in patients with bicuspid aortic valve. Biochem Biophys Res Commun 2006;345:1460-5.

[39] Martin LJ, Ramachandran V, Cripe LH, et al. Evidence in favor of linkage to human chromosomal regions 18q, 5q and 13q for BAVand associated cardiovascular malformations. Hum Genet 2007;121:275–84.

[40] Guo DC, Pannu H, Tran-Fadulu V, et al. Mutations in smooth muscle alpha-actin [ACTA2] lead to thoracic aortic aneurysms and dissections. Nat Genet 2007;39:1488–93.

[41] Mohamed SA, Hanke T, Schlueter C, et al.Ubiquitin fusion degradation 1-like gene dysregulation in bicuspid aortic valve. The Journal of thoracic and cardiovascular surgery 2005;130:1531-36.

[42] Yamagishi C, Hierck BP, Gittenberger-De Groot AC, et al. Functional attenuation of UFD1l, a 22q11.2 deletion syndrome candidate gene, leads to cardiac outflow septation defects in chicken embryos. Pediatric Research 2003;53:546-553.

[43] Warnes CA, Williams RG, Bashore TM, et al. ACC/AHA 2008 guidelines for the management of adults with congenital heart disease: a report of the American College of Cardiology/American Heart Association Task Force on Practice Guidelines [Writing Committee to Develop Guidelines on the Management of Adults With Congenital Heart Disease]. J Am Coll Cardiol 2008;52:e1–121.

[44] Novaro GM, Griffin BP. Congenital BAVand rate of ascending aortic dilatation. Am J Cardiol 2004;93:525–6.

[45] Emanuel R, Withers R, O'Brien K, et al. Congenitally bicuspid aortic valves: clinicogenetic study of 41 families. Br Heart J 1978; 40: 1402-7.

[46] Clementi M, Notari L, Borghi A, et al. Familial congenital bicuspid aortic valve: a disorder of uncertain inheritance. Am J Med Genet 1996; 62: 336-8.

[47] P. Mills, G. Leech, M. Davies, et al. The natural history of a non-stenotic bicuspid aortic valve. British Heart Journal 1978;40:951-957.

[48] K. L. Chan, W. A. Stinson, J. P. Veinot. Reliability of transthoracic echocardiography in the assessment of aortic valve morphology: pathological correlation in 178 patients. Canadian Journal of Cardiology 1999;15:48-52.

[49] R. Tanaka, K. Yoshioka, H. Niinuma,et al. Diagnostic value of cardiac CT in the evaluation of bicuspid aortic stenosis: comparison with echocardiography and operative findings. American Journal of Roentgenology 2010;195:895-899.

[50] Samuel C. Siu, Candice K. Silversides.BAVDisease. J Am Coll. Cardiol 2010;55;2789-2800.

[51] Bonow RO, Carabello BA, Kanu C, et al. ACC/AHA 2006 guidelines for the management of patients with valvular heart disease: a report of the American College of Cardiology/American Heart Association Task Force on Practice Guidelines [Writing Committee to Revise the 1998 Guidelines for the Management of Patients With Valvular Heart Disease]. J Am Coll Cardiol 2006;48:e1–148.

[52] S. C. Malaisrie, J. Carr, I. Mikati et al. Cardiac magnetic resonance imaging is more diagnostic than 2-dimensional echocardiography in determining the presence of bicuspid aortic valve. The Journal of Thoracic and Cardiovascular Surgery.

[53] Hiratzka LF, Bakris GL, Beckman JA, et al. 2010 ACCF/AHA/AATS/ACR/ASA/SCA/ SCAI/SIR/STS/SVM Guidelines for the diagnosis and management of patients with thoracic aortic disease. A Report of the American College of Cardiology Foundation/

American Heart Association Task Force on Practice Guidelines, American Association for Thoracic Surgery, American College of Radiology,American Stroke Association, Society of Cardiovascular Anesthesiologists, Society for Cardiovascular Angiography and Interventions, Society of Interventional Radiology, Society of Thoracic Surgeons,and Society for Vascular Medicine. J Am Coll Cardiol. 2010 6;55[14]:e27-e129

[54] Karayel F, Ozaslan A, Turan AA, et al. Sudden death in infancy due to bicuspid aortic valve. J Forensic Sci. 2006;51[5]:1147-50.

[55] Lamas CC, Eykyn SJ. Bicuspid aortic valve–A silent danger: analysis of 50 cases of infective endocarditis.Clin Infect Dis 2000; 30: 336–41.

[56] Michelena HI, Desjardins VA, Avierinos JF, et al. Natural history of asymptomatic patients with normally functioning or minimally dysfunctional BAVin the community. Circulation 2008; 117:2776-84.

[57] J. J. Fenoglio Jr, H. A. McAllister, C. M. DeCastro. Congenital BAVafter age 20. Am J Cardiol 1977;39:164–169.

[58] Schaefer BM, Lewin MB, Stout KK, et al. The bicuspid aortic valve: an integrated phenotypic classification of leaflet morphology and aortic root shape. Heart 2008;94:1634-1638.

[59] Hoffman JI. Congenital heart disease: incidence and inheritance. Pediatr Clin North Am 1990;37:25-43.

[60] H. I. Michelena, V. A. Desjardins, J. F. Avierinos et al. Natural history of asymptomatic patients with normally functioning or minimally dysfunctional BAVin the community. Circulation 2008;117:2776-2784.

[61] H. I. Michelina, A. D. Khanna, D. Mahoney et al. Incidence of aortic complications in patients with bicuspid aortic valves.The Journal of the American Medical Association. 2011;306:1104–1112.

[62] Tzemos N, Therrien J, Yip J, et al. Outcomes in adults with bicuspid aortic valves. JAMA 2008;300:1317–25.

[63] Michelena HI, Desjardins VA, Avierinos JF, et al. Natural history of asymptomatic patients with normally functioning or minimally dysfunctional BAVin the community. Circulation 2008;117:2776–84.

[64] Turina J, Turina M, Krayenbühl HP. [Significance of the BAVin the incidence of aortic valve defects in adults]. Schweiz Med Wochenschr. 1986;116[44]:1518-23.

[65] Matsumura T, Ohtaki E, Misu K, et al. Etiology of aortic valve disease and recent changes in Japan: a study of 600 valve replacement cases. Int J Cardiol. 2002;86[2-3]: 217-23.

[66] Wallby L, Janerot-Sjoberg B, Steffensen T, et al. T lymphocyte infiltration in non-rheumatic aortic stenosis: a comparative descriptive study between tricuspid and bi-cuspid aortic valves. Heart 2002;88:348–51.

[67] Fenoglio JJ Jr, McAllister HA Jr, DeCastro CM, et al. Congenital BAVafter age 20. Am J Cardiol. 1977;39[2]:164-9.

[68] Roman MJ, Devereux RB, Niles NW, et al. Aortic root dilatation as a cause of isolat-ed, severe aortic regurgitation. Prevalence, clinical and echocardiographic patterns, and relation to left ventricular hypertrophy and function. Ann Intern Med 1987;106:800-7.

[69] Roberts WC, Morrow AG, McIntosh CL,et al. Congenitally BAVcausing severe, pure aortic regurgitation without superimposed infective endocarditis. Analysis of 13 pa-tients requiring aortic valve replacement. Am J Cardiol 1981;47:206-9.

[70] Morishita A, Shimakura T, Nonoyama M, et al. Ascending aorta dissection associated with bicuspid aortic valve. Considerations 4 years after combined coronary artery bypass grafting and mitral valve replacement. Jpn J Thorac Cardiovasc Surg. 2001;49[6]:368-72.

[71] Hahn RT, Roman MJ, Mogtader AH, et al. Association of aortic dilation with regurgi-tant, stenotic and functionally normal bicuspid aortic valves. J Am Coll Cardiol. 1992;19[2]:283-8.

[72] Collins MJ, Dev V, Strauss BH, Fedak PW, Butany J. Variation in the histopathologi-cal features of patients with ascending aortic aneurysms: a study of 111 surgically ex-cised cases. J Clin Pathol. 2008;61[4]:519-23.

[73] Cotrufo M, Della Corte A, De Santo LS, et al. Different patterns of extracellular ma-trix protein expression in the convexity and the concavity of the dilated aorta with bicuspid aortic valve:preliminary results. J Thorac Cardiovasc Surg. 2005;130:504-11.

[74] Edwards WD, Leaf DS, Edwards JE. Dissecting aortic aneurysm associated with con-genital bicuspid aortic valve. Circulation. 1978;57[5]:1022-5.

[75] N. Tzemos, E. Lyseggen, C. Silversides et al. Endothelial function, carotid-femoral sti ∙ ness, and plasma matrix metalloproteinase-2 in men with BAVand dilated aor-ta," Journal of the American College of Cardiology 2010;55:660-668.

[76] Ando M, Okita Y, Matsukawa R, et al. Surgery for aortic dissection associated with congenital bicuspid aortic valve. Jpn J Thorac Cardiovasc Surg. 1998;46[11]:1069-73.

[77] Fedak PW, de Sá MP, Verma S, et al. Vascular matrix remodeling in patients with BAVmalformations: implications for aortic dilatation. J Thorac Cardiovasc Surg. 2003;126[3]:797-806.

[78] McKusick VA. Association of congenital BAVand erdheim's cystic medial necrosis. Lancet.1972;1[7758]:1026-7.

[79] Keane MG, Wiegers SE, Plappert T, Pochettino A, Bavaria JE, Sutton MG. Bicuspid aortic valves are associated with aortic dilatation out of proportion to coexistent valvular lesions.Circulation. 2000;102[19 Suppl 3]:III35-9.

[80] Sá M, Moshkovitz Y, Butany J, David TE. Histologic abnormalities of the ascending aorta and pulmonary trunk in patients with BAVdisease: clinical relevance to the Ross procedure. J Thorac Cardiovasc Surg.1999;118[4]:588-94.

[81] Schmid FX, Bielenberg K, Holmer S, et al. Structural and biomolecular changes in aorta and pulmonary trunk of patients with aortic aneurysm and valve disease: implications for the Ross procedure. Eur J Cardiothorac Surg. 2004;25[5]:748-53.

[82] Nistri S, Sorbo MD, Basso C, Thiene G. Bicuspid aortic valve: abnormal aortic elastic properties. J Heart Valve Dis. 2002 May;11[3]:369-73.

[83] Parai JL, Masters RG, Walley VM, Stinson WA, Veinot JP. Aortic medial changes associated with bicuspid aortic valve: myth or reality? Can J Cardiol 1999; 15:1233–8.

[84] De Backer JF, Devos D, Segers P, Matthys D, Francois K, Gillebert TC et al.Primary impairment of left ventricular function in Marfan syndrome. Int J Cardiol 2006;112:353–8.

[85] Bonderman D, Gharehbaghi-Schnell E, Wollenek G, et al. Mechanisms underlying aortic dilatation in congenital aortic valve malformation. Circulation.1999;99:2138 2143.

[86] Pape LA, Tsai TT, Isselbacher EM, et al., on behalf of International Registry of Acute Aortic Dissection [IRAD] Investigators. Aortic diameter >5.5 cm is not a good predictor of type A aortic dissection: observations from the International Registry of Acute Aortic Dissection [IRAD]. Circulation 2007;116:1120–7.

[87] W. M. Gersony, C. J. Hayes, D. J. Driscoll et al., "Bacterial endocarditis in patients with aortic stenosis, pulmonary stenosis, or ventricular septal defect," Circulation, vol. 87, no.2, pp. I121–I126, 1993.

[88] Lamas CC, Eykyn SJ. Bicuspid aortic valve--A silent danger: analysis of 50 cases of infective endocarditis. Clin Infect Dis. 2000;30[2]:336-41.

[89] Nishimura RA, Carabello BA, Faxon DP, et al. ACC/AHA 2008 guideline update on valvular heart disease: focused update on infective endocarditis: a report of the American College of Cardiology/American Heart Association Task Force on Practice Guidelines.J Am Coll Cardiol 2008;52:676–85.

[90] Johnson AD, Detwiler JH, Higgins CB. Left coronary artery anatomy in patients with bicuspid aortic valves. Br Heart J. 1978;40[5]:489-93.

[91] Labombarda F, Legallois D, Sabatier R. Spontaneous coronary artery dissection and bicuspid aortic valve. Arch Cardiovasc Dis. 2009;102[12]:857-8.

[92] Yokoyama S, Ashida T, SugiyamaT, et al. An autopsied case with a BAVwho had progressive angina pectoris and heart failure during follow-up of 27 years. Nippon Ronen Igakkai Zasshi 2002;39:444-447.

[93] Yuan SM, Jing H, Lavee J.The BAVand its relation to aortic dilation. Clinics [Sao Paulo] 2010;65:497-505.

[94] Shi-Min Yuan, Hua Jing. The BAVand related disorders. Sao Paulo Med J. 2010; 128[5]:296-301.

[95] Chuangsuwanich T, Warnnissorn M, Leksrisakul P, et al. Pathology and etiology of 110 consecutively removed aortic valves. J Med Assoc Thai. 2004;87[8]:921-34.

[96] Pleet AB, Massey EW, Vengrow ME. TIA, stroke, and the bicuspid aortic valve. Neurology.1981;31[12]:1540-2.

[97] Mahajan N, Khetarpal V, Afonso L. Stroke secondary to calcific bicuspid aortic valve: Case report and literature review. J Cardiol. 2009;54[1]:158-61.

[98] Shores J, Berger KR, Murphy EA, et al. Progression of aortic dilatation and the benefit of long-term beta-adrenergic blockade in Marfan's syndrome. N Engl J Med 1994;330:1335–41.

[99] Stewart BF, Siscovick D, Lind BK, et al. Clinical factors associated with calcific aortic valve disease. Cardiovascular Health Study. J Am Coll Cardiol 1997;29:630–4.

[100] H. M. Rosenfeld, M. J. Landzberg, S. B. Perry, et al. Balloon aortic valvuloplasty in the young adult with congenital aortic stenosis. Am J Cardiol 1994;73:1112-1117.

[101] David TE, Omran A, Ivanov J, et al. Dilation of the pulmonary autograft after the Ross procedure. J Thorac Cardiovasc Surg 2000;119:210–20.

[102] Silversides CK, Colman JM, Sermer M, et al.Early and intermediate-term outcomes of pregnancy with congenital aortic stenosis. Am J Cardiol 2003;91:1386-9.

[103] Tzemos N, Silversides CK, Colman JM, et al. Late cardiac outcomes after pregnancy in women with congenital aortic stenosis. Am Heart J 2009;157:474–80.

[104] Lambert EC, Menon VA, Wagner HR, Vlad P. Sudden unexpected death from cardiovascular disease in children. A cooperative international study. Am J Cardiol 1974;34:89-96.

[105] Graham TP Jr, Driscoll DJ, Gersony WM, et al.Task Force 2: congenital heart disease. J Am Coll Cardiol 2005;45:1326-33.

Chapter 2

Bicuspid Aortic Valve

George Tokmaji, Berto J. Bouma,
Dave R. Koolbergen and Bas A.J.M. de Mol

Additional information is available at the end of the chapter

1. Introduction

Bicuspid aortic valve (BAV) disease is one of the most frequent observed congenital heart abnormalities affecting 0.5-1.4% of the general population and has a 3:1 male predominance [1-4]. Although some genes have been described that found to be responsible for the abnormal valvulogenesis, little is known about BAV disease with respect to the genetic and embryological insight of calcification and why patients with BAV disease develop aortic valve calcification including severe aortic valve stenosis (AS) at an earlier age compared with degenerative tricuspid valve. BAV disease is also associated with several cardiovascular abnormalities including coarctation of the aorta (COA) and Turner Syndrome. While patients with BAV disease are often asymptomatic during the childhood, BAV disease is generally diagnosed in the adulthood using echocardiography when aortic stenosis with or without valve calcification, infective endocarditis, aortic regurgitation (AR), and proximal thoracic aortic dilatation are detected, often necessitating surgical intervention [5]. Patients with BAV disease require close observation before complications as heart failure and aortic dissection may occur. In this chapter, the contemporary knowledge regarding BAV disease will be discussed.

2. Anatomy and pathology

The anatomic features of BAV are characterized by smooth cusps margins and the fusion of two cusps of unequal size. These cusps often include a central raphé or false commissure which are usually in the centre of the larger cusp [Figure 2]. The main difference between a commissure and a raphé is that the commissure does not completely span into the cusp [6]. The raphé is to be considered as a hypoplastic commissure between two partially fused cusps. The most commonly seen variant of BAV is the fusion of the left and right coronary cusps (L-R BAV) also known as the latero-lateral cusps position which is seen in 70-86% of the BAV cases, whereas the fusion of the right and noncoronary cusps (R-N BAV; antero-posterior cusps position) are observed in 12-28% and the left and noncoronary cusps (L-N BAV) in 0.5-3% of the cases [7-11] [Figure 1]. R-N BAVs and asymmetrical sized cusps are relative risk factors that seem to accelerate the stenosis with 27 mm Hg per decade and are therefore more often associated with AS [12]. BAV with equal cusps and absence of raphé have also been reported [6, 7]. In some cases, the raphé can have a quite deep indentation, which could give a false echocardiographic image of a normal tricuspid aortic valve [13]. Calcium depositions are often confined to the raphé and the base of the cusps [7]. AS tend to develop in BAVs which contain no redundant cusp tissue whereas AR tend to develop in BAVs due to the different dimensions of the two cusps, valve prolapse or redundancy of one cusp [14-16]. Histological examination demonstrates that the raphé does not contain fibrous valve tissue but rather include elastin fibers [17]. BAV should also be distinguished from unicommisural valves that tend to calcify and degenerate even earlier in life. Unicommissural valves includes one commissure with normal height and two raphe's that are much lower height, while there is one large cusp, more or less moving like a bicuspid valve. Up to 90% of the individuals with normal tricuspid valve have right coronary artery dominance whereas 29% to 57% of the patients with BAV disease present with left coronary artery dominance. The average length of the left main stem for individuals with BAV and tricuspid valve is less than 5 mm (90% of the cases) and 10 mm in length, respectively. Recognition of these associations with BAV is mandatory due to the increased risk of perioperative myocardial infarction and a potential risk of insufficient myocardial preservation at the time of aortic valve replacement (AVR) [18, 19, 20]. L-R BAVs are often associated with right coronary artery taking its origin from the right sinus of Valsalva, while in the R-N BAVs, both coronary arteries derive from the anterior sinus [21]. The vast majority of the patients with COA present with a L-R BAV (66-90%) [9, 135, 136].

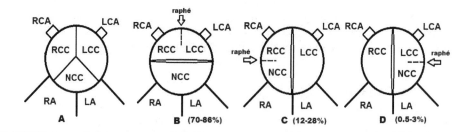

Figure 1. Schematic illustration of the anatomic variations of BAV. (A) normal tricuspid aortic valve. (B) Bicuspid aortic valve, fusion of the left and right coronary cusps. (C) Bicuspid aortic valve, fusion of the right and noncoronary cusps. (D) Bicuspid aortic valve, fusion of the left and noncoronary cusps.

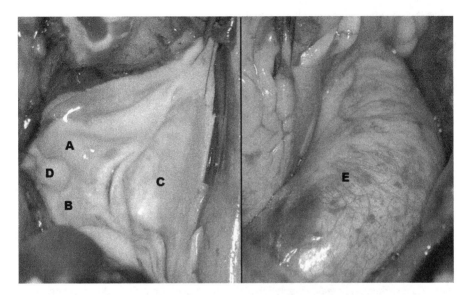

Figure 2. Macroscopic illustration of a bicuspid aortic valve with the fusion of the right and noncoronary cusps (left image) and a dilated ascending aorta (right image). A: Non coronary cusp, B: Right coronary cusp, C: Left coronary cusp, D: Raphé, E: Ascending aorta (dilated).

3. Morphologenesis

The embryogenesis of BAV is still not fully understood. It seems that both genetic predisposition and environmental factors, which could influence the valve morphogenesis, play an important role in the pathogenesis of BAV disease. Initially, the major factor in the formation of BAV is the fusion of the two cusps at the early foundation of the valvulogenesis [22]. The valve morphogenesis occurs in the early stage of foetal development. The heart is one of the first organs to develop through the specification and migration of the anterior lateral plate mesoderm cells which later forms the cardiac crescent [23]. At 3 weeks of gestation in humans, the cardiac progenitors migrate along the ventral midline where they fuse and form a linear heart tube. This beating heart tube is composed of an inner endocardial cell layer which is separated by the extracellular matrix (ECM). Cardiac looping occurs at 4 to 5 weeks of gestation which brings the atrial region of the linear tube into the posterior position of the common ventricles. This is followed by the increase of ECM production which causes the tissue to swell at several areas of the primitive heart, which leads to the formation of the endocardial cushions at the outflow tract (OFT) and atrioventricular (AV) canal. The inner endocardial cells transform into mesenchymal cells, also known as the epithelial-to-mesenchymal transformation (EMT). EMT initiates the formation of the aortic valve in the OFT. Afterwards, the cushions undergo massive cell proliferation, as a result growing towards each other with cushion fusion being the outcome. Subsequently, the endocardial cushions develop into thin protruding leaflets that are composed of endocardial cells and ECM which remodels the valves. This complex development is reliant on apoptosis, ECM remodeling and cell differentiation. The main contributors for the aortic valve in the OFT are the mesenchymal cells that reach the OFT cushions in association with the endocardial derived mesenchymal cells [24, 25]. Therefore, any disorder in the endocardial cushion development could lead to potential valve disorder including BAV. A disturbance in the neural crest migration which could lead to the fusion of the aortic valve cushions is thought to be a possible embryological explanation for the pathogenesis of BAV disease [22, 26-28]. Several aneurysms which originate from the neural crest including intracranial aneurysms, aortic aneurysms, and cervicocephalic aneurysm have also been observed in patients with BAV disease [29, 30]. Endothelial nitric oxide synthase is a vital protein for valve formation during embryogenesis. Knockout mice lacking this protein showed a high predisposition for BAV due to the fact that malformation in this protein could lead to disturbance of the intricate cell signals which are essential for valvulogenesis [31]. Moreover, it seems that L-R BAV and R-N BAV have different etiological attributes and genotypes. The pathogenesis of R-N BAV is most likely the result of morphogenetic defect which occurs before the OFT septation and is dependent on an aggravated nitric oxide–dependent epithelial-to-mesenchymal transformation. In contrast, L-R BAV is most probably the outcome from the anomalous septation of the proximal portion of the OFT which is caused by distorted activities of neural crest cells [32].

4. Genetics

Genetic burden also seem to contribute to the pathogenesis of BAV disease. It appears that BAV disease has a male-to-female ratio of roughly 3:1 [1-4]. Although some anatomical risk factors have been described, little is known about BAV disease with respect to the genetic insight of calcification process and why patients with BAV disease develop aortic valve calcification including stenosis at an earlier age compared with degenerative tricuspid valve. Chromosomal linkage with BAV disease has been discovered in chromosomal regions 5q, 13q and 18q [36]. Genetic mutations in the NOTCH 1 gene, which is situated at chromosome 9q seems to be one of the major genetic contributors in the pathogenesis of BAV disease. NOTCH 1 gene contributes to the pathogenesis of BAV disease through the pathological acceleration of aortic valvular calcium deposition by the increase of the osteogenesis due to the abnormalities in the signalling pathways [37]. Also, genetic mutations in the ACTA2 gene which is located at chromosome 10q, is associated not only with BAV disease, but also with familial thoracic aortic aneurysms [38]. ACTA2 gene encodes for the smooth muscle protein α-actin which is an important element of the contractile apparatus. Several familial clusters associated with BAV disease with an estimated prevalence of 24% of aortic valve disorder were found in relatives with more than one member with aortic valve disorder [33]. Additionally, an estimated BAV disease prevalence of up to 9% in first-degree family members of patients with BAV disease has been reported [34, 35]. Based on this known data, it is advisable for first-degree family members of BAV patients to receive an echocardiographic screening to exclude any potential congenital heart disease including thoracic aortic aneurysms [39, 67, 68].

5. Congenital associated cardiovascular malformations

Although the vast majority of BAV disease are isolated cases, patients with BAV could also present with additional congenital cardiovascular malformations [40-43]. BAV associated anomalies are illustrated in Table 1. Whereas most associated anomalies need treatment early in life, BAV often contributes to morbidity at an older age. COA and Turner Syndrome will be further discussed in this chapter.

5.1. Coarctation of the aorta

COA is a commonly seen congenital abnormality with an incidence of 50 of 100.000 births, whereby the aorta is narrowed in the region where the ductus arteriosus enters [figure 3]. COA can present itself as a simple or complex COA with simple COA referring to COA being an isolated defect and complex COA referring to a combination of COA with other cardiac defects. Congenital BAV is present in around 57% of the COA cases [44]. In the vast majority of the cases, COA in combination with BAV is observed with the fusion of left and right coronary cusps [9]. Patients with both BAV and COA have an increased risk for developing several aortic complications including aortic dissection, AS, AR, and aortic aneurysms [16, 44, 46, 49]. The overwhelming majority of BAV patients present with a L-R BAV (66-90%) [9, 135, 136].

Patients with both BAV and COA receive surgical intervention at a relative young age. Surgical options, mostly depending of the type of lesion include bypass of the coarctation, patch aortoplasty, aneurysm replacement, arch and descending aorta replacement, subclavian artery patch aortoplasty, tube graft replacement, ascending aorta–to– descending aorta bypass or 2-stage combined BAV surgery [69]. Endovascular balloon dilatation and stent placement are currently becoming successful novel interventional options to conventional open surgical treatment [70]. Around 11% to 14% of the patients require a reoperation somewhere in the adulthood [50]. A large cohort study showed that up to 41% of the patients who had a COA required a valve related re-operation [9]. Thus, long-term follow-up in (all) patients with COA including the evaluation of the function of the aortic valve, but also to trace re-coarctation and dilatation of the ascending aorta with routine MRI or echocardiographic evaluation is obligatory.

5.2. Turner Syndrome

Turner Syndrome is a gonadal dysgenesis with complete or partial absence of one of the X chromosome. Cardiovascular defects are frequently observed in Turner Syndrome patients. Turner Syndrome is characterized as neck webbing, short stature, low hairline, and a shield-like chest. BAV disease is the most frequently seen cardiovascular abnormality in Turner Syndrome patients [51, 52]. In Turner Syndrome patients, cardiovascular abnormalities are often the primary cause of mortality including the increase risk of aortic dissection due to aortic root dilatation and therefore responsible for a much lower life expectancy in this subgroup of BAV disease [53, 54]. Due to the relative small body size, Turner Syndrome patients require an elective ascending aortic aneurysm replacement at a much smaller absolute size [54]. Moreover, it should be noted that the aortic size has to be properly indexed to the body surface area. Therefore, proper follow-up and evaluation of the cardiovascular lesions including imaging of the heart and the aorta for evidence of BAV disease or dilatation of the ascending aorta is mandatory. When imaging appears to be without any lesions and there are no additional risk factors for aortic dissection present, a repeated imaging should be conducted every 5 to 10 years or otherwise clinically indicated. In contrast, when abnormal imaging is present, regular imaging at smaller intervals should be made with echocardiography or CMRI [67].

• Coarctation of the Aorta	• Ascending Aortic Aneurysm
• Turner Syndrome	• Coronary Artery Anomalies
• Patent Ductus Arteriosus	• Sinus of Valsalva Aneurysm
• William's Syndrome	• Supravalvular Aortic Stenosis
• Ventricular Septal Defect	• Aortic Dissection
• Shone's Syndrome	

Table 1. Known cardiovascular abnormalities related to BAV disease.

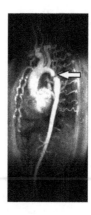

Figure 3. Sagittal plane cardiac magnetic resonance imaging illustrating coarctation of the aorta. Typical post ductal stenosis (arrow).

6. Diagnosis

6.1. Clinical examination

AS or AR can present themselves with significant symptoms in patients with BAV disease during activity, stress or rest including angina, shortness of breath, syncope or dizziness. In many cases, clinical examination reveals an ejection sound during auscultation at the apex. When AS is present, an ejection click can be often heard at the S1. The S2 is often simultaneously with P2 when AS is present. A diastolic murmur can often be heard when an AR is present. Heart failure of unknown cause could also be present during clinical examination. The ejection sound in BAV patients is most likely associated with anterior movement of the dome shaped BAV, and in rare cases heart failure could also be present during clinical examination in case of rapid deterioration [55]. AS, mitral valve prolapsed, AR, and COA are several associated pathological findings which have to be considered with BAV when a murmer is present.

6.2. Echocardiography

The current golden standards for diagnosing, surveilling and monitoring BAV disease are echocardiography and cardiac magnetic resonance imaging (CMRI) [39].

Both transthoracic echocardiography (TTE) and transesophageal echocardiography (TEE) can be used in the diagnosis of BAV disease. TTE has a sensitivity of 78% to 87% and a specificity of 91% to 96% for the diagnosis of BAV disease whereas TEE has a sensitivity and specificity of 87% and 96%, respectively [56, 57, 58]. However, up to 25% of TTE have non-diagnostic findings for aortic valve morphology due to severe valvular calcification [57].

The features of BAV on a TTE include systolic doming, an eccentric closure line in the parasternal long axis views, presence of a single commissural line in the diastolic phase with the occurrence of two cusps and the occurrence of two commisures in the parasternal short axis views [figure 4] [59, 60].

Moreover, both preoperative echocardiography and intraoperative TEE are essential for surgical preparation. When BAV disease is present, the degree of AS and AR should be determined with the help of Doppler analysis. After determining the severity of the AR, to ascertain the indication for surgery, especially TEE is needed to clarify the mechanisms that are responsible for AR. This is required to estimate the chance of successful repair and indispensible in surgical preparation. Moreover, any associated cardiovascular abnormalities or complications should be considered. Aortic diameters should therefore also be measured at several levels including valvular insertion, sinuses of Valsalva, sino-tubular junction and the ascending aorta. It should also be noted that in order to measure the severity of the AS by echocardiography- Doppler analysis, the aortic valve area and mean gradient should be applied rather than measuring only on peak systolic gradient, sequentially to prevent overestimation of the severity of the AS [39]. Also, aortic valve area should always be indexed to body surface area in order to correct for different habitus and body sizes, especially in Turner Syndrome patients [39, 54].

6.3. Cardiac magnetic resolution imaging

CMRI as a noninvasive diagnostic tool appears to have a high diagnostic sensitivity and specificity. CMRI showed a sensitivity of 100% and a specificity of 95% with steady state free-precession (SSFP) cine [61]. It seems that CMRI is more reliable than the standard TTE in diagnosing BAV [Figure 5]. When TTE is found to be non-diagnostic for aortic valve morphology, particularly in patients with severe AS, CMRI can be conducted as a complementary test [62].

When the diagnostic results of AR with the use of echocardiography is indefinite or at borderline, CMRI can be used to quantify the AR more accurately [39]. In addition, the valve can be visualized with any correlated lesion of the ascending aorta. This could be used for proper evaluation of the entire aortic and to prepare complex surgical interventions for both the aorta valve and the surrounding cardiovascular structures including the ascending aorta and the aortic root. Of importance, all patients with evidence of BAV should have the aortic root and ascending aorta inspected for indication of aortic dilatation with echocardiography or MRI [67].

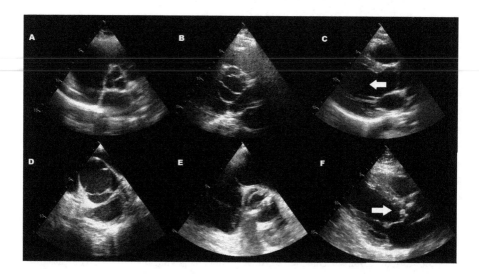

Figure 4. (A) Transthoracic echocardiography short axis view illustrating a normal tricuspid aortic valve. (B) Transthoracic echocardiography short axis view illustrating a bicuspid aortic valve with fusion of the left and right coronary cusps. (C) Transthoracic echocardiography long axis view illustrating a dilated ascending aorta (Arrow). (D) Transthoracic echocardiography short axis view illustrating a bicuspid aortic valve with fusion of the right and non coronary coronary cusps. (E) Transthoracic echocardiography short axis view illustrating a severe calcified bicuspid aortic valve with fusion of the right and non coronary coronary cusps. (F) Transthoracic echocardiography long axis view illustrating a severe calcified bicuspid aortic valve.

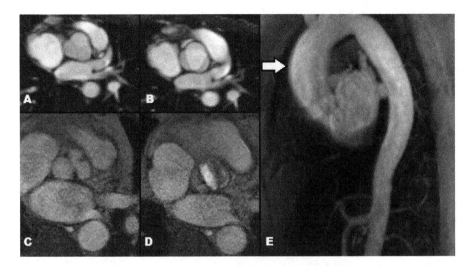

Figure 5. Panel (A, B) Cardiac magnetic resonance imaging in the axial plane illustrating a normal tricuspid valve in the diastolic (A) and systolic phase (B). (Panel C, D) Bicuspid aortic valve with fusion of the right coronary cusp and the non coronary cusp in the diastolic (C) and systolic (D) phase. (Panel E) Sagittal plane illustrating a dilatation of the ascending aorta (Arrow).

7. Complications associated with BAV

7.1. Aortic stenosis

Up to 50% of the adults who present with AS show evidence of BAV disease [71]. BAV degeneration is due to both fibrosis and calcification and is age related [16, 72, 73]. Additionally, the incidence of BAV related AS that is observed in patients with the age of under 60 years, 60 to 75 years, and more than 75 years are 59%, 40% and 32%, respectively [74].

Patients with BAV generally require AVR 5 years earlier compared with the patients who have an AS of the tricuspid valve [75]. Three-quarters of the patient with BAV who underwent AVR showed to have an isolated AS [7]. Both fibrosis and cusp calcifications occur in an accelerated pattern in BAV compared with tricuspid aortic valve [Figure 4, E &F] [76]. Moreover, several valve related factors seem to accelerate the calcification in BAV including larger sized cusp, presence of raphé and the overall BAV anatomy. It seems that sclerosis of the aortic valve starts in the second decade whereas calcification tends to develop around the fourth decade onwards with a 18 mmHg per decade increase of the average aortic valve gradient [75, 12]. Both R-N BAVs and asymmetrical sized cusps seem to contribute to the acceleration of the stenosis due to the progressive calcification and fibrosis with 27 mm Hg per decade [9, 45, 12]. It has to be noted that smoking and a poor lipid panel are both modifiable independent risk factors that could have a great impact on BAV degeneration [77]. In children, BAV with stenosis can sometimes be treated with balloon valvuloplasty whereas in other cases surgical commissur-otomy is indicated [75, 78-80]. Severe fibrosis of the cusp tissue and calcified degeneration, which is found in the older population, make surgical repair difficult or impossible in most cases. AVR is therefore the primary surgical treatment of BAV with severe stenosis in adults.

7.2. Aortic regurgitation

AR most often involves patients with a young age and is less frequently seen than AS with prevalence ranging from 7% to 20% [15, 78, 81, 82]. AR can occur in the isolated form due to the prolapse of one of the cusps, but it could also occur due to and in combination with endocarditis, COA, and proximal aortic root dilatation [16, 25]. The presence of AR could have severe consequences for the patient's morbidity including the increased risk of heart failure, endocarditis and arrhythmia [80]. Aortic root dilatation is found in nearly half of the young adults with BAV disease, thus increasing the risk for AR [83]. In selected cases, patients with BAV disease and isolated AR can be a candidate for aortic valve repair [84].

7.3. Aortic dilatation and dissection

BAV disease is linked with dilatation of the proximal aortic root and ascending aorta and develops independently from stenotic or regurgitant aortic valvular lesions [91]. This process eventually leads to dissection or rupture of the aortic wall with potentially fatal consequences. Several molecular pathways have been discovered, possibly of genetic basis, which suggest that histopathologic modifications in the extracellular matrix of the dilated proximal aortic wall are a key pathogenesis of aortic dilatation in BAV patients. This includes the loss of smooth muscle cells, cystic medial necrosis and elastic fibre fragmentation [92, 93]. Furthermore, morphometric analysis of the aortic media showed deformities of the elastic lamellae and less elastic tissue in BAV patients in comparison with patients with tricuspid aortic valves [93, 94]. It appears that apoptosis is a key mechanism for the loss of the smooth muscle cells in the ascending aorta of BAV patients which can eventually lead to cardiovascular complications [95, 96, 97]. In addition, regarding the remodeling of the extracellular matrix, fibrillin-1 microfibrils were significantly reduced while the matrix metalloproteinase-2 and -9 activities were significantly increased in the aortic media of BAV patients. When fibrillin-1 deficiency is present, the release of enzymes, also known as matrix metalloproteinases, will increase and weaken the aortic wall by degrading elastic matrix components, thus resulting in aortic dilatation and degeneration [98, 99, 100].

Approximately 40% of the BAV cases develop proximal aortic root dilatation while an estimation of 6% lifetime risk is observed for aortic dissection [101].

Risk factors for developing an adverse aortic complications such as rupture or dissection in BAV patients include positive family history of aortic aneurism, dilatation of the sinotubular junction, the presence of AR, young age (<40 years), and aortic dilatation greater than 50 mm [101, 102]. Aortic dissection occurs most commonly in young adults with an asymptomatic medical history of BAV. A severe risk for aortic dissection is present when the aortic diameter surpasses 50 mm. [102]. When BAV is present in combination with aortic dilatation, the risk of aortic dissection is increased 9 fold compared with tricuspid valve cases [16]. Additionally, the area of the aortic dilation also varies among BAV patients. Some patients have a dilatation of the proximal ascending aorta dilation, while others have a dilation of the sinuses of Valsalva and yet other patients present with a dilatation of the transverse arch or a combination of these locations [103].

Aortic dilatation of the sinuses of Valsalva is often seen in patients with L-R BAV, whereas patients with R-N BAV present with the dilatation of the ascending aorta [10]. Of note, aortic dilatation and thoracic aortic aneurysm formation could also occur in BAV patients or related family members with the absence of significant valve pathology in the form of AS or AR [51, 68].

7.4. Infective endocarditis

Infective endocarditis is a condition high risk on mortality and morbidity which effects 10% to 30% of the BAV patients with actual risk assessment of 0.3% to 2% per patient-years in adults. Although these estimations are based on selected cases, the true incidence of BAV related infective endocarditis is most likely lower. [16, 85, 86]. Moreover, one-fourth of the infective endocarditis cases are a complication due to BAV. Infective endocarditis is frequently seen in young adults and adolescents rather than in elderly patients, particularly the male gender [16]. Almost three-quarters of the endocarditis related BAV cases are caused by *Viridans streptococci* and *Staphylococci* [87]. Poor dental hygiene, presence of a dialysis shunt and venous catheters are major independent risk factors for developing infective endocarditis due to the high risk of contamination [88]. Several complications due to infective endocarditis in BAV patient can occur including heart failure, the formation of myocardial or valvular abscess, and mortality within 6 month after hospital admission [89]. Antibiotic prophylaxis is nowadays no longer recommended for patients with BAV and with calcified aortic stenosis, except in BAV patients with a prior history of infective endocarditis, prosthetic heart valves, or prosthetic material used for heart valve repair [90].

8. Interventions

Surgical intervention is the key treatment option for patients with symptomatic BAV disease and the related aortic dilatation. Several factors are dependent on the surgical treatment management including the location and the severity of the aortic dilatation and the performance status of BAV.

8.1. Surgical indications for aortic valve repair/replacement

Surgical intervention for patients with BAV disease occurs at a relative earlier age than for degenerative tricuspid aortic valve disease [71]. In a study of 212 asymptomatic community residents, an average age for surgical intervention was reported for BAV disease versus degenerative tricuspid valve disease of 40± 20 years and 67 ± 16 years, respectively [85]. In Scheme 1, indications for surgical intervention in patients with BAV disease including AR, AS and/or proximal ascending aorta dilation are described. In adults with BAV disease, surgical intervention in the form of AVR is recommended when severe AS, chronic AR and left ventricle dysfunction (LV) with a LV ejection fraction (EF) of < 50% is present. Furthermore, adolescents and young adults with severe AR who have developing symptoms, persistent LV dysfunction with LV EF < 50%, or progressive LV dilatation, are also suitable candidates for AVR [39]. Several factors has to be kept in mind when choosing a patient tailored intervention namely, the risk for reoperation with bioprosthetic valves due to valve degeneration, and the necessity of lifelong anticoagulation with mechanical valve replacement. In athletic patients, bleeding risks due to chronic use of anticoagulation should be discussed, as well as the potential risk of teratogenic dangers of warfarine for women who desire pregnancy in the future. The discussion of the risk and benefits for both procedures is therefore mandatory.

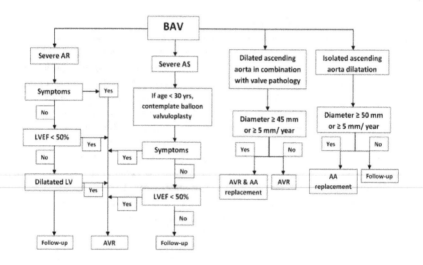

Scheme 1. Indication for cardiac surgical intervention in patients with bicuspid aortic valve disease including aortic regurgitation (AR), aortic stenosis (AS), and/or aortic dilatation. LVEF = left ventricle ejection fraction; LV dilatation = Left ventricle dilatation (End-systolic diameter > 55mm or end-diastolic diameter > 75 mm); Clinical symptoms include dyspnoea, angina, or syncope; Severe AS = jet velocity > 4 m/s, mean gradient. 40 mm Hg, valve area < 1 cm²; severe AR = jet width < 65% of LOVT, vena contracta width > 0.6 cm, regurgitant volume > 60 mL, regurgitant fraction > 60%, regurgitant orifice area >0.3 cm². AVR = aortic valve replacement (Data derived from Bonow *et al.* [39]).

8.2. Surgical indications for ascending aorta dilation

As mentioned earlier, BAV disease is associated with aortic dilatation. BAV patients with the presence of AR or AS should receive surgical intervention of the ascending aorta when an aortic diameter of ≥ 45 mm is present. Conversely, BAV patients with absence of additional risk factors and co morbidities should receive surgical intervention at an aortic root or ascending aorta dilatation of ≥ 50 mm or a aortic dilatation expansion rate of ≥ 5 mm per year [39]. However, it seems that aortic size relative to body size could be a more superior novel technique to define high risk patients requiring surgical intervention [104]. Proper routine evaluation of the aortic root and ascending aorta is therefore mandatory in patients with BAV with echocardiography or MRI to determine the potential presence of an aortic dilatation [67].

8.3. Pharmacological treatment options

Systematic high blood pressure is an independent risk factor for developing complications including aorta dissection in patients with stenotic BAV with aortic root dilatation. B-blocker therapy is therefore advisable for patients with BAV disease [39]. Moreover, osteogenic and proteolytic activities,which is a precursor to atherosclerotic and calcified degenerative AS, have been revealed in early aortic valve disease with the use of multimodality molecular imaging [115]. However, lipid lowering therapy didn't reduce calcific valve progression with respect to moderate to severe AS [116, 134]. Although, little evidence have acknowledged the beneficial use of statins in BAV disease, patients with BAV disease who have risk factors for atherosclerosis should receive statins with the purpose of reducing the degenerative risk in the aorta and potentially preventing atherosclerosis. Long-term vasodilator therapy is only recommended in BAV patients with AR if systematic hypertension is present [39]. Despite this, there is currently no concrete evidence suggesting that pharmacological treatments could alter the natural history or halt the development BAV calcifiation.

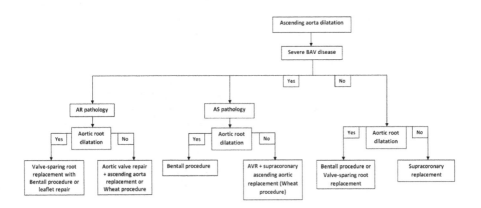

Scheme 2. Cardiac surgical options for aortic dilatation in patients with bicuspid aortic valve disease. AR = aortic re-gurgitation, AS = Aortic stenosis.

8.4. Surgical options

The surgical options are illustrated in Scheme 2 for BAV disease with aortic dilatation. When patients require an intervention of the aortic valve with an aortic diameter < 45 mm, the main surgical option is a bioprosthetic AVR, mechanical AVR, the Ross procedure which is contra-indicated in older patients with BAV and onset of aortic dilatation, or aortic valve repair in selected cases of AR. In patients with > 45 mm ascending aorta root dilatation with significant aortic valve pathology, aortic root replacement therapy, (Bentall procedure) is the main surgical option.

8.5. Valve repair

Surgical repair can be considered when BAV disease is presented without any significant signs of calcification or valve thickening [105]. Several surgical repair options are available including raphé resection with or without leaflet placation, shortening or reinforcement of the free margin, augmentation of the pericardial patch cusp, aortic root repair, and subcommissural annuloplasty [105, 106]. Patients with BAV disease show evidence of sclerosis after the second decade and calcification associated with increasing stenosis at the fourth decade [12, 75]. This raises the question with respect to valve sparing replacement of a dilated aorta, especially in young patients. Although, it appears that the need for reoperation is greater in the surgical repair group for AR, this surgical option still remains attractive in both young adults with AR and women with BAV disease who want to become pregnant.

8.6. Ross procedure

The Ross procedure, also known as the pulmonary autograft, is a cardiac surgical procedure in which the pathological aortic valve is replaced with a patient's own pulmonary valve after which a pulmonary allograft is performed with a valve from a donor which is then used to substitute the patient's own pulmonary valve. Several benefits have been reported with the Ross procedure including the absence of anticoagulation, reduced endocarditis risk, and encouraging valve hemodynamic gradients [107]. However, major concerns have been raised including the most important concern regarding the durability of the autograft and allograft. In addition, another key concern is that histopathologic alterations of the pulmonary trunk may occur, after which the pulmonary trunk can show resemblances of the proximal aorta, thus increasing the risk for aortic aneurysms with a reoperation being the most likely end result [108]. The Ross procedure has no beneficial benefits over conventional AVR in adult patients with respect to hemodynamics or postoperative outcomes. Nevertheless, the Ross procedure offers adolescents, young adults and women with BAV disease who want to become pregnant, an adequate solution in the first decade after the operation. However, limitation with respect to the durability is evident by the end of the first postoperative decade, especially in younger patients [109]. Ross procedure in the setting of BAV disease still remains controversial and should only be performed in selected cases in specialized centres.

8.7. Bentall procedure

Due to the risk of aortic dilatation in patients with BAV disease, the majority of the surgeons evaluate the option of reinforcing or replace the ascending aorta with at the time of the valve surgery. The Bentall procedure is a widely used surgical procedure for patients with BAV and aortic root dilatation. This procedure includes the replacement of the aortic valve, aortic root and ascending aorta with the reimplantation of the coronary arteries [110]. Excellent long-term results have been observed with the Bentall procedure with respect to survival in patients with aortic valve disease and aorta dilatation [111]. This procedure is a suitable intervention in older patients with severe BAV pathology with normal-sized sinuses and dilatation of the supra-coronary ascending aorta.

8.8. Yacoub and David procedure

Valve sparing aortic root replacement procedure may be an alternative to Bentall procedures in selected BAV patients such as young adults who present with aortic root lesion with normally functioning aortic valve including the absence of calcified aortic valves, multileaflet prolapsed and annular dilatation [112]. Two variations for this procedure have been described namely the remodeling (Yacoub) procedure and the re-implantation (David) procedure [113, 114]. The coronary artery ostia are removed as buttons in both procedures followed by reimplantation of a Dacron aortic graft with additional leaflet repair, if required. However, in the David procedure, the aortic root is mobilized to below the plane of the ventriculo-aortic junction followed by a Dacron graft replacement which is telescoped down outside the aortic root to provide a functional aortic annuloplasty. It seems that there is no significant difference between these two procedures in BAV patients. Valve sparing procedures are more surgically changeling than the traditional Bentall procedure and are only conducted in specialized aortic centres. When tubular ascending aorta dilatation is present with no root or valve pathology, supracoronary ascending aortic replacement is required in BAV patients. When valve pathology is present with this anatomical lesion, a Wheat procedure should be preformed. This procedure includes separate AVR or repair leaving the sinus segment intact. However, due to the fact that in most cases sclerosis of the aortic valve starts in the second decade and calcification begins to develop around the fourth decade, serious consideration have to be made with respect to valve-sparing replacement of a dilated aorta in young adults with normally functioning BAV [12, 75].

8.9. Balloon valvuloplasty

Due to the growth of adolescents during childhood, prosthetic valve insertion is unsatisfactory. Balloon valvuloplasty is therefore a successful treatment option because of the fact the aortic valve is not calcified at this age of the child and the fact that valvuloplasty disrupts the commissural fusion and reduces the obstruction when implemented. Balloon valvuloplasty is indicated in young adults and adolescents without significantly calcified BAV and no AR who experience symptoms with a peak-to-peak gradients of > 50 mm Hg. Also, asymptomatic adolescents who develop ST- or T wave changes with exercise or rest or demonstrate a peak-to-peak gradient of > 60 mm Hg should be considered candidates for balloon valvuloplasty. Additional indications for balloon valvuloplasty are asymptomatic adolescent or young adult who are interested in sport activities or becoming pregnant with a peak-to-peak gradient > 50 mm Hg. When severe AR is evident after balloon valvulplasty, AVR should be considered. Conversely, valvuloplasty is seldom performed in old adults due to often severe calcification of the aortic valve [39, 86]. However, balloon valvuloplasty should be considered as a bridge to surgery in adults with AS who have a high risk for AVR, who are hemodynamically unstable, or when AVR is not possible to perform due to secondary co morbidities. Excellent mid-term results have been observed after balloon valvuloplasty at experienced centres [117-119].

8.10. Transcatheter aortic valve implantation

Transcatheter aortic valve implantation (TAVI) is a novel minimally invasive technique indicated for patients who are contraindicated for cardiac surgery due to associated comorbilities or who have a high risk of perioperative mortality. TAVI is an alternative treatment for patients with valve disease in which a valve replacement is introduced through the femoral artery via a small incision or in some cases, an incision into the chest after which the catheter is inserted into the left ventricular apex, also known as the transapical approach. Other methods include subclavian in which the catheter is inserted beneath the collar bone and direct aortic incision in which the catheter is inserted directly into the aorta via a minimally invasive incision in the chest [120]. Due to the asymmetric anatomy which is observed with BAV disease, the TAVI device could potentially be affected to a noncircular expansion, thus creating an elevated risk of paravalvular leak [121]. Due to this major concern, BAV is considered a contraindication with respect to TAVI. BAV have been overall excluded in all the major TAVI trials in which little clinical experience is now known with regard to TAVI in BAV cases. However, several centres showed acceptable results in selected BAV patients with AS [121-123]. A high risk of suboptimal device seating has been observed in BAV patients with asymmetric valvular anatomy, AR, and bulky leaflets. Whether novel valve designs could improve TAVI performance in the BAV group, still remains uncertain.

9. Surveillance

All patients with BAV disease whether AS, AR, operated or not, should receive lifelong serial follow-up depending on symptoms and degree of the functional disorder. Moreover, serial follow-up with imaging assessment with respect to the cardiac and aortic anatomy including valve function, LV function, diameter of both ascending aorta, sinotublular junction, sinuses of Valsvalva and the annulus should be performed in BAV patients regardless the severity of the pathology. TTE is a reliable diagnostic tool to monitor the aortic valve and ascending aorta. However, it should be noted that it is difficult to obtain adequate imaging with the TTE regarding the mid and distal ascending aorta and arch, especially in BAV patients with large body index, in which MRI or CT scan should be used.

The occurrence of imaging should depend on the size of the aortic root at the initial assessment. If the aortic root is < 40 mm with no clinical symptom alternations, the ascending aorta should be reimaged every 2 years. Whereas, if the aortic root is ≥ 40 mm, it is should be reimaged annually or even more often if progression of the aortic root dilatation is present or whenever a change in clinical symptoms and/or findings occur with echocardiography or MRI [39]. Also of importance, first degree family members of patients with BAV disease should receive echocardiographic screening due to the increased risk of cardiovascular abnormalities [39].

10. Sport participation

The vast majority of young adults with BAV disease are asymptomatic. Little is known regarding the risks of aortic dissection and sudden cardiac death in young adults with BAV who participate in athletic activity. Also, the severity of the valve pathology and aortic root dilatation in this subgroup of BAV patients influence the clinical decision making with respect to strategy and recommendations for sport activity.

No restrictions are necessary with respect to BAV patients with an athletic lifestyle who present with a mild AS. However, asymptomatic BAV patients with moderate AS can only conduct low-intensity athletic competitive activities. Exercise stress testing is mandatory for BAV patients with moderate AS to detect any additional risk factors including unusual blood pressure during exercise, onset of symptoms during exercise or pathological arrhythmias, which could eventually alter the clinical strategy and recommendations. In addition, BAV patients with symptomatic moderate or severe AS should receive immediate surgical intervention and should therefore not participate in any form of competitive sport activities upon surgery [124].

BAV patients with mild enlargement of the left ventricular end-diastolic dimension and mild to moderate AR have no restriction in participating in all forms of athletic activity. Also in this case, an exercise stress testing should be performed to estimate the risk. Patients with BAV disease who have a definite LV enlargement of ≥ 60 mm, pulmonary hypertension, or any degree of LV systolic dysfunction at rest should avoid any form of competitive sport activities [124]. BAV patients who underwent an AVR should avoid any form of contact sport.

Also, BAV patients with severe AR and left ventricular end-diastolic diameter > 65 mm should avoid any form of competitive sport activities. This also includes BAV patients with mild-to-moderate AR associated with positive symptoms for valve disease [124]. Young adults with uncalcified AS with a peak-to-peak gradient > 50 mm Hg should who play competitive sports are candidates for aortic balloon valvuloplasty [39]. The recommendation for sport activity for BAV patients with respect to dilatation of the proximal aortic root depends on the level of severity the aortic dilatation. BAV patients with an aortic root diameter of 40 to 45 mm should only perform low to moderate intensity sport activity and preferably avoid any form of contact sport. Moreover, BAV patients with an aortic root diameter of > 45 mm are allowed to conduct low-intensity sport activity due to due to the potential risk of aortic root dissection [125].

11. Pregnancy

Although, the vast majority of pregnancies with congenital AS go through labour uncomplicated, some pregnancies with severe AS have a higher risk rate of morbidity, although the mortality rates still remains rare [126, 127].

Severe AS is not well tolerated in pregnant women and is associated with high peripartum complications [75]. Around one-third of the pregnant women with maternal congenital AS showed clinical complications with a significant rate of abortion [128]. Of note, it is recommended that women with AS who are considering becoming pregnant receive prepregnancy counselling [39].

Nevertheless, mild-to-moderate AS is well tolerated by pregnant women and show no complications with respect to labour compared to pregnant women with severe AS who had a deterioration rate of 10% [126].

Asymptomatic severe AR is well endured by pregnant women unlike severe AS [129]. A possible explanation for this phenomenon is because of pregnancy related physiologic changes which presents with an afterload decrease and heart rate increase with a shortening of the diastole, thus reducing the level of AR.

Of note, several recommendations has to be considered in pregnant women with severe BAV pathology with symptoms including pre-pregnancy counselling, foetal echocardiography during the second trimester to investigate whether cardiac defects is present in the foetus, and close cardiac follow-up in the form of echocardiography to monitor changes in symptoms and further valve deterioration [39]. Several side effects have been reported when cardiac surgery requiring cardiopulmonary bypass is used including the potential risk of fetal distress, fetal wastage and growth retardation [130, 131]. Therefore, it should be noted that women with a high risk for complications during pregnancy should abstain from pregnancy until the valve pathology is properly surgically treated [124]. Moreover, parents should receive proper clinical counselling with respect to the genetic predisposition and the risk of congenital cardiac defect in their children [132].

Encouraging results have been observed with the balloon valvuloplasty during pregnancy including successful completion of the pregnancy [133]. However, concerns have been raised regarding symptomatic AR after balloon valvuloplasty which is also a burden for pregnant patients. Therefore, balloon valvuloplasty should be considered as a bridge to surgery in pregnant women with severe AS. When an unplanned pregnancy occurs in women with severe aortic pathology with symptoms, physical restriction with close cardiac follow-up are obligated. Furthermore, vasodilatation and volume depletion medicine should be avoided at all time. Due to the compression of the inferior vena cava by the gravid uterus, it is recommended that the delivery should be performed in the left lateral decubitus position.

12. Conclusion

BAV disease is a frequently seen congenital cardiac defect, complicated with proximal thoracic aortic aneurysm and associated with other cardiovascular malformations including Turner Syndrome and COA. Although little is known about the pathogenesis of BAV disease, it seems that BAV disease is linked with both genetic predisposition and defects in the early valvulogenesis. Further investigation is required with respect to the basic genetic and embryological defects associated with BAV disease and the proximal aortic dilatation including the cellular mechanisms and signalling pathways. This will give us more understanding regarding the background of the degeneration and calcification of the bicuspid valve, and the development of aortic aneurysm. This could offer new pharmacological targets to prevent calcification, degeneration and aortic dilatation.

The dilatation of the proximal thoracic aorta may lead to complications including ascending aortic aneurysm and dissection. Early detection, vigilant patient assessment and frequent follow-up by imaging including echocardiography, CT and CMRI can potentially persevere both long-term survival and quality of life in patients affected by BAV disease.

Several interventional options are available for patients with BAV disease and aortic dilatation. Balloon valvuloplasty is indicated in young adults and adolescents without significantly BAV calcification. Surgical repair (Yacoub and David procedure) should be considered when BAV disease is presented without any significant signs of calcification or valve thickening. In contrast, when calcified BAV disease is present, AVR, Bentall procedure or Ross procedure is necessary. Although in some cases these procedures are performed in valves without calcification. TAVI is relatively contraindicated due to the asymmetric anatomy which is observed patients with BAV disease. The TAVI device could potentially be affected to a noncircular expansion with the risk of paravalvular leak. BAV patients were excluded in the major TAVI studies. Future research should focus on novel valve designs.

Despite the fact that limited data exist with respect to prophylactic interventions, BAV disease associated aortic dilatation with absence of additional risk factors and co morbidities is indicated when the diameter is ≥ 50 mm or an aortic dilatation expansion rate of ≥ 5 mm per year. In patients with BAV disease with additional risk factors, such as COA, Turner Syndrome and a family history of aortic dissection, replacement should be considered when a diameter of ≥ 45 mm is present. Patients with symptoms of BAV disease due to AR or AS, or asymptomatic LV dysfunction all require surgery. If the ascending aorta exceeds 45 mm, the root should be replaced as well. Valve sparing aortic root replacement procedure is recommended in young patients who present with aortic root lesion with normally functioning aortic valve including the absence of calcified aortic valves, multileaflet prolapsed and annular dilatation. Future studies are mandatory, not only to predict the optimal timing for AVR when symptoms occur, but also to investigate whether prophylactic intervention of the ascending aorta at the time of AVR is necessary. Also, additional studies are required to determine the risks factors for aortic dissection and the optimal diameter at which replacement of the ascending aorta should be performed in patients with BAV disease. Future studies should also focus on sudden cardiac death in young adults with BAV disease who participate in athletic activity.

Author details

George Tokmaji[1], Berto J. Bouma[2], Dave R. Koolbergen[1,3] and Bas A.J.M. de Mol[1]

1 Department of Cardiothoracic Surgery, Academic Medical Center, Amsterdam, The Netherlands

2 Department of Cardiology, Academic Medical Center, Amsterdam, The Netherlands

3 Department of Cardiothoracic Surgery, Leiden University Medical Center, Leiden, The Netherlands

References

[1] Tadros TM, Klein MD, Shapira OM. Ascending aortic dilatation associated with bicuspid aortic valve. Pathophysiology, molecular biology, and clinical implications. Circulation 2009;119:880-890.

[2] Nistri S, Basso C, Marzari C, et al. Frequency of bicuspid aortic valve in young male conscripts by echocardiogram. Am J Cardiol. 2005;96:718–21.

[3] Tutar E, Ekici F, Atalay S, et al. The prevalence of bicuspid aortic valve in newborns by echocardiographic screening. Am Heart J. 2005;150:513–5.

[4] Basso C, Boschello M, Perrone C, et al. An echocardiographic survey of primary school children for bicuspid aortic valve. Am J Cardiol. 2004;93:661–3.

[5] Yener N, Oktar GL, Erer D, Yardimci MM, Yener A. Bicuspid aortic valve. Ann Thorac Cardiovasc Surg 2002;8:264–7.

[6] Roberts WC. The congenitally bicuspid aortic valve. A study of 85 autopsy cases. Am J Cardiol. 1970;26 (1):72–83.

[7] Sabet HY, Edwards WD, Tazelaar HD, Daly RC. Congenitally bicuspid aortic valves: a surgical pathology study of 542 cases (1991 through 1996) and a literature review of 2,715 additional cases. Mayo Clin Proc. 1999;74(1):14–26.

[8] Sievers HH, Schmidtke C. A classification system for the bicuspid aortic valve from 304 surgical specimens. J Thorac Cardiovasc Surg. 2007;133(5):1226–33.

[9] Fernandes SM, Sanders SP, Khairy P, Jenkins KJ, Gauvreau K, Lang P, et al. Morphology of bicuspid aortic valve in children and adolescents. J Am Coll Cardiol. 2004;44(8):1648–51.

[10] Schaefer BM, Lewin MB, Stout KK, Gill E, Prueitt A, Byers PH, et al. The bicuspid aortic valve: an integrated phenotypic classification of leaflet morphology and aortic root shape. Heart. 2008;94(12):1634–8.

[11] Russo CF, Cannata A, LanfranconiM, Vitali E, Garatti A, Bonacina E. Is aortic wall degeneration related to bicuspid aortic valve anatomy in patients with valvular disease? J Thorac Cardiovasc Surg. 2008;136(4):937–42.

[12] Beppu S, Suzuki S, Matsuda H, et al. Rapidity of progression of aortic stenosis in patients with congenital bicuspid aortic valve. Am J Cardiol 1993;71:322–7.

[13] Mancuso D, Basso C, Cardaioli P, Thiene G. Clefted bicuspid aortic valve. Cardiovasc Pathol 2002; 11:217–220.

[14] Peacock TB. Valvular disease of the heart. London: Churchill, 1865:2–33.

[15] Olson LJ, Subramanian R, Edwards WD. Surgical pathology of pure aortic insufficiency: a study of 225 cases. Mayo Clin Proc 1984;59:835–41.

[16] Ward C. Clinical significance of the bicuspid aortic valve. Heart 2000; 83:81–85.

[17] Johnson AD, Detwiler JH, Higgins CB. Left coronary artery anatomy in patients with bicuspid aortic valves. Br Heart J. 1978;40(5):489–93.

[18] Hutchins GM, Nazarian IH, Bulkley BH. Association of left dominant coronary arterial system with congenital bicuspid aortic valve. Am J Cardiol. 1978;42:57–9.

[19] Higgins CB,Wexler L. Reversal of dominance of the coronary arterial system in isolated aortic stenosis and bicuspid aortic valve. Circulation 1975;52:292–6.

[20] Murphy ES, Rosch J, Rahimtoola S. The frequency and significance of coronary arterial dominance in isolated aortic stenosis. Am J Cardiol 1977;39:505–9.

[21] Roberts WC. The structure of the aortic valve in clinically isolated aortic stenosis. An autopsy of 162 patients over 15 years of age. Circulation 1970; 42:91–97.

[22] Sans-Coma V, Fernandez B, Duran AC, Thiene G, Arque JM, Munoz- Chapuli R, Cardo M. Fusion of valve cushions as a key factor in the formation of congenital bicuspid aortic valves in Syrian hamsters. Anat Rec 1996; 244:490–498.

[23] R. Abu-Issa and M. L. Kirby, "Heart field: frommesodermto heart tube," Annual Review of Cell and Developmental Biology, vol. 23, pp. 45–68, 2007.

[24] R. R.Markwald, T. P. Fitzharris, and F. J.Manasek, "Structural development of endocardial cushions," American Journal of Anatomy, vol. 148, no. 1, pp. 85–119, 1977.

[25] A. D. Person, S. E. Klewer, and R. B. Runyan, "Cell biology of cardiac cushion development," International Review of Cytology, vol. 243, pp. 287–335, 2005.

[26] Duran AC, Frescura V, Sans-Coma V, et al. Bicuspid aortic valves in hearts with other congenital heart disease. J Heart Valve Dis 1995;4:581-90.

[27] Fernández B, Fernandez MC, Durán AC, et al. Anatomy and formation of congenital bicuspid and quadricuspid pulmonary valves in Syrian hamsters. Anat Rec 1998;250:70-9.

[28] Kappetein AP, Gittenberger-de Groot AC, Zwinderman AH, et al. The neural crest as a possible pathogenetic factor in coarctation of the aorta and bicuspid aortic valve. J Thorac Cardiovasc Surg 1991;102:830-6.

[29] Schievink WI, Mokri B. Familial aorto-cervicocephalic arterial dissections and congenitally bicuspid aortic valve. Stroke 1995;26: 1935– 40.

[30] Schievink WI, Mokri B, Piepgras DG, Gittenberger-de Groot AC. Intracranial aneurysms and cervicocephalic arterial dissections associated with congenital heart disease. Neurosurgery 1996;39:685–9, discussion 689–90.

[31] Lee TC, Zhao YD, Courtman DW, Stewart DJ. Abnormal aortic valve development in mice lacking endothelial nitric oxide synthase. Circulation 2000;101:2345– 8.

[32] Fernández B, Durán AC, Fernández-Gallego T, Fernández MC, Such M, Arqué JM, Sans-Coma V. Bicuspid aortic valves with different spatial orientations of the leaflets are distinct etiological entities. J Am Coll Cardiol. 2009 Dec 8;54(24):2312-8.

[33] Glick BN, Roberts WC. Congenitally bicuspid aortic valve in multiple family members. Am J Cardiol. 1994 Feb 15;73(5):400-4.

[34] Cripe L, Andelfinger G, Martin J, et al. Bicuspid aortic valve is heritable. J Am Coll Cardiol. 2004;44:138–43.

[35] Huntington K, Hunter AG, Chan KL. A prospective study to assess the frequency of familial clustering of congenital bicuspid aortic valve. J Am Coll Cardiol. 1997;30:1809–12.

[36] Martin LJ, Ramachandran V, Cripe LH, et al. Evidence in favor of linkage to human chromosomal regions 18q, 5q and 13q for bicuspid aortic valve and associated cardiovascular malformations. Hum Genet. 2007;121:275–84.

[37] Garg V, Muth AN, Ransom JF, et al. Mutations in NOTCH 1 cause aortic valve disease. Nature. 2005;437:270–4.

[38] Guo DC, Pannu H, Tran-Fadulu V, et al. Mutations in smooth muscle alpha-actin (ACTA2) lead to thoracic aortic aneurysms and dissections. Nat Genet. 2007;39:1488–93.

[39] Warnes CA, Williams RG, Bashore TM, et al. ACC/AHA 2008 guidelines for the management of adults with congenital heart disease: a report of the American College of Cardiology/American Heart Association Task Force on Practice Guidelines (Writing Committee to Develop Guidelines on the Management of Adults With Congenital Heart Disease). J Am Coll Cardiol 2008;52:e1–121.

[40] Bolling SF, Iannettoni MD, Dick M. Shone's anomaly: operative results and late outcome. Ann Thorac Surg 1990;49:887-93.

[41] Oppenheimer-Dekker A, Gittenberger-de Groot AC, Bartelings MM. Abnormal architecture of the ventricles in hearts with an overriding aortic valve and a perimembranous ventricular septal defect. Int J Cardiol 1985;9:341-55.

[42] Neumayer U, Stone S, Somerville J. Small ventricular septal defects in the adult. Eur Heart J 1998;9:1573-82.

[43] Sugayama SM, Moises RL, Wagenfur J, Ikari NM, Abe KT, Leone C, et al. Williams-Beuren syndrome: cardiovascular abnormalities in 20 patients diagnosed with fluorescence in situ hybridization. Arq Bras Cardiol. 2003;81(5):462–73.

[44] Oliver JM, Gallego P, Gonzalez A, et al. Risk factors for aortic complications in adults with coarctation of the aorta. J Am Coll Cardiol 2004;44:1641-7.

[45] Kuboki K. Clinicopathologic study of congenital bicuspid aortic valve in the aged. Cardio 2000; 35:287–296.

[46] Abbott ME. Coarctation of the aorta of adult type; statistical study and historical retrospect of 200 recorded cases with autopsy; of stenosis or obliteration of descending arch in subjects above age of two years. Am Heart J 1928;3:574.

[47] Luijendijk P, Franken RJ, Vriend JW, Zwinderman AH, Vliegen HW, Winter MM, Groenink M, Bouma BJ, Mulder BJ. Increased risk for ascending aortic dilatation in patients with complex compared to simple aortic coarctation. Int J Cardiol. 2012 Feb 25

[48] Attenhofer Jost CH, Schaff HV, Connolly HM, et al. Spectrum of reoperations after

[49] air of aortic coarctation: importance of an individualized approach because of

[50] xistent cardiovascular disease. Mayo Clin Proc 2002;77:646-53.

[51] Roos-Hesselink JW, Scholzel BE, Heijdra RJ, et al. Aortic valve and aortic arch pathology after coarctation repair. Heart 2003;89:1074-7.

[52] Miller MJ, Geffner ME, Lippe BM, et al. Echocardiography reveals a high incidence of bicuspid aortic valve in Turner syndrome. J Pediatr 1983;102:47-50.

[53] Price WH, Clayton JF, Collyer S, et al. Mortality ratios, life expectancy, and causes of death in patients Turner's syndrome. J Epidem Comm Health 1986;40:97-102.

[54] Matura LA, Ho VB, Rosing D, et al. Aortic dilation and dissection in Turner syndrome. Circulation 2007;116:1e7.

[55] Perloff, JK. The Clinical Recognition of Congenital Heart Disease, 4th ed. Philadelphia, PA: W.B. Saunders, 1994.

[56] Espinal M, Fuisz AR, Nanda NC, Aaluri SR, Mukhtar O, Sekar PC. Sensitivity and specificity of transeophgeal echocardiography for determination of aortic valve morphology. A Heart J. 2000;139 (6):1071-6.

[57] Brandenburg Jr RO, Tajik AJ, Edwards WD, Reeder GS, Shub C, Seward JB. Accuracy of 2-dimensional echocardiographic diagnosis of congenitally bicuspid aortic valve: echocardiographic-anatomic correlation in 115 patients. Am J Cardiol. 1983;51(9): 1469–73.

[58] Espinal M, Fuisz AR, Nanda NC, Aaluri SR, Mukhtar O, Sekar PC. Sensitivity and specificity of transesophageal echocardiography for determination of aortic valve morphology. Am Heart J. 2000;139 (6):1071–6.

[59] Fowles RE, Martin RP, Abrams JM, et al. Two dimensional echocardiographic features of bicuspid aortic valve. Chest 1979;75:434-40.

[60] Nanda NC, Gramiak R. Echocardiographic recognition of the congenital bicuspid aortic valve. Circulation 1974;49:870-5.

[61] Gleeson TG,Mwangi I, Horgan SJ,Cradock A, Fitzpatrick P, Murray JG. Steady-state free-precession (SSFP) cine MRI in distinguishing normal and bicuspid aortic valves. J Magn Reson Imaging. 2008;28(4):873–8.

[62] Malaisrie SC, Carr J, Mikati I, Rigolin V, Yip BK, Lapin B, McCarthy PM. Cardiac magnetic resonance imaging is more diagnostic than 2-dimensional echocardiography in determining the presence of bicuspid aortic valve. J Thorac Cardiovasc Surg. 2012 Aug;144(2):370-6.

[63] McElhinney DB, Lock JE, Keane JF, et al. Left heart growth, function, and reintervention after balloon aortic valvuloplasty for neonatal aortic stenosis. Circulation 2005; 111:451.

[64] Maskatia SA, Ing FF, Justino H, et al. Twenty-five year experience with balloon aortic valvuloplasty for congenital aortic stenosis. Am J Cardiol 2011; 108:1024.

[65] Rehnström P, Malm T, Jögi P, Fernlund E, Winberg P, Johansson J, Johansson S. Outcome of surgical commissurotomy for aortic valve stenosis in early infancy. Ann Thorac Surg. 2007 Aug;84(2):594-8.

[66] Alexiou C, Langley SM, Dalrymple-Hay MJ, Salmon AP, Keeton BR, Haw MP, Monro JL. Open commissurotomy for critical isolated aortic stenosis in neonates. Ann Thorac Surg. 2001 Feb;71(2):489-93.

[67] Hiratzka LF, Bakris GL, Beckman JA, et al. 2010 ACCF/AHA/AATS/ACR/ASA/SCA/ SCAI/SIR/STS/SVM Guidelines for the diagnosis and management of patients with thoracic aortic disease. A Report of the American College of Cardiology Foundation/ American Heart Association Task Force on Practice Guidelines, American Association for Thoracic Surgery, American College of Radiology,American Stroke Association, Society of Cardiovascular Anesthesiologists, Society for Cardiovascular

Angiography and Interventions, Society of Interventional Radiology, Society of Thoracic Surgeons,and Society for Vascular Medicine. J Am Coll Cardiol. 2010 Apr 6;55(14):e27-e129.

[68] Loscalzo ML, Goh DL, Loeys B, et al. Familial thoracic aortic dilation and bicommissural aortic valve: a prospective analysis of natural history and inheritance. Am J Med Genet A. 2007;143A:1960–7.

[69] Svensson LG, Crawford ES. Cardiovascular and Vascular Disease of the Aorta. Philadelphia, PA: WB Saunders Co; 1997.

[70] Kutty S, Greenberg RK, Fletcher S, et al. Endovascular stent grafts for large thoracic aneurysms after coarctation repair. Ann Thorac Surg. 2008;85:1332– 8.

[71] Roberts WC, Ko JM. Frequency by decades of unicuspid, bicuspid, and tricuspid aortic valves in adults having isolated aortic valve replacement for aortic stenosis, with or without associated aortic regurgitation. Circulation 2005; 111:920–925.

[72] Wallby L, Janerot-Sjoberg B, Steffensen T, et al. T lymphocyte infiltration in non-rheumatic aortic stenosis: a comparative descriptive study between tricuspid and bicuspid aortic valves. Heart 2002;88:348-51.

[73] Subramanian R, Olson LJ, Edwards WD. Surgical pathology of pure aortic stenosis: a study of 374 Cases.Mayo Clin Proc 1984;59:683–90.

[74] Pomerance A. Pathogenesis of aortic stenosis and its relation to age. Br Heart J 1972;34:569–74.

[75] Mautner GC, Mautner SL, Cannon RD, et al. Clinical factors useful in predicting aortic valve structure in patients >40 years of age with isolated valvular aortic stenosis. Am J Cardiol 1993;73:194–8.

[76] Wallaby L, Janerot-Sjoberg B, Steffensen T, Broqvist M. T-lymphocyte infiltration in non-rheumatic aortic stenosis: a comparative descriptive study between tricuspid and bicuspid aortic valves. Heart 2002; 88:348–351.

[77] Chan KL, Ghani M, Woodend K, Burwash IG. Case-controlled study to assess risk factors for aortic stenosis in congenitally bicuspid aortic valve. Am J Cardiol 2001; 88:690–693.

[78] Pachulski RT, Chan KL. Progression of aortic valve dysfunction in 51 adult patients with congenital bicuspid aortic valve: assessment and follow-up by Doppler echocardiography. Br Heart J 1993; 69:237–240.

[79] Yotsumoto G, Moriyama Y, Toyohira H, Shimokawa S, Iguro Y, Watanabe S, et al. Congenital bicuspid aortic valve: analysis of 63 surgical cases. J Heart Valve Dis 1998; 7:500–503.

[80] Fedak PWM, Verma S, Tirone ED, Leask RL, Weisel RD, Butany J. Clinical and pathophysiological implications of a bicuspid aortic valve. Circulation 2002; 106:900–904.

[81] Roberts WC, Morrow AG, McIntosh CL, Jones M, Epstein SE. Congenitally bicuspid aortic valve causing severe, pure aortic regurgitation without superimposed infective endocarditis. Analysis of 13 patients requiring aortic valve replacement. Am J Cardiol. 1981;47(2):206–9.

[82] Lewin MB, Otto CM. The bicuspid aortic valve: adverse outcomes from infancy to old age. Circulation. 2005;111(7):832–4.

[83] Nistri S, Sorbo MD, Marin M, et al. Aortic root dilatation in young men with normally functioning bicuspid aortic valves. Heart 1999;82:19–22.

[84] Cosgrove DM, Valvuloplasty for aortic insufficiency. J Thorac Cardiovasc Surg 1991, 102, 571–576.

[85] Michelena HI, Desjardins VA, Avierinos JF, et al. Natural history of asymptomatic patients with normally functioning or minimally dysfunctional bicuspid aortic valve in the community. Circulation 2008; 117:2776–84.

[86] Tzemos N, Therrien J, Yip J, et al. Outcomes in adults with bicuspid aortic valves. JAMA 2008;300:1317–25.

[87] Thiene G, Basso C Pathology and pathogenesis of infective endocarditis in native heart valves. Cardiovasc Pathol 2006, 15, 256–263.

[88] Habib G, Hoen B, Tornos P, et al. Guidelines on the prevention, diagnosis, and treatment of infective endocarditis (new version 2009): the Task Force on the Prevention, Diagnosis, and Treatment of Infective Endocarditis of the European Society of Cardiology (ESC). Endorsed by the European Society of Clinical Microbiology and Infectious Diseases (ESCMID) and the International Society of Chemotherapy (ISC) for Infection and Cancer. Eur Heart J. 2009 Oct;30(19):2369-413.

[89] Lamas GC, Eykyn SJ. Bicuspid aortic valve—a silent danger: analysis of 50 cases of infective endocarditis. Clin Infect Dis 2000;30:336-41.

[90] Nishimura RA, Carabello BA, Faxon DP et al. ACC/AHA 2008 guideline update on valvular heart disease: focused update on infective endocarditis: a report of the American College of Cardiology/American Heart Association Task Force on Practice Guidelines: endorsed by the Society of Cardiovascular Anesthesiologists, Society for Cardiovascular Angiography and Interventions, and Society of Thoracic Surgeons. Circulation. 2008 Aug 19;118(8):887-96.

[91] Keane MG, Wiegers SE, Plappert T et al. (2000) Bicuspid aortic valves are associated with aortic dilatation out of proportion to coexistent valvular lesions. Circulation, 102, III35–III39.

[92] Niwa K, Perloff JK, Bhuta SM, Laks H, Drinkwater DC, Child JS, Miner PD. Structural abnormalities of great arterial walls in congenital heart disease. Light and electron microscopic analyses. Circulation 2001; 103:393– 400.

[93] Parai JL, Masters RG, Walley VM, Stinson WA, Veinot JP. Aortic medial changes associated with bicuspid aortic valve: myth or reality? Can J Cardiol 1999; 15:1233–1238.

[94] Bauer M, Pasic M, Meyer R. Morphometric analysis of aortic media in patients with bicuspid and tricuspid aortic valve. Ann Thorac Surg 2002; 74:58–62.

[95] Bonderman D, Gharehbaghi-Schnell E, Wollenek G, Maurer G, Baumgartner H, Lang IM. Mechanisms underlying aortic dilatation in congenital aortic valve malformation. Circulation 1999; 99:2138–2143.

[96] Schmid FX, Bielenberg K, Schneider A, Haussler A, Keyser A, Birnbaum D. Ascending aortic aneurysm associated with bicuspid and tricuspid aortic valve: involvement and clinical relevance of smooth muscle cell apoptosis and expression of cell death-initiating proteins. Eur J Cardiothorac Surg 2003; 23:537–543.

[97] Nataatmadja M, West M, West J, Summers K, Walker P, Nagata M, Watanabe T. Abnormal extracellular matrix protein transport associated with increased apoptosis of vascular smooth muscle cells in Marfan syndrome and bicuspid aortic valve thoracic aortic aneurysm. Circulation 2003; 108 (suppl II):329–334.

[98] Fedak PW, de Sa MP, Verma S, Nili N, Kazemian P, Butany J, et al. Vascular matrix remodeling in patients with bicuspid aortic valve malformations: implications for aortic dilatation. J Thorac Cardiovasc Surg 2003; 126:797–806.

[99] Boyum J, Fellinger EK, Schmoker JD, Trombley L, McPartland K, Ittleman FP, Howard AB. Matrix metalloproteinase activity in thoracic aortic aneurysms associated with bicuspid and tricuspid aortic valves. J Thorac Cardiovasc Surg 2004; 127:686–691.

[100] Koullias GJ, Korkolis DP, Ravichandran P, Psyrri A, Hatzaras I, Elefteriades JA. Tissue microarray detection of matrix metalloproteinases, in diseased tricuspid and bicuspid aortic valves with or without pathology of the ascending aorta. Eur J Cardiothorac Surg 2004; 26:1098–1103.

[101] El-Hamamsy I, Yacoub MH. A measured approach to managing the aortic root in patients with bicuspid aortic valve disease. Curr Cardiol Rep. 2009;11 (2):94–100.

[102] Roberts CS, Roberts WC (1991) Dissection of the aorta associated with congenital malformation of the aortic valve. J Am Coll Cardiol, 17, 712–716.

[103] Fazel SS, Mallidi HR, Lee RS, Sheehan MP, Liang D, Fleischman D, Herfkens R, Mitchell RS, Miller DC: The aortopathy of bicuspid aortic valve disease has distinctive patterns and usually involves the transverse aortic arch. J Thorac Cardiovasc Surg 2008, 135 (4):901–907, 907 e901-902.

[104] Davies RR, Gallo A, Coady MA, Tellides G, Botta DM, Burke B, Coe MP, Kopf GS, Elefteriades JA. Novel measurement of relative aortic size predicts rupture of thoracic aortic aneurysms. Ann Thorac Surg. 2006 Jan;81(1):169-77.

[105] Borger MA, David TE. Management of the valve and ascending aorta in adults with bicuspid aortic valve disease. Semin Thorac Cardiovasc Surg. 2005;17(2):143–7.

[106] El Khoury G, Vanoverschelde JL, Glineur D, Pierard F, Verhelst RR, Rubay J, et al. Repair of bicuspid aortic valves in patients with aortic regurgitation. Circulation. 2006;114(1 Suppl):I610–1616.

[107] Cameron DE, Vricella LA. What is the proper place of the Ross procedure in our modern armamentarium? Curr Cardiol Rep. 2007;9(2):93–8.

[108] de Sa M, Moshkovitz Y, Butany J, David TE. Histologic abnormalities of the ascending aorta and pulmonary trunk in patients with bicuspid aortic valve disease: clinical relevance to the ross procedure. J Thorac Cardiovasc Surg. 1999;118(4):588–94.

[109] Takkenberg JJ, Klieverik LM, Schoof PH, van Suylen RJ, van Herwerden LA, Zondervan PE, Roos-Hesselink JW, Eijkemans MJ, Yacoub MH, Bogers AJ. The Ross procedure: a systematic review and meta-analysis. Circulation. 2009 Jan 20;119(2):222-8.

[110] Bentall H, De Bono A. A technique for complete replacement of the ascending aorta. Thorax. 1968;23 (4):338–9.

[111] Etz CD, Bischoff MS, Bodian C, et al. The Bentall procedure: is it the gold standard? A series of 597 consecutive cases. Ann Thorac Cardiovasc Surg. 2010;140:S64–71.

[112] Schmitto JD, Mokashi SA, Chen FY, Chen EP. Aortic valve-sparing operations: state of the art. Curr Opin Cardiol. 2010 Mar;25(2):102-6.

[113] David TE, Feindel CM. An aortic valve-sparing operation for patients with aortic incompetence and aneurysm of the ascending aorta. J Thorac Cardiovasc Surg 1992; 103:617–621.

[114] Sarsam MA, Yacoub M. Remodeling of the aortic valve annulus. J Thorac Cardiovasc Surg 1993; 105:435–438.

[115] Aikawa E, Nahrendorf M, Sosnovik D, et al. Multimodality molecular imaging identifies proteolytic and osteogenic activities in early aortic valve disease. Circulation. 2007;115:377– 86.

[116] Cowell SJ, Newby DE, Prescott RJ, et al. A randomized trial of intensive lipid-lowering therapy in calcific aortic stenosis. N Engl J Med. 2005 Jun 9;352(23):2389-97

[117] Moore P, Egito E, Mowrey H, Perry SB, Lock JE, Keane JF. Midterm results of balloon dilation of congenital aortic stenosis: predictors of success. J Am Coll Cardiol 1996;27:1257– 63.

[118] McCrindle BW, for the Valvuloplasty and Angioplasty of Congenital Anomalies (VACA) Registry Investigators. Independent predictors of immediate results of percutaneous balloon aortic valvotomy in children. Am J Cardiol 1996;77:286 –93.

[119] Rosenfeld HM, Landzberg MJ, Perry SB, Colan SD, Keane JF, Lock JE. Balloon aortic valvuloplasty in the young adult with congenital aortic stenosis. Am J Cardiol 1994;73:1112-7.

[120] Holmes DR Jr, Mack MJ, Kaul S, et al. 2012 ACCF/AATS/SCAI/STS expert consensus document on transcatheter aortic valve replacement. J Am Coll Cardiol. 2012 Mar 27;59(13):1200-54.

[121] Wijesinghe N, Ye J, Rodes-Cabau J, et al. Transcatheter aortic valve implantation in patients with bicuspid aortic valve stenosis. J Am Coll Cardiol Intv. 2010;3:1122-5.

[122] Delgado V, Tops LF, Schuijf JD, et al. Successful deployment of a transcatheter aortic valve in bicuspid aortic stenosis: role of imaging with multislice computed tomography. Circ Cardiovasc Imaging. 2009;2: e12-3.

[123] Chiam PT, Chao VT, Tan SY, et al. Percutaneous transcatheter heart valve implantation in a bicuspid aortic valve. J Am Coll Cardiol Intv. 2010;3:559-61.

[124] Bonow RO, Carabello BA, Kanu C, et al. ACC/AHA 2006 guidelines for the management of patients with valvular heart disease: a report of the American College of Cardiology/American Heart Association Task Force on Practice Guidelines (Writing Committee to Revise the 1998 Guidelines for the Management of Patients With Valvular Heart Disease). J Am Coll Cardiol 2006;48:e1–148.

[125] Bonow RO, Cheitlin MD, Crawford MH, Douglas PS. Task Force 3: valvular heart disease. J Am Coll Cardiol. 2005;45(8):1334-40.

[126] Silversides C, Colman JM, Sermer M, et al. Early and intermediate-term outcomes of pregnancy with congenital aortic stenosis. Am J Cardiol 2003;91:1386-9.

[127] Hameed A, Karaalp IS, Tummala PP, et al. The effect of valvular heart disease on maternal and fetal outcome of pregnancy. J Am Coll Cardiol. 2001;37:893–9.

[128] Lao TT, Sermer M, Magee L, et al. Congenital aortic stenosis. Am J Obstet Gynecol 1993;169:540-5.

[129] Elkayam U, Bitar F. Valvular heart disease and pregnancy part I: native valves. J Am Coll Cardiol. 2005 Jul 19;46(2):223-30.

[130] Sullivan HJ. Valvular heart surgery during pregnancy. Surg Clin North Am 1995;75:59-75.

[131] Goldstein I, Jakobi P, Gutterman E, et al. Umbilical artery flow velocity during maternal cardiopulmonary bypass. Ann Thorac Surg 1995;60:1116-8.

[132] Brickner ME. Valvar aortic stenosis. In: Gatzoulis MA, Webb GD, Daubeney PE, editors. Diagnosis and Management of Adult Congenital Heart Disease. Philadelphia, PA: Churchill Livingstone, 2003.

[133] Banning AP, Pearson JF, Hall RJ. Role of balloon dilatation of the aortic valve in pregnant patients with severe aortic stenosis. Br Heart J 1993;70:544-5.

[134] Teo KK, Corsi DJ, Tam JW, Dumesnil JG, Chan KL Lipid lowering on progression of mild to moderate aortic stenosis: meta-analysis of the randomized placebo-controlled clinical trials on 2344 patients. Can J Cardiol. 2011 Nov-Dec;27(6):800-8.

[135] Ciotti GR, Vlahos AP, Silverman NH. Morphology and function of the bicuspid aortic valve with and without coarctation of the aorta in the young. Am J Cardiol. 2006 Oct 15;98(8):1096-102.

[136] Wendell DC, Samyn MM, Cava JR et al. Including aortic valve morphology in computational fluid dynamics simulations: Initial findings and application to aortic coarctation. Med Eng Phys. 2012 Aug 20.

Current Treatment Approaches

Chapter 3

Current Treatment Options in Aortic Stenosis

Fahrettin Oz, Fatih Tufan, Ahmet Ekmekci,
Omer A. Sayın and Huseyin Oflaz

Additional information is available at the end of the chapter

1. Introduction

There is a trend towards a worldwide aging in the last decades and diseases which are common in the elderly people would take important place in clinical practice. Although patients with aortic stenosis (AS) usually remain asymptomatic for a long time, once the classic triad of angina, syncope, and exertional dyspnea develop, the prognosis becomes dramatically worse. Accurate diagnosis and efficient treatment are getting more important as aortic valve replacement is the treatment of choice for severe AS.

We present a detailed description of the different therapeutic procedures that are being developed and increasingly used as an alternative to standard surgical treatment. However special surgical techniques as low-profile mechanical prosthesis, biological prosthesis (both stented and stentless), homograft and Ross technique (pulmonary autograft in aortic position and homograft in pulmonary position) will also be discussed in this chapter. We would also like to mention special considerations about treatment in special groups such as elderly.

2. Medical treatment

The standard therapy for symptomatic patients with severe aortic stenosis (AS) due to any cause is replacement of the valve. Since the prognosis dramatically worsens once the symptoms of AS develop, this is a late stage for an effective medical treatment. Patient education regarding the disease course and typical symptoms is an important priority. Current management of patients with AS comprises monitoring disease progression. Unfortunately, in patients with AS medical therapy may not prolong life nor improve progression and has limited utility in alleviating symptoms. Severe AS is adversely affected by changes in preload and afterload. In patients with severe AS, drugs that reduce preload or afterload should be used with caution because any medical treatment option used in these patients may worsen the patients' conditions. Meanwhile, there is a growing body of evidence about TAVI which is currently used mainly in patients with multi-morbidity and high surgical risk. In patients with rheumatic valve disease, rheumatic fever prophylaxis is strongly recommended to prevent repetitive valve scarring [1]. It has been hypothesized that some of the risk factors and pathophysiologic mechanisms in atherosclerosis play an important role in the development of calcific AS. Therefore theoretically, anti-inflammatory and anti-proliferative agents might slow or prevent disease progression. Because patients with severe AS are mostly older adults, some important and common issues like kidney insufficiency (KI), autonomic dysfunction, conduction disturbances, propensity to falls, and osteoporosis should always be kept in mind in the medical management of these patients.

2.1. Hypertension

Hypertension is not uncommon in patients with AS and approximately 40 percent of patients have hypertension [2]. In patients with concomitant hypertension and AS, left ventricular afterload is elevated as result of the "double-load" of increased systemic vascular resistance and valve stenosis [3]. For this reason reducing afterload may improve the degree of valvular opening and stroke volume. Therefore treatment of hypertension is recommended in patients with asymptomatic AS by many clinicians. There are a few studies assessing the safety of anti-hypertensive treatment in patients with AS [4]. Angiotensin converting enzyme (ACE) inhibitors seem to be well tolerated both in patients with mild-to-moderate and severe AS [5, 6]. Recently, ACE inhibitors and angiotensin receptor blockers (ARBs) were reported to be associated with improved survival and reduced cardiovascular (CV) events [7]. On the other hand, the recently published Simvastatin and Ezetimibe in Aortic Stenosis (SEAS) study reported an increased risk of CV events associated with antihypertensive treatment. However, this study was not a dedicated study on HT in AS and the only type of anti-hypertensive drug group associated with increased CV events was alpha-blockers [4]. This finding is in accordance with the results of Antihypertensive and Lipid-Lowering Treatment to Prevent Heart Attack Trial [8]. Blood pressure lowering agents should be initiated at low doses and gradually titrated with frequent monitoring, especially in older patients with increased risk of falls and osteoporotic fractures. Especially older patients given alpha blockers or diuretics should be informed about orthostatic hypotension to avoid falls.

2.2. Coronary artery disease

Coronary artery disease (CAD) is rather common in patients with AS and evaluation regarding conventional atherosclerotic risk factors is recommended in these patients. Tobacco use should be discouraged. The current US Preventive Services Task Force recommends usage of low dose aspirin for primary prevention when CV risk outweighs the risk of gastrointestinal hemorrhage in men between 45-79 years and when the risk of ischemic stroke outweighs the risk of gastrointestinal hemorrhage in women between 55-79 years [9]. It is also stated that the current evidence is insufficient to assess the balance of benefits and harms of aspirin in patients 80 years or older [9]. A recently published article reported the outcomes of percutaneous coronary intervention (PCI) in patients with concomitant severe AS and CAD [10]. In this well-matched trial, 30-day mortality after PCI was similar in patients with and without severe AS. In this study AS patients with low EF (≤30) and high Society of Thoracic Surgeons score (≥10) were associated with significantly increased 30-day mortality after PCI. Patients with mild AS should not be restricted from physical activity. Patients with severe AS should avoid competitive or vigorous activities that involve high dynamic and static muscular demands, although other forms of exercise are safe. Exercise may also improve functional capacity and may prevent skeletal muscle mass loss (i.e. sarcopenia).

2.3. Atrial fibrillation

Valvular heart disease, particularly left-sided valvular lesions precipitate the development of atrial fibrillation (AF). Although it has been less well studied in AS compared to mitral valve disorders, AF often complicates uncorrected aortic valve disorders [11]. In the recently published SEAS study, baseline or prior was present in approximately 9% of patients with mild-to-moderate AS [12]. The study excluded the patients with baseline and prior AF and sought the effect of simvastatin plus ezetimibe on new-onset AF. During an average of 4.3±0.8 years of follow up, 6% of the patients developed AF and the rate was similar between the simvastatin plus ezetimibe and placebo groups. In this study, increased age and left ventricular mass index were independent predictors of new onset AF. New-onset AF was associated with two-fold higher risk of AF related outcomes and four-fold higher risk of nonfatal nonhemorrhagic stroke. In a previously asymptomatic patient, new onset AF may cause overt heart failure symptoms due to the noncompliant left ventricle which is associated with a relative shift of left ventricular filling to the later part of diastole with a greater dependence upon atrial contraction. Similar treatment approaches for AF in patients with AS can be used as in patients without AS. Heart rate control is important to enable an adequate diastolic filling time. Although guidelines generally recommend rate control over rhythm control in patients with AS, there is a trend towards preference of rhythm control with the benefits of early rhythm control and options of left atrial catheter ablation and new anti-arrhythmic drugs [13, 14]. Within the current ECS guidelines on AF, severe AS is stated as a contraindication for verkalant usage [14]. It is also important to screen for coronary disease in patients with AS before the initiation of class Ic anti-arrhythmic drugs for rhythm control for AF [11]. Significant ventricular hypertrophy or dysfunction increases the risk of proarrhythmia associated with class Ic and most class III anti-arrhythmic drugs. In such patients amidodarone is the preferred agent [11]. However, when medications for heart rate control such as beta blockers and non-dihydropridine calcium channel blockers are used, their potential to depress LV systolic function and cause clinical deterioration should be kept in mind. Specific considerations about drug choices to control heart-rate are depicted in the following specific drug classes section. Specific considerations about warfarin treatment are depicted in the following specific drug classes section.

2.4. Heart failure

In patients with severe AS, aortic valve replacement (AVR) is indicated when symptomatic heart failure develops. Even when severe AS is present, transvalvular pressure gradients may not be found high because of left ventricular systolic dysfunction. Reduced EF is associated with worse clinical outcome. A recent study compared the outcomes of severe AS patients with an EF of ≤30 or >30 who was followed with medical treatment or underwent TAVI [15]. While an EF of ≤30 was associated with worse prognosis in the medically treatment group, TAVI was associated with an improvement in EF and functional class and patients who underwent TAVI had better prognoses irrespective of their baseline EF. When patients with mild or moderate AS have HF, there is generally other causes of HF like coronary heart disease and medical therapy of HF is preferable to AVR. Vasodilator therapy and beta blockers may be started with careful dose titration and closely monitoring. Volume status of patients should also be determined and followed up carefully [3, 16].

Invasive hemodynamic monitoring in the intensive care unit should be considered for decompensated patients with severe AS [3]. Nitroprusside rapidly and markedly improves cardiac function in patients with decompensated HF due to severe left ventricular systolic dysfunction and severe AS. It provides a safe and effective bridge to AVR or oral vasodilator therapy in these critically ill patients [17].

Phosphodiesterase type 5 inhibition had beneficial effects on pressure overload in preclinical models and a preliminary study of oral sildenafil in 20 patients with severe symptomatic AS showed that it was associated a reduction in systemic and pulmonary vascular resistance and pulmonary artery and wedge pressures [18]. Although sildenafil was also resulted in 11% decrease in mean systemic arterial pressure, it was not associated with any episodes of symptomatic hypotension.

2.5. Metabolic syndrome

Metabolic syndrome (MS) is a worldwide problem with increased risk of CV events. The results of Multi-Ethnic Study of Atherosclerosis (MESA) and another recent prospective trial suggest that MS is independently associated with progression of AS, particularly in younger individuals [19, 20]. Although these findings need to be confirmed in larger studies, studies assessing the effects of lifestyle modification and reduction of insulin resistance on the incidence and progression rate of AS could be of value.

2.6. Malnutrition

Malnutrition is a common and important health problem in the older adults and being underweight is associated with a worse prognosis than being overweight in this population [21]. Association of malnutrition and heart valve disorders is rarely reported in the literature. Otto et al reported increased long-term mortality independently associated with cachexia in 674 elderly patients who underwent balloon aortic valvuloplasty for AS [22]. Another observational study showed association of heart valve calcification with malnutrition in patients on hemodialysis [23]. In this study evaluation of malnutrition was done only with albumin level which is not specific for malnutrition. Wang et al demonstrated the correlation of fetuin-A, which has recently been identified as an important circulating inhibitor of calcification, with the presence and degree of malnutrition in patients on peritoneal dialysis [24].

There is also data indicating undernutrition is associated with worse outcomes after cardiac valve surgery. In a retrospective study, impact of BMI and albumin levels on morbidity and mortality after cardiac surgery was assessed in 5168 patients undergoing coronary artery bypass or valve operations [25]. Preoperative low albumin (<2.5 g/dl) and low BMI (<20 kg/m2) were independently associated with increased postoperative mortality. Tepsuwan et al. assessed the impact of cardiac cachexia retrospectively in 353 patients who underwent cardiac valve surgery [26]. The study population was relatively young and mitral stenosis and mitral regurgitation were the most frequent valve disorders. They found significant association between cachexia and worse New York Heart Association functional class and worse postoperative outcomes. Thourani et al investigated the impact of body mass index (BMI) on outcomes after cardiac valve surgery in 4247 patients [27]. Most of the procedures were isolated AVR (47.2%). They showed increased in-hospital and all-cause long-term mortality in patients with a BMI of less than 25 compared to patients with a BMI of 25-35 or higher than 35. In this study, no laboratory or clinical data about nutritional status was reported.

Patients with AS may suffer from dietary restriction due to reduced physical capacity and depressive mood. When concomitant mesenteric vessel atherosclerosis is present, abdominal angina may cause avoidance from eating. All these factors may render these patients susceptible to infectious diseases, osteoporosis, skeletal muscle loss (i.e. sarcopenia) and fall related fractures. Unfortunately, there is no study evaluating the role of nutritional intervention, which may potentially improve muscle and bone mass, muscle functions, and functional capacity, on clinical outcomes in patients with AS.

2.7. Depression

Later-life depression (LLD) is associated with disability and poor outcomes [28]. Among various chronic medical conditions, cardiac disease and arthritis are the most commonly ones associated with depression [29]. Underlying medical problems may affect the prognosis of depression and depression may decrease compliance to medical treatment thus delay recovery from medical illnesses [28]. The importance of screening for depression in patients with heart disease is well established, but identifying patients with depression may be difficult. Organic somatic symptoms possibly unrelated to mood may increase the score on depression scales and patients with depression may deny and do not report their depressive symptoms [28]. Furthermore, there are many shared symptoms of heart disease and depression like insomnia, fatigue, shortness of breath, weight loss, palpitations, and exercise intolerance. Vascular depression is associated with late onset, treatment-resistant symptoms, vascular disease, vascular risk factors, and extensive cerebrovascular lesions [28]. Although there is no specific data about the association of vascular depression and AS in the elderly, atherosclerosis has pivotal role in the pathogenesis of both.

Beta blocker treatment, which is being used commonly in patients with heart disease, may potentially precipitate depression. Although there is conflicting data about the association of beta blockers and depression, and individual susceptibility to depression may be important, patients with risk factors for depression should be followed up in terms of development of depression [30]. Lipophilic beta blockers like propranolol, timolol, pindolol, metoprolol, carvedilol and nebivolol are more strongly associated with depression than hydrophilic beta blockers like atenolol, nadolol, practolol and sotalol [30]. When there are strong indications like CAD and CHF for beta blocker treatment are present, depression should not be considered as an absolute contraindication. SSRI are among the most commonly used medications in the treatment of depression. There is some data that indicate use of SSRI in patients with CAD and depression may improve CV outcomes [31]. Because treatment with SSRI may reduce platelet functions as severe AS do, bleeding complications of surgical procedures may be increased in patients with severe AS under SSRI treatment. Sodium levels should be monitored in older patients under SSRI treatment, especially if concomitant diuretic use is present because both of them may be associated with hyponatremia.

2.8. Perioperative medical treatment

Careful manipulation of hemodynamics in the perioperative period is crucial in patients with AS [32]. Maintaining sinus rhythm, a relatively slow heart rate, and adequate preload and afterload are important goals to minimize the perioperative CV risk [32]. Ideal heart rate is between 60 and 70 beats per minute and bradicardia should be avoided. Careful assessment of hydration status and providing adequate hydration is also important to maintain preload which these patients are dependent upon. Careful monitoring of the arterial blood and central venous pressures is also important. Hypotension should be controlled with pure α agonists because they do not cause tachycardia. Routine antibiotic prophylaxis is not recommended unless the patient has a previous history of infective endocarditis [33]. Severe AS may be associated with markedly reduced platelet functions. One recent double-blind placebo controlled trial investigated effects of infusion of desmopressin (0.3 µg/kg) on platelet functions and postoperative blood loss [34]. The authors recommend assessing of platelet functions in the preoperative period in patients with severe AS and usage of desmopressin to avoid increased blood loss in patients with reduced platelet functions.

Delirium is rather common after cardiac valve surgery and is independently associated with increased risk of short and long term morbidity and mortality [35, 36]. Hyperactive delirium is easily recognized because of agitation, hallucinations and delusions. Routine assessment of attention and orientation is crucial to detect hypoactive delirium because it is easily and frequently overlooked. Providing adequate volume status, following up of renal functions and electrolyte levels, controlling postoperative pain and rational selection of medications may reduce the risk of delirium. Many drugs like anticholinergics, antihistaminics, narcotics and central acting drugs may precipitate delirium. Maldonado et al. investigated the effects of postoperative sedation on the development of delirium in patients undergoing cardiac valve surgery [35]. In this open label study, dexmedetomidine was associated with a significantly decreased rate of delirium with compared to propofol and midazolam (rates of delirium 3%, 50% and 50% respectively).

2.9. Perioperative medical treatment for non-cardiac surgery

Beta blocker treatment is recommended in patients with CAD or more than one of the cardiac risk factors which are listed in Table 1 [37]. However, the multicenter POISE trial showed an increased rate of death associated with perioperative beta blocker treatment despite a significant reduction in the primary composite endpoint of CV death, nonfatal MI or nonfatal cardiac arrest [38]. This trial resulted in the following recommendation in the current guidelines: "Routine administration of high-dose beta blockers in the absence of dose titration is not useful and may be harmful to patients not currently taking beta blockers who are undergoing noncardiac surgery" [37]. Titration of beta blockers to heart rate and blood pressure is recommended if the patient will undergo high- or intermediate-risk surgery [37]. Like it is recommended for many drug classes, starting beta blockers in low doses and careful titration is important in elderly patients who are at increased risk for bradycardia and hypotension. The role of beta blockers in intermediate- and low-risk patients is not well known. Optimal type, dose, timing, duration, and titration of beta blockers are also lacking [37]. Withdrawal of beta blockers in the preoperative period may be associated with adverse events and should not be performed unless necessary. Metformin and renin-angiotensin-aldosterone system (RAS) blockers increase the risk of postoperative lactic acidosis and KI respectively and it is recommended to stop them before the surgery.

History of ischemic heart disease
History of compensated or prior heart failure
History of cerebrovascular disease
Diabetes Mellitus
Renal insufficiency (defined as a preoperative serum creatinine of greater than 2 mg/dL)

Table 1. Clinical risk factors for perioperative cardiovascular complications

2.10. Specific drug classes

2.10.1. Statins

It has been considered that the valve lesion in calcific AS might share similar pathogenetic mechanisms with atherosclerosis and progression may be related to known atherosclerotic risk factors [39]. Statins are now well established in the primary and secondary prevention of CAD. Several studies have suggested that statins may cause regression of CAD and reduce the calcific volume of coronary plaques [40]. In accordance with this finding, presence and progression of aortic valve calcification are reported to be increased in patients with a serum LDL cholesterol >130 mg/dL [41].

While some earlier studies indicate that statin therapy is associated with a slower rate of hemodynamic progression of AS [42-45], some more recent trials have inconsistent results of different statin preparations on the progression of AS [46-49]. SALTIRE (Scottish aortic stenosis and lipid lowering therapy, impact on regression) trial was the first double blind randomized controlled trial of lipid lowering treatment in patients with calcific AS. This trial of 155 adults with calcific AS showed that, although atorvastatin 80 mg daily, more than halved serum LDL cholesterol concentrations, there was no difference in the rate of increase in aortic jet velocity or of progression of aortic valve calcification as measured by Doppler echocardiography or helical computed tomography [46]. The prospective open-label RAAVE study (The Rosuvastatin Affecting Aortic Valve Endothelium) comprised of 121 consecutive patients with moderate to severe AS. Treatment with rosuvastatin 20 mg was given when LDL-cholesterol was greater than 130 mg/dL and no statin therapy was given when LDL-cholesterol was less than 130 mg/dL. Patients treated with rosuvastatin had significantly attenuated rates of deterioration in mean aortic valve area and aortic jet velocity compared to patients who did not receive rosuvastatin [47]. The prospective and placebo controlled SEAS trial sought the effect of statins on calcific AS. In this study, 1873 adults (mean age 68) with mild-to-moderate AS were enrolled and randomly assigned to treatment with simvastatin plus ezetimibe or placebo [48]. At median follow-up of 52 months there were no differences in the peak aortic jet velocity or valve area noted between the 2 groups. There was also no difference in CV death, aortic valve replacement, non-fatal myocardial infarction, hospitalized unstable angina pectoris, and heart failure due to progression of AS, coronary artery bypass grafting, percutaneous coronary interventions, or non-hemorrhagic stroke. Although there were fewer ischemic events in the treatment group, this difference was only due to a lower rate of coronary bypass grafting at the time of aortic valve surgery so the clinical relevance of this finding is unclear. SEAS study results show that the effect of statin therapy on disease process does not provide convincing evidence [48]. The investigators of SEAS study recently reported the results of simvastatin plus ezetimibe on new-onset AF in 1421 patients with asymptomatic mild-to-moderate AS [6]. The rate of new-onset AF was similar in the simvastatin plus ezetimibe group compared to placebo group. Aortic Stenosis Progression Observation (ASTRONOMER) is the most recently published trial regarding effect of statins on AS. This double-blind prospective trial randomized 269 younger asymptomatic patients with mild to-moderate AS with no indications for lipid-lowering agents to rosuvastatin 40 mg daily (134 patients) or placebo (135 patients). Unlike earlier trials in which bicuspid aortic valve was rare, a bicuspid valve was present in nearly half of the subjects in this study. After a mean follow-up of 3.5 years, there were no significant differences in the transaortic gradient or aortic valve area in the rosuvastatin group compared to placebo [49].

At present, if atherosclerotic vascular disease or other indications do not coexist, statin therapy solely for AS cannot be recommended. It should be noted that effect of therapy has not been evaluated in earlier stages of the disease.

2.10.2. Angiotensin converting enzyme inhibitors

Although expression of angiotensin II has not been shown the in normal valves, sclerotic aortic valve tissues demonstrably express angiotensin II and angiotensin converting enzyme (ACE). Therefore it may contribute to valve inflammation, calcification, and disease progression [50]. It has been shown that ACE inhibitors suppress ventricular fibrosis and inhibit angiotensin II type 1 receptor in the cardiomyocytes and therefore decrease systolic and diastolic dysfunction in patients with left ventricular hypertrophy and AS [51]. For these reasons ACE inhibitors may have a role in the management of patients with AS. Two preliminary observational studies examined the effect of ACE inhibitors in patients with AS in preventing further changes in the valve leaflets. Rosenhek et al showed that hemodynamic progression of AS did not occur in 211 patients with moderate AS after at least 6 months of treatment with the ACE inhibitors. Furthermore, the presence of hypertension did not appear to influence the outcome [44]. Another retrospective study by Obrien et al of 123 patients evaluated the aortic valve calcium score by electron beam computed tomographic scans. The study showed that ACE inhibitor treatment was associated with a 71% reduction in the progression of aortic valve calcification in 123 patients with AS [52]. At the present, there are no published randomized prospective studies using ACE inhibitors to delay the progression of calcific AS. Some potential targets for therapy in AS such as the pathways involved in inflammation and tissue calcification have not yet been studied. ACE inhibitors have beneficial effects on ventricular systolic and diastolic functions and are well tolerated, increase exercise capacity, and reduce dyspnea in symptomatic patients with mild to moderate AS [6]. ACE inhibitors may provide symptomatic relief when patients with severe AS who are not good candidates for surgery develop symptoms of left heart failure. It should also be kept in mind that ACE inhibitors may increase the transvalvular gradient by reducing afterload or preload and cause sudden clinical deterioration in patients with severe AS. In older adults, ACE inhibitors should be initiated at low doses and gradually increased to avoid hypotension and fall related fractures. Because elderly patients with severe AS generally have extensive atherosclerosis, before initiation of ACE inhibitors bilateral renal artery stenosis should be considered and investigated if suspected.

2.10.3. Angiotensin receptor blockers

Angiotensin receptor blockers have similar hemodynamic effects like ACE inhibitors. A recently published observational study indicates that both ACE inhibitors and ARBs are associated with lower mortality and CV events in patients with AS [7]. However, prospective and controlled studies are needed to test this finding. Although similar precautions as in ACE inhibitors should be considered when starting and maintaining ARBs, they have some benefits like less incidence of cough. Because compelling evidence does not exist for neither ACE inhibitors nor ARBs for these patients, when RAS blockage is planned ACE inhibitors may be selected in the first step and switching to ARBs may be considered if adverse effects like chronic cough develop.

2.10.4. Beta blockers

Beta blockers are a not part of routine medical treatment. Because beta blockers may aggravate the symptoms of HF, patients with symptoms and signs of HF are not good candidates for this treatment option. Beta blockers may be used in AS patients with angina pectoris or AF with rapid ventricular response. Because older adults are at increased risk for hypotension, bradycardia, conduction disturbances and diabetes, a close follow-up should be performed when patients with AS are given beta blocker treatment.

2.10.5. Diuretics

Diuretics are not indicated in patients without signs of congestion because of their potential for reducing preload, which may lead to fall in cardiac output and exacerbation in symptoms of HF. Therefore, diuretics are not first-line treatment options in hypertensive patients with severe AS without findings of congestion. Diuretics may improve symptoms of HF by reducing left ventricular end-diastolic pressure in patients with lung congestion, ascites or edema. Older patients may not excrete free water effectively, and they may more easily develop hyponatremia after diuretic treatment [53]. Thiazide diuretics cause hyponatremia more frequently than loop diuretics [54]. These older patients also have increased tendency to diuretic induced hyponatremia, because concomitant use of other medications like selective serotonin reuptake inhibitors (SSRI), which precipitate hyponatremia, is common. Because of disruption of normal circadian rhythm of antidiuretic hormone, nocturia is frequently seen in elderly patients and may be bothersome and increase the risk of falls when evening or night doses of diuretics are used [55]. Administration of diuretics in earlier hours of the day may be safer. Patients with urgency incontinence may need urinary anti-cholinergics under diuretic treatment to avoid urgency induced falls and significant physical exertion. Diuretics also lead to orthostatic hypotension by inducing volume depletion. Because falls are more frequent and are associated with great morbidity and mortality in these older patients, monitoring of blood pressure at home and avoidance of hypotension is crucial.

2.10.6. Nitrates

Nitrates may be used in symptomatic treatment of angina pectoris in patients with severe AS. They should be initiated at low doses and gradually increased to avoid sudden hypotension. Concomitant use of phosphodiesterase inhibitors for erectile dysfunction should be avoided to prevent substantial hypotension.

2.10.7. Digoxin

Digoxin has a narrow therapeutic index and the risk of adverse events associated with it may be more common in older patients [56]. Digoxin levels may be increased in older patients with impaired kidney functions. Because creatinine levels may be normal or minimally increased in older adults with impaired kidney functions when significant loss of muscle mass (i.e. sarcopenia) is present. It is recommended in the recent ACC/AHA guideline that an initial dose of 0.125 mg daily or every other day is chosen if the patient is older than 70 years old, has impaired kidney function, or has a low lean body mass [57]. Digoxin above 0.125 mg/d is also listed among the potentially inappropriate medications (PIMs) list in the recent Beers criteria [58]. Because digoxin concentrations above 1 ng/ml are not associated with better clinical outcomes and may adversely increase morbidity and mortality, a target digoxin concentration of 0.5-1 ng/ml is recommended despite conventional therapeutic serum concentration is defined as 0.8-2 ng/ml [56, 57]. When there is concomitant hypokalemia, hypomagnesemia or hypothyroidism, digoxin toxicity may occur in lower concentrations [57]. Older patients under digoxin treatment may develop adverse effects like anorexia, nausea, vomiting, confusion, visual problems, and rhythm and conduction disturbances more commonly [56]. Clarithromycin, erythromycin, amiodarone, itraconazole, cyclosporine, verapamil, and quinidine can increase serum digoxin concentrations [57]. Digoxin should not be used in patients with severe AS and sinus rhythm. Digoxin may be used to reduce the ventricular rate in patients with AF and a rapid ventricular rate especially when hemodynamic deterioration is present. When these harms are taken into consideration, should be used with caution as an adjunctive agent for heart rate control. Alternatively, beta blockers, which are associated with improved survival in patients with HF and may effectively control heart rate alone, may be used as first line agents in these patients. However, when hypotension and significant HF signs are present, digoxin may be a better agent for symptomatic treatment.

2.10.8. Calcium channel blockers

Although published data regarding anti-hypertensive drugs in patients with AS is limited, calcium channel blockers like amlodipine do not appear to depress LV function and may be safe to use in patients with AS. Non-dihydropridine agents like diltiazem and verapamil may influence left ventricular systolic functions and may cause clinical deterioration.

2.10.9. Alpha blockers

Peripheral alpha blocker use may possibly lead to hypotension or syncope, decreased coronary perfusion due to reduced afterload and should generally be avoided. Alpha blockers are listed among the PIMs in the recent Beers criteria and routine use for the treatment of hypertension is not recommended [58]. Alpha blockers are also listed among the PIMs in patients with a history of syncope [58].

2.10.10. Warfarin

Warfarin treatment is generally recommended in patients with AS and AF to decrease the incidence of stroke and systemic arterial embolism. Assessing the risk of embolism associated with AF and bleeding associated with warfarin treatment should be carefully performed. It is very important to educate the patient and his/her relatives about the benefits and risks of warfarin treatment and the details of follow-up. Integration of the patients' relatives in the treatment plan is crucial especially in older adults with significant cognitive problems. A meta-analysis which was published in 2007 indicated that aspirin was associated with a 22% reduction in the rate of stroke, while warfarin was associated with 64% reduction [59]. Because warfarin is associated with a significantly lower risk of stroke than aspirin, simply prescribing aspirin without discussing the benefits and risks of warfarin treatment with the patients and their relatives would be therapeutic nihilism. Although there are newer anticoagulant medications like dabigatran which do not require therapeutic monitoring, we need more data especially in the older individuals in order to prescribe them instead of warfarin. For instance, dabigatran is associated with greater risk of bleeding than with warfarin in patients ≥ 75 years and efficacy and safety is not known in patients with a creatinine clearance below 30 ml/min [58].

Warfarin is also the drug of choice in patients with AVR with mechanical prostheses. To date there is no alternative for warfarin for these patients and a higher international normalized ratio (2.5-3.5) is targeted. This translates into increased risk of bleeding associated with warfarin especially in the older patients. These patients may also have other bleeding risk factors like concurrent anti-platelet, SSRI or ginkgo biloba use and platelet dysfunction associated with KI or significant AS. Whether warfarin treatment is appropriate for the patient, may even determine if AVR might be performed and if a mechanical prosthesis might be used. Patients, in whom warfarin treatment is planned, should also be carefully assessed about the risk of falls which may lead to significant bleeding, most importantly to intracranial hemor-rhage. If warfarin is started, ensuring precautions by educating the patients and their relatives to avoid falls is also crucial.

3. Transcathater aortic valve implantation

Surgical AVR is currently the gold-standard treatment for patients with severe symptomatic AS. Without surgery, the prognosis is extremely poor, with a 3-year survival rate of <30%.How-ever, in the huge Euro Heart multinational registry in Europe, 33% of symptomatic patients over the age of 65 years were not referred for surgery [60]. The reasons for not planning surgery were not always the co morbidities. David Bach's series showed the same issue and 33% of symptomatic patients were not referred for surgery, some of whom had a low Euro Score risk [61]. Balloon aortic valvuloplasty, which was described in the 1980s, was the first alternative to surgical therapy [62]. Despite high rates of initial procedural success, restenosis is frequently encountered in the long term. The procedure has generally been abandoned in adult patients except as a palliative procedure often prior to surgical AVR [63]. Trans-catheter aortic valve implantation (TAVI) was first described by Andersen et al in 1992 [64]. They implanted an expandable aortic valve by a catheter technique in a closed chest pig model. The first attempt to use TAVI in man was in 2002 by Cribier et al [65]. A percutaneous bioprosthesis was successfully implanted within the diseased native aortic valve through an antegrade trans-septal approach. In more recent years, the technology has developed very rapidly and, to date, more than 40,000 transcathater valves have been implanted worldwide. The results of several large multicenter registries and randomized Placement of Aortic Transcathater Valves (PARTNER) trial, TAVI is now the standard of care for extremely high risk or 'inoperable ' patients and is a valid alternative to surgery for selected high-risk but ' operable ' patients with symptomatic AS [66-68].

Patients might be considered candidates for TAVI if they fulfill the following criteria: symp-tomatic severe AS, a life expectancy of >1year, contraindications for surgery, high risk for surgery (clinical judgment plus Euro Score (logistic) >20%; STS Score>10%), and/or porcelain aorta, history of thoracic irradiation, severe thoracic deformity, patent coronary bypass, cachexia, recurrent pulmonary emboli, right ventricular insufficiency and cirrhosis.

Contraindications for TAVI are as follows: an aortic annulus of <18 mm or >27 mm, bicuspid valves or unicuspid or noncalcified valve, severe aortic regurgitation or mitral regurgitation, estimated life expectancy < 12 months, evidence of an acute myocardial infarction within one month, MRI confirmed CVA within six months, ejection fraction < 20 %, heavy calcification in front of LM, presence of LV thrombus and need for CABG

Risk Estimation: Accurate estimation of the risk of SAVR performed by an experienced cardiothoracic surgeon and cardiologist is vital to appropriate evaluation of potential candidates for TAVI. Some risk score algorithms like Ambler score, logistic EuroSCORE and Society of Thoracic Surgeons Predicted Risk of Mortality (STS-PROM) are widely used to identify patients at high risk for cardiac surgery. Ambler score was dedicated to predict in-hospital mortality after heart valve surgery [69]. EuroSCORE integrates increased age, female gender, chronic pulmonary disease, extracardiac arteriopathy, neurological dysfunction, previous cardiac surgery, increased serum creatinine, active endocarditis, critical perioperative state, unstable angina, LV dysfunction, recent MI, and pulmonary hypertension as patient and cardiac related factors and some operation related factors like emergency, other than isolated CABG, surgery on thoracic aorta, and postinfarct septal rupture. An online calculator is available in their official website (http://www.euroscore.org/). Logistic EuroSCORE appears to overestimate mortality risk in patients undergoing high-risk aortic valve replacement. The STS-PROM risk scoring which is more complicated integrates age, gender, race, weight, creatinine level, various chronic cardiac and non-cardiac diseases, previous cardiovascular interventions, perioperative cardiac status, hemodynamic status, and operative risk factors. This scoring estimates the rates of postoperative morbidity, mortality, permanent stroke, prolonged ventilation, renal failure, and reoperation. It is updated regularly and calculation can be performed only via the online calculator (http://www.sts.org/). However the STS-PROM model may provide more accurate risk stratification than other scores, more appropriate scoring systems are not currently available. In clinical practice, it seems reasonable that high –risk patients should be evaluated using clinical judgment and a combination of several scores [70, 71].

4. Overview of procedure

4.1. Approaches used for TAVI

Stented valves placed either transapically or percutaneously are garnering much attention. In the percutaneous approach, the valve is deployed either antegradely via the transseptal route,or retrogradely across the native aortic valve.

Transfemoral Approach: The transfemoral approach is simper and quick to access the aortic valve. This route is the first choice of approach in the vast majority of centers performing TAVI procedures. Although surgical cutdown was the technique used for the transfemoral approach at the beginning of the TAVI experience, most centers are now using a fully percutaneous technique. The aortic valve is corossed and a stiff wire is placed in the LV with a large loop. Within these procedures, firstly balloon aortic valvotomy is undertaken and a stented bioprosthesis is then deployed over a balloon intothe aortic annulus. Inflation of the balloon anchors the valve in place in the annulus,effectively achieving AVR. Some specific contraindications for transfemoral approach are; narrow peripheral arteries (diameter < 8-9 mm), severe tortuousity or calcification, history of aorto-femoral by pass, aneurysm of abdominal aorta with thrombosis, and severe atheroma of the arch.

Transapical approach: Transapical approach necessitates a thoracotomy but the valve is deployed into the beating heart and extracorporeal circulation is not performed. This approach is particularly suited to patients with severe peripheral artery disease and heavily calcified ascending aorta and arch. The transapical approach includes the following other benefit: no stored tension in the delivery system, more reliable device control and feedback and no size limitations. The main disadvanteges are the need for thoracotomy; a greater degree of myocardial injury and the potentially life threating bleeding complications associated with the surgical repair.

Subclavian Approach: A subclavian approach allows patient with unfavorable iliofemoral artery anatomy or extensive disease to be treated with TAVI. A surgical cutdown is needed to isolate the subclavian artery. However no specific complications for subclavian access reported, any injury of the subclavian artery would translate into a major intrathoracic bleeding that might be difficult control.

Transaortic approach: In 2009 and 2010, transaortic approach with direct access to the ascending aorta though an anterior minithorocatomy has been advocated. Altough requiring sternotomy, avoidance of LV apical injury and avoidance of the use of large cathaters are potential advantages of this novel approach.

4.2. TAVI systems and placement

Currently two valve systems are approved for TAVI: the balloon expandable Edwards valve-the first generation Cribier-Edwards, second generation Edwards SAPİEN, and the third generation Edwards SAPIEN XT versions and the self expandable CoreValve (Medtronic CV) system.

The EdwardsSAPİEN System consists of a trileaflet pericardial bovine valve mounted in a stainless steel,and it is available in three sizes: 23 mm, 26 mm and 29 mm for transfemoral, transapical and subclavian approaches [Fig1]. The third generation SAPİEN XT calve is available in 20 mm, 23 mm, and 29 mm sizes and is introduced via an 18 F sheath.

The CoreValve ReValving System consist of three porcine pericardial leaflets mounted in a self expandable nitinol frame housed within a percutaneus delivery catheter. This system is available two sizes, 26 mm and 29 mm. The valve is introduced via an 18 F sheath [Fig 2].

Balloon aortic valvuloplasty is systematically performed before valve implantation to facilitate passage of the prosthesis through the stenotic native valve. Although, Grube at al. have suggested direct implantation of the CoreValve system with no prior balloon valvuloplasty [72]. The balloon expandable valve is positioned using fluoroscopy and echocardiography, and ventricular burst pacing is used at balloon inflation to decrease transvalvular flow and avoid expulsion of the system toward the aorta. The self-expandable valve is deployed without burst pacing, by the retracting the outer sheath of the delivery catheter.

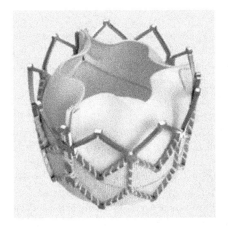

Figure 1. The EDWARS SAPİEN system

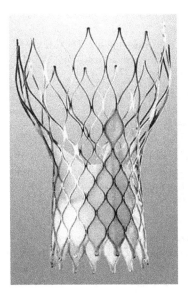

Figure 2. The CoreValve ReValving System

5. Outcomes

Overall, the procedural success rate was >90% in all studies. Valve embolization or conversion to open heart surgery occurred in ~1% of the patients (0.3–3.0% for valve embolization; 0.5–2.3% for conversion to open heart surgery) [73].

5.1. Mortality

In the multicenter registries and series, mortality was systematically <10% in patients treated using the transfemoral approach and ranged from 11.3% to 16.9% in patients treated using the transapical approach, probably owing to the higher risk profile of the patients treated via the latter route [73-74].At 1-year follow-up, the survival rates were ~80% (75–85%) for the transfemoral approach and ~70% (63–78%) for the transapical approach.

As the first of two parallel trials was completed, the results of PARTNER IB showed that TF TAVI was superior to standard therapy in patients not deemed candidates for surgery [73]. The primary endpoint of all-cause mortality was markedly reduced by 46% (P, 0.001). Recently reported 2-year outcomes showed continued encouraging results. At 2 years, the primary endpoint of all-cause mortality was reduced from 67.6% in the standard treatment arm to 43.3% in the TAVI arm (P, 0.001). The PARTNER cohort IA compared TAVI with SAVR and met its non-inferiority endpoint: the all-cause 1-year mortality in the TAVI group was non-inferior to the SAVR group (24.2 vs. 26.8%;P: 0.44; P: 0.001 for non-inferiority) [74]. Some concerns were raised with regard to neurologic events that were somewhat higher with TAVI than SAVR at 30 days (5.5 vs. 2.4%; P: 0.04) and 1 year (8.3 vs. 4.3%; P: 0.04). Although the recently published 2-year results showed that stroke rates were similar for TAVI and SAVR during 1 and 2 years with a hazard ratio of 1.22 (95% CI 0.67–2.23, P: 0.52), the issue of stroke warrants further investigation and should not be underestimated The rate of the composite of all-cause death and stroke was encouragingly nearly identical after TAVI (37.1%) and SAVR (36.4%) at 2 years (P: 0.85)[73-74]

Predictors of mortality — Risk factors for early and late mortality were identified in a study of 663 patients undergoing TAVR with CoreValve. Intraprocedural mortality was 0.9 percent. Mortality was 5.4 percent at 30 days and 15 percent at one year. Independent predictors of mortality at 30 days included certain procedural complications (conversion to open heart surgery, cardiac tamponade, major vascular or access site complications) as well as baseline characteristics (left ventricular ejection fraction <40 percent, prior balloon valvuloplasty, and diabetes mellitus). Independent predictors of mortality between 30 days and one year included prior stroke, postprocedural paravalvular leak ≥2+, prior acute pulmonary edema, and chronic kidney disease.

Indeed, in the past few years, 1-year survival rates from some registries have been reported to be ≥80%, and we can expect better survival rates at the 2-year and 3-year follow-ups in the coming years. Importantly, no structural failures of the transcatheter valves have been seen in studies with a follow-up of more than 1 year [73-74].

In addition to baseline and procedural factors, the learning-curve phenomenon and the improvements in valve prosthesis and delivery catheters have also been associated with a substantial improvement in the results obtained with TAVI.

5.2. Symptom improvement

Three-year follow-up data have been published and are consistent with lasting improvement in cardiac symptoms [72]. While 86% of patients were in NYHA class III or IV at baseline, 93%

of surviving patients were in NYHA class I/II at 3-year follow-up. Similarly, the PARTNER trial showed that patients treated with TAVI compared with patients treated with standard medical therapy have better symptom control at 1 year. Indeed, the 1-year rate of NYHA class III or IV was 25.2% for the TAVI group compared with 58.0% for the standard medical therapy group (P, 0.001).

6. Complications

Stroke: The occurrence of stroke is one of the most –fearing complication of TAVI. The most frequent etiology of procedural stroke is likely to be atheroembolism from the ascending aorta or the aortic arh. Other several factors include manipulation of a wire, positioning of device, performance of the balloon aortic valvuloplasty, air embolism, dissection of the arc vessels and inadequate blood flow to brain during rapid pacing. Reported 30 day stroke rate was 3.5 (ranging from 1.2% to 6.7%) [76]. Additionaly Kahlert et al observed that using diffusion-weighed MRI has underlined this issue, demonstrating multiple embolic cerebral lesion in all patients after TAVI. Although most of these lesions were clinically silent, silent cerebral infarcts are associated with subtle cognitive change. Efforts have been directed towards prevention of stroke. Procedural anticoagulation to reach a target activated clotting time over 250 s is suggested. Empiric dual antiplatelet therapy is recommended for 3 to 6 months followed by long-term daily low dose aspirin. Additionally less traumatic valve delivery system and embolic protection devices (Embrella embolic deflector system) currently under devolepment might lower the risk of stroke. However some authors have suggested that stroke risk might be lower with transapical access, this has not been a universal finding.

Vascular Complication: Common vascular complication arterial dissection, closure device failure, arterial stenosis, haematoma in the accsess site. Artery avulsion, vessel perforation, annulus rupture represent more severe complications which are fatal if not rapidly treated. In the SOURCE registry, 10.6 % of patients had major vascular complication and major vascular complications were less frequent in the transapical approach (2.4 %) [73-74]. Small vessel diameter, severe atherosclerosis, bulky calcification, and tortusosity are the main determinats of vascular complications. In the future delivery catheter and sheath size will likely decrease which should be associated with reductions in the risk of vascular injury. Additionally, for patients with unsuitable access, alternatives include apical, axillar/subclavian or transaortic approaches, or treatment of iliofemoral lesion with stents or grafts.

Coronary obstruction and myocardial infarction: Coronary ostia obstruction (especially of the left main coronary artery) might occur if an obstructive portion of the valve frame or the sealing cuff is placed directly over a coronary ostium however this is very rare but potentially fatal event [77]. Some cases may require immediate coronary angioplasty or coronary artery bypass graft operation. TAVI has been associated with a variable rate of myocardial infarction, ranging from 0% to 16.3% [73-74] Myocardial infarction could be explained by myocardial tissue compression, hypotension due to rapid pacing, atheroembolism and mechanic complication such as coronary ostia obstruction. Additionally myocardial infarction was associated with an increased cardiac mortality at midterm follow up

Heart Block: High grade atrioventricular block and consecutive pacemaker implantation are frequent (especially in CoreValve) complications following TAVI. CoreValve implantation is associated with a need for permanent pacemaker in 20 % of patients compared with in 5 % of patients implanted with the balloon expandable valves [78]. Potential risk factors include aggressive over sizing, low implantation of the prosthesis, small annulus diameter, using CoreValve and the presence of preexisting infranodal block such as RBBB [79, 80].

Cardiogenic Schock and low cardiac output: This complication may be induced by ischemia, rapid pacing, volume depletion, anesthesia and interruption in cardiac output during valve implantation. Vasopresor agents and intraaortic balloon support to maintain adequate perfusion pressure are often helpful. Rarely elective femoral cardiopulmonary bypass is an option for patients at hemodynamic instability.

Paravalvuler Regurgitation: However paravalvuler aortic regurgitation is common, occurring in about 85 %, Grade > 2 + regurgitation is found in 7-24 % [72,73].Trivial, mild and even moderate degrees of regurgitation seem well tolerated, although grade > 2+ regurgitation associated with increased short and long term mortality [81]. Causes of paravalvular regurgitation include a heavily calcified annulus,large annulus size, an undersized prosthesis, device failure and inadequate balloon aortic valvuloplasty. Redilatation or implantation of a second, overlapping transcathater valve can often correct the problem.

Acute Kidney Injury: Angiographic contrast injection, hypotension, atheroembolism, periprocedural blood transfusion might contribute to acute renal failure. The incidence of acute kidney injury after TAVI has been reported with incidence of 8 %. Additionally need for hemodialysis has ranged from 1.4% to 15.7 %, respectively [82]. Predictors of acute kidney injury include hypertension, decrease baseline renal function, previous myocardial infarction, high logistic EuroSCORE and chronic obstructive pulmonary disease [83].

Other Complication: Other significant and very rare complications include aortic rupture, aortic dissection, periaortic hematoma, ventricular or aortic embolization of valve, structural valve failure, cardiac tamponade and acute mitral regurgitation due to mitral valve apparatus damage [73-74].

Valve-in-valve — A valve-in-valve procedure involves catheter-based valve implantation inside an already implanted bioprosthetic valve. This approach may provide an alternative to replacement of a degenerated surgically-implanted valve, or a means of salvaging suboptimal implantation of a catheter-based valve during the initial implantation procedure.

Conclusion: Despite continual technical advancement of TAVI devices and procedures, the combined mortality and morbidity is still high in the range of 5-10%, especially when we are facing a group of high surgical risk patients. In addition TAVR offered no survival benefit compared to standard therapy in patients with an STS score of > 15 % because of high degree of comorbid conditions in these patients. In the future when it is a safer and more reliable procedure and further refinement of the device (i.e. smaller size delivery systems and multiple valve size options) is done, utilization of the procedure in patients with lower surgical risk may be possible.

7. Surgery

In 1912, Theodore Tuffier was the first to attempt opening AS using his finger. Russel Brock and then Bailey used dilatators for stenotic aortic valves. Today more than 1000 patients have aortic valve surgery per year and surgery for AS is more common than it is for aortic insufficiency [84]. Aortic valve surgery has been improved with the developments of new technologies in cardiopulmonary bypass techniques and valve industry. Approximately 2% to 5% of elderly individuals aged 75 years present with signs of severe AS and they are scheduled for elective AVR. AVR is the treatment of choice for patients with severe degenerative AS, offering both symptomatic relief and a potential for improved long term survival [85].

It's obvious that AVR is indicated in all symptomatic patients and asymptomatic patients with severe AS undergoing open heart surgery. The surgery should immediately be programmed if the patient becomes symptomatic. Despite LV dysfunction, the risk of aortic valve replacement for AS was satisfactory and related to meanaortic gradient and additional coronary artery disease, and long-term survival was related to also coronary disease and cardiac output [86].

5-year survival for adults after aortic valve replacement is 80-90%. The results of the conventional surgery for octogenarians are also satisfactory and 5% to 10% of mortality is noted for isolated AVR (2). On the other hand, elderly patients stay longer in the hospitals and intensive care units during the postoperative period [87]. United Kingdom heart valve registry observed 1100 elderly patients (56% women) who underwent AVR that the 30-day mortality was 6.6% [88]. The actuarial survival was 89% at 1 year, 79% at 3 years, 69% at 5 years, and 46% at 8 years. The mortality is rising up to 10% per year for the patient becoming symptomatic. The indications for AVR in patients with AS according to the current ACC/AHA guidelines are listed in Table 2 [89]. Although the surgery for the asymptomatic patients is preferred due to sudden death, surgery for asymptomatic octogenarians is controversial. The complex cardiac procedures have high risks for elderly patients.

The mortality rate of valve surgery and risk of sudden death without surgery have to be carefully considered. Postoperatively symptoms diminish and quality of life is improved in the majority of patients ≥75 years who had undergone aortic valve surgery, but long term survival was not affected [90].

AVR usually performed under general anesthesia using conventional techniques of open heart surgery with median sternotomy. Minimally invasive surgery has continued to be an evolving concept after the first publication of Cosgrove in 1996 [91] Minimally invasive procedures are associated with acceptable mortality and morbidity rates even in high risk patients. 30-day in-hospital mortality was 0.8% for 1,103 minimally invasive aortic valve procedures [92].

The major advantages of minimally access surgeries are improved cosmesis with reduced insicion size, decreased surgical trauma, less pain, better respiratory function and early return to work [92].

These procedures can be performed through different approaches. These are upper mini sternotomy, transverse sternotomy and right parasternal or anterolateral mini thoracotomy,

Class I
AVR is indicated for symptomatic patients with severeAS.* *(Level of Evidence: B)*
AVR is indicated for patientswith severe AS* undergoing coronaryartery bypass graft surgery(CABG). *(Level of Evidence: C)*
AVR is indicated for patientswith severe AS* undergoing surgeryon the aorta or other heartvalves. *(Level of Evidence: C)*
AVR is recommended for patientswith severe AS* and LV systolicdysfunction (ejection fractionless than 0.50). *(Level of Evidence: C)*

Class IIa
AVR is reasonable for patients with moderate AS*undergoingCABG or surgery on the aorta or other heart valves(see Section3.7 on combined multiple valve disease and Section10.4 on AVRin patients undergoing CABG). *(Level of Evidence: B)*

Class IIb
AVR may be considered for asymptomatic patientswith severeAS* and abnormal response to exercise (e.g., developmentofsymptoms or asymptomatic hypotension). *(Level of Evidence: C)*
AVR may be considered for adults with severe asymptomaticAS* if there is a high likelihood of rapid progression (age,calcification, and CAD) or if surgery might be delayed at thetime of symptom onset. *(Level of Evidence: C)*
AVR may beconsidered in patients undergoing CABG who havemild AS* whenthere is evidence, such as moderate to severevalve calcification,that progression may be rapid. *(Level of Evidence: C)*
AVRmay be considered for asymptomatic patients with extremelysevereAS (aortic valve area less than 0.6 cm^2, mean gradientgreaterthan 60 mm Hg, and jet velocity greater than 5.0 m persecond)when the patient's expected operative mortalityis 1.0%or less. *(Level of Evidence: C)*

Class III
AVR is not useful for the prevention of sudden deathin asymptomaticpatients with AS who have none of the findingslisted underthe class IIa/IIb recommendations. *(Level of Evidence: B)*

Table 2. Indications for Aortic Valve Replacement.

using port access technique or not. Although mini sternotomy is the most common approach, the outcomes after right anterior thoracotomy have satisfactory results [93]. The arterial cannulation sites are either aorta or femoral artery. The venous cannulation sites are right atrium, femoral vein or percutanous supeior vena cava with femoral vein. The incisions differ from 5 to 10 cm and small incisions may provide low infection rates [94]. This procedure has advantages such as less 1 surgical trauma, decreased pain and faster recovery. It reduces blood transfusions and shortens the length of hospital and ICU stay [95]. It is a safe operation and results lower incidence of atelectasis inthe cardiac ICU [96]. Port access aortic surgery also allows patients to be extubated earlier [97]. Avoidance of full sternotomy for patients prompts a comfortable postoperative period. Although the number of the aortic valve procedures increase worldwide, the ideal valve choice is still a debate. There are several options for valves. These are mechanical valve prosthesis, stented and stentless bioprosthetic valves, aortic homograft and pulmonary autograft. The use of these valves differs from patient to patient due to comorbidities and anticoagulant needs. The bioprosthetic valves are good alternatives for elderly patients and women who want to be pregnant because long term anticoagulation use is not required. The other situation for the patients undergoing AVR is the injurious effects of Cardiopulmonary bypass to the life organs. This results as a systemic inflammatory response and this may affect the post-operative course of the patients. Paroxysmal or chronic AF is a risk factor for mortality in patients with severe AS and a LVEF <35% undergoing AVR. Of 83 elderly patients with severe AS and an LVEF <35%, 29 (35%) had paroxysmal or chronic AF [86]. The perioperative mortality was 24% in the group with AF versus 5,5% in the group without AF.

The Ross procedure is another surgical technique for aortic valve replacement. This is more commonly used in pediatric cases but also good alternative for especially young adult patients and women want have child. In this operation the patient's own pulmonary valve and main pulmonary artery are used as an autograft and they are implanted to the aortic position, with reimplantation of coronary arteries.

The primary indication for the Ross procedure is to provide a permanent valve replacement among younger patients who will grow potentially. Other possible indications include complex left ventricular outflow obstructive disease, native or prosthetic valve endocarditis, and adult aortic insufficiency with a dilated aortic annulus [98].

One of the most commonly seen complications of Ross procedure is autograft regurgitation and sinus or ascending aortic dilatation, which can usually be corrected with a valve-sparing root replacement. In a study 212 patients underwent Ross aortic valve replacement; 51% were older than 19 years old. There were just 2 early deaths. At 15 years, freedom from autograft sinus or ascending aortic dilatation was 79%, autograft dysfunction, 91%. And actuarial survival was 98% [99].

Recent years aortic valve repair also become popular when valve morphology is amenable to repair. But this is a limited procedure among patients who have aortic regurgitation (AR) without aortic stenosis. Aortic valve repair is commonly indicated commonly in patients with a dilated aortic annulus without any degeneration of the leaflets [100]

Author details

Fahrettin Oz[1], Fatih Tufan[2], Ahmet Ekmekci[3], Omer A. Sayın[4] and Huseyin Oflaz[1]

1 Istanbul University, Istanbul School of Medicine, Department of Cardiology, Turkey

2 Istanbul University, Istanbul School of Medicine, Department of Internal Medicine, Division of Geriatrics, Turkey

3 Istanbul University, Istanbul School of Medicine, Department of Internal Medicine, Turkey

4 Istanbul University, Istanbul School of Medicine, Department of Cardiovascular Surgery, Turkey

References

[1] Gerber MA, Baltimore RS, Eaton CB, Gewitz M, Rowley AH, Shulman ST, Taubert KA. Prevention of rheumatic fever and diagnosis and treatment of acute Streptococcal pharyngitis: a scientific statement from the American Heart Association Rheumatic Fever, Endocarditis, and Kawasaki Disease Committee of the Council on Cardiovascular Disease in the Young, the Interdisciplinary Council on Functional Genomics and Translational Biology, and the Interdisciplinary Council on Quality of Care and Outcomes Research: endorsed by the American Academy of Pediatrics. Circulation. 2009;119(11):1541-51.

[2] Antonini-Canterin F, Huang G, Cervesato E, Faggiano P, Pavan D, Piazza R, Nicolosi GL. Symptomatic aortic stenosis: does systemic hypertension play an additional role? Hypertension. 2003;41(6):1268-72.

[3] Zile MR, Gaasch WH. Heart failure in aortic stenosis - improving diagnosis and treatment. N Engl J Med. 2003;348(18):1735-6.

[4] Rieck ÅE, Cramariuc D, Boman K, Gohlke-Bärwolf C, Staal EM, Lønnebakken MT, Rossebø AB, Gerdts E. Hypertension in aortic stenosis: implications for left ventricular structure and cardiovascular events. Hypertension. 2012;60(1):90-7.

[5] O'Brien KD, Zhao XQ, Shavelle DM, Caulfield MT, Letterer RA, Kapadia SR, Probstfield JL, Otto CM. Hemodynamic effects of the angiotensin-converting enzyme inhibitor, ramipril, in patients with mild to moderate aortic stenosis and preserved left ventricular function. J Investig Med. 2004;52(3):185–191.

[6] Chockalingam A, Venkatesan S, Subramaniam T, Jagannathan V, Elangovan S, Alagesan R, Gnanavelu G, Dorairajan S, Krishna BP, Chockalingam V. Safety and efficacy of angiotensin-converting enzyme inhibitors in symptomatic severe aortic stenosis: Symptomatic Cardiac Obstruction-Pilot Study of Enalapril in Aortic Stenosis (SCOPE-AS). Am Heart J. 2004;147(4):E19.

[7] Nadir MA, Wei L, Elder DH, Libianto R, Lim TK, Pauriah M, Pringle SD, Doney AD, Choy AM, Struthers AD, Lang CC. Impact of renin-angiotensin system blockade therapy on outcome in aortic stenosis. J Am Coll Cardiol. 2011;58(6):570–576.

[8] ALLHAT Collaborative Research Group. Major cardiovascular events in hypertensive patients randomized to doxazosin vs chlorthalidone: the Antihypertensive and Lipid-Lowering Treatment to Prevent Heart Attack Trial (ALLHAT). JAMA. 2000;283(15):1967–1975.

[9] U.S. Preventive Services Task Force. The Guide to Clinical Preventive Services 2010 - 2011: Recommendations of the U.S. Preventive Services Task Force. Rockville (MD): Agency for Healthcare Research and Quality (US); 2010 Aug.

[10] Goel SS, Agarwal S, Tuzcu EM, Ellis SG, Svensson LG, Zaman T, Bajaj N, Joseph L, Patel NS, Aksoy O, Stewart WJ, Griffin BP, Kapadia SR. Percutaneous coronary inter-

vention in patients with severe aortic stenosis: implications for transcatheter aortic valve replacement. Circulation. 2012 Feb 28;125(8):1005-13.

[11] Darby AE, Dimarco JP. Management of atrial fibrillation in patients with structural heart disease. Circulation. 2012;125(7):945-57.

[12] Bang CN, Greve AM, Boman K, Egstrup K, Gohlke-Baerwolf C, Køber L, Nienaber CA, Ray S, Rossebø AB, Wachtell K. Effect of lipid lowering on new-onset atrial fibrillation in patients with asymptomatic aortic stenosis: the Simvastatin and Ezetimibe in Aortic Stenosis (SEAS) study. Am Heart J. 2012;163(4):690-6.

[13] Camm AJ, Savelieva I. Atrial fibrillation: the rate versus rhythm management controversy. J R Coll Physicians Edinb. 2012;42 Suppl 18:23-34.

[14] Authors/Task Force Members, Camm AJ, Lip GY, De Caterina R, Savelieva I, Atar D, Hohnloser SH, Hindricks G, Kirchhof P; ESC Committee for Practice Guidelines (CPG), Bax JJ, Baumgartner H, Ceconi C, Dean V, Deaton C, Fagard R, Funck-Brentano C, Hasdai D, Hoes A, Kirchhof P, Knuuti J, Kolh P, McDonagh T, Moulin C, Popescu BA, Reiner Z, Sechtem U, Sirnes PA, Tendera M, Torbicki A, Vahanian A, Windecker S; Document Reviewers, Vardas P, Al-Attar N, Alfieri O, Angelini A, Blömstrom-Lundqvist C, Colonna P, De Sutter J, Ernst S, Goette A, Gorenek B, Hatala R, Heidbüchel H, Heldal M, Kristensen SD, Kolh P, Le Heuzey JY, Mavrakis H, Mont L, Filardi PP, Ponikowski P, Prendergast B, Rutten FH, Schotten U, Van Gelder IC, Verheugt FW. 2012 focused update of the ESC Guidelines for the management of atrial fibrillation: An update of the 2010 ESC Guidelines for the management of atrial fibrillation * Developed with the special contribution of the European Heart Rhythm Association. Europace. 2012 Aug 24. [Epub ahead of print] No abstract available.

[15] Pilgrim T, Wenaweser P, Meuli F, Huber C, Stortecky S, Seiler C, Zbinden S, Meier B, Carrel T, Windecker S. Clinical outcome of high-risk patients with severe aortic stenosis and reduced left ventricular ejection fraction undergoing medical treatment or TAVI. PLoS One. 2011;6(11):e27556.

[16] Chockalingam A, Venkatesan S, Subramaniam T, Jagannathan V, Elangovan S, Alagesan R, Gnanavelu G, Dorairajan S, Krishna BP, Chockalingam V; Symptomatic Cardiac Obstruction-Pilot Study of Enalapril in Aortic Stenosis. Safety and efficacy of angiotensin-converting enzyme inhibitors in symptomatic severe aortic stenosis: Symptomatic Cardiac Obstruction-Pilot Study of Enalapril in Aortic Stenosis (SCOPE-AS). Am Heart J. 2004;147(4):E19.

[17] Khot UN, Novaro GM, Popović ZB, Mills RM, Thomas JD, Tuzcu EM, Hammer D, Nissen SE, Francis GS. Nitroprusside in critically ill patients with left ventricular dysfunction and aortic stenosis. N Engl J Med. 2003;348(18):1756-63.

[18] Lindman BR, Zajarias A, Madrazo JA, Shah J, Gage BF, Novak E, Johnson SN, Chakinala MM, Hohn TA, Saghir M, Mann DL. Effects of phosphodiesterase type 5 inhibi-

tion on systemic and pulmonary hemodynamics and ventricular function in patients with severe symptomatic aortic stenosis. Circulation. 2012;125(19):2353-62.

[19] Katz R, Budoff MJ, Takasu J, Shavelle DM, Bertoni A, Blumenthal RS, Ouyang P, Wong ND, O'Brien KD. Relationship of metabolic syndrome with incident aortic valve calcium and aortic valve calcium progression: the Multi-Ethnic Study of Atherosclerosis (MESA). Diabetes. 2009;58(4):813-9

[20] Capoulade R, Clavel MA, Dumesnil JG, Chan KL, Teo KK, Tam JW, Côté N, Mathieu P, Després JP, Pibarot P; ASTRONOMER Investigators. Impact of metabolic syndrome on progression of aortic stenosis: influence of age and statin therapy. J Am Coll Cardiol. 2012;60(3):216-23.

[21] Berrington de Gonzalez A, Hartge P, Cerhan JR, Flint AJ, Hannan L, MacInnis RJ, Moore SC, Tobias GS, Anton-Culver H, Freeman LB, Beeson WL, Clipp SL, English DR, Folsom AR, Freedman DM, Giles G, Hakansson N, Henderson KD, Hoffman-Bolton J, Hoppin JA, Koenig KL, Lee IM, Linet MS, Park Y, Pocobelli G, Schatzkin A, Sesso HD, Weiderpass E, Willcox BJ, Wolk A, Zeleniuch-Jacquotte A, Willett WC, Thun MJ. Body-mass index and mortality among 1.46 million white adults. N Engl J Med. 2010;363(23):2211-9.

[22] Otto CM, Mickel MC, Kennedy JW, Alderman EL, Bashore TM, Block PC, Brinker JA, Diver D, Ferguson J, Holmes DR Jr, Lambrew CT, McKay CR, Palacios IF, Powers ER, Rahimtoola SH, Weiner BH, Davis KB. Three-year outcome after balloon aortic valvuloplasty. Insights into prognosis of valvular aortic stenosis. Circulation. 1994;89(2):642-50.

[23] Ikee R, Honda K, Oka M, Maesato K, Mano T, Moriya H, Ohtake T, Kobayashi S. Association of heart valve calcification with malnutrition-inflammation complex syndrome, beta-microglobulin, and carotid intima media thickness in patients on hemodialysis. Ther Apher Dial. 2008;12(6):464-8.

[24] Wang AY, Woo J, Lam CW, Wang M, Chan IH, Gao P, Lui SF, Li PK, Sanderson JE. Associations of serum fetuin-A with malnutrition, inflammation, atherosclerosis and valvular calcification syndrome and outcome in peritoneal dialysis patients. Nephrol Dial Transplant. 2005;20(8):1676-85.

[25] Engelman DT, Adams DH, Byrne JG, Aranki SF, Collins JJ Jr, Couper GS, Allred EN, Cohn LH, Rizzo RJ. Impact of body mass index and albumin on morbidity and mortality after cardiac surgery. J Thorac Cardiovasc Surg. 1999;118(5):866-73.

[26] Tepsuwan T, Schuarattanapong S, Woragidpoonpol S, Kulthawong S, Chaiyasri A, Nawarawong W. Incidence and impact of cardiac cachexia in valvular surgery. Asian Cardiovasc Thorac Ann. 2009;17(6):617-21.

[27] Thourani VH, Keeling WB, Kilgo PD, Puskas JD, Lattouf OM, Chen EP, Guyton RA. The impact of body mass index on morbidity and short- and long-term mortality in cardiac valvular surgery. J Thorac Cardiovasc Surg. 2011;142(5):1052-61.

[28] Maixner SM, Struble L, Blazek M, Kales HC. Later-life depression and heart failure. Heart Fail Clin. 2011;7(1):47-58.

[29] Bisschop MI, Kriegsman DM, Deeg DJ, Beekman AT, van Tilburg W. The longitudinal relation between chronic diseases and depression in older persons in the community: the Longitudinal Aging Study Amsterdam. J Clin Epidemiol. 2004;57(2): 187-94.

[30] Verbeek DE, van Riezen J, de Boer RA, van Melle JP, de Jonge P. A review on the putative association between beta-blockers and depression. Heart Fail Clin. 2011;7(1): 89-99.

[31] Kimmel SE, Schelleman H, Berlin JA, Oslin DW, Weinstein RB, Kinman JL, Sauer WH, Lewis JD. The effect of selective serotonin re-uptake inhibitors on the risk of myocardial infarction in a cohort of patients with depression. Br J Clin Pharmacol. 2011;72(3):514-7.

[32] Frogel J, Galusca D. Anesthetic considerations for patients with advanced valvular heart disease undergoing noncardiac surgery. Anesthesiol Clin. 2010;28(1):67-85.

[33] Nishimura RA, Carabello BA, Faxon DP, Freed MD, Lytle BW, O'Gara PT, O'Rourke RA, Shah PM. ACC/AHA 2008 Guideline update on valvular heart disease: focused update on infective endocarditis: a report of the American College of Cardiology/ American Heart Association Task Force on Practice Guidelines endorsed by the Society of Cardiovascular Anesthesiologists, Society for Cardiovascular Angiography and Interventions, and Society of Thoracic Surgeons. J Am Coll Cardiol. 2008;52(8): 676-85.

[34] Steinlechner B, Zeidler P, Base E, Birkenberg B, Ankersmit HJ, Spannagl M, Quehenberger P, Hiesmayr M, Jilma B. Patients with severe aortic valve stenosis and impaired platelet function benefit from preoperative desmopressin infusion. Ann Thorac Surg. 2011;91(5):1420-6.

[35] Maldonado JR, Wysong A, van der Starre PJ, Block T, Miller C, Reitz BA. Dexmedetomidine and the reduction of postoperative delirium after cardiac surgery. Psychosomatics. 2009;50(3):206-17.

[36] Giltay EJ, Huijskes RV, Kho KH, Blansjaar BA, Rosseel PM. Psychotic symptoms in patients undergoing coronary artery bypass grafting and heart valve operation. Eur J Cardiothorac Surg. 2006;30(1):140-7.

[37] Fleisher LA, Beckman JA, Brown KA, Calkins H, Chaikof EL, Fleischmann KE, Freeman WK, Froehlich JB, Kasper EK, Kersten JR, Riegel B, Robb JF. 2009 ACCF/AHA focused update on perioperative beta blockade incorporated into the ACC/AHA 2007 guidelines on perioperative cardiovascular evaluation and care for noncardiac surgery: a report of the American college of cardiology foundation/American heart association task force on practice guidelines. Circulation. 2009;120(21):e169-276.

[38] POISE Study Group, Devereaux PJ, Yang H, Yusuf S, Guyatt G, Leslie K, Villar JC,
      Xavier D, Chrolavicius S, Greenspan L, Pogue J, Pais P, Liu L, Xu S, Málaga G, Ave-
      zum A, Chan M, Montori VM, Jacka M, Choi P. Effects of extended-release metopro-
      lol succinate in patients undergoing non-cardiac surgery (POISE trial): a randomised
      controlled trial. Lancet. 2008;371(9627):1839-47.

[39] Agmon Y, Khandheria BK, Meissner I, Sicks JR, O'Fallon WM, Wiebers DO, Whisn-
      ant JP, Seward JB, Tajik AJ. Aortic valve sclerosis and aortic atherosclerosis: different
      manifestations of the same disease? Insights from a population-based study. J Am
      Coll Cardiol. 2001;38(3):827-34.

[40] Callister TQ, Raggi P, Cooil B, Lippolis NJ, Russo DJ. Effect of HMG-CoA reductase
      inhibitors on coronary artery disease as assessed by electron-beam computed tomog-
      raphy. N Engl J Med. 1998;339(27):1972-8.

[41] Pohle K, Mäffert R, Ropers D, Moshage W, Stilianakis N, Daniel WG, Achenbach S.
      Progression of aortic valve calcification: association with coronary atherosclerosis
      and cardiovascular risk factors. Circulation. 2001;104(16):1927-32.

[42] Novaro GM, Tiong IY, Pearce GL, Lauer MS, Sprecher DL, Griffin BP.Effect of hy-
      droxymethylglutaryl coenzyme a reductase inhibitors on the progression of calcific
      aortic stenosis. Circulation. 2001;104(18):2205-9.

[43] Bellamy MF, Pellikka PA, Klarich KW, Tajik AJ, Enriquez-Sarano M. Association of
      cholesterol levels, hydroxymethylglutaryl coenzyme-A reductase inhibitor treatment,
      and progression of aortic stenosis in the community. J Am Coll Cardiol 2002;
      40:1723-30.

[44] Rosenhek R, Rader F, Loho N, Gabriel H, Heger M, Klaar U, Schemper M, Binder T,
      Maurer G, Baumgartner H. Statins but not angiotensin-converting enzyme inhibitors
      delay progression of aortic stenosis. Circulation 2004; 110:1291-5.

[45] Aronow WS, Ahn C, Kronzon I, Goldman ME. Association of coronary risk factors
      and use of statins with progression of mild valvular aortic stenosis in older persons.
      Am J Cardiol 2001; 88:693-5.

[46] Cowell SJ, Newby DE, Prescott RJ, Bloomfield P, Reid J, Northridge DB, Boon NA;
      Scottish Aortic Stenosis and Lipid Lowering Trial, Impact on Regression (SALTIRE)
      Investigators. A randomized trial of intensive lipid-lowering therapy in calcific aortic
      stenosis. N Engl J Med 2005; 352:2389-97.

[47] Moura LM, Ramos SF, Zamorano JL, Barros IM, Azevedo LF, Rocha-Gonçalves F, Ra-
      jamannan NM. Rosuvastatin affecting aortic valve endothelium to slow the progres-
      sion of aortic stenosis. J Am Coll Cardiol 2007; 49:554-61.

[48] Rossebø AB, Pedersen TR, Boman K, Brudi P, Chambers JB, Egstrup K, Gerdts E,
      Gohlke-Bärwolf C, Holme I, Kesäniemi YA, Malbecq W, Nienaber CA, Ray S,

Skjaerpe T, Wachtell K, Willenheimer R; SEAS Investigators. Intensive lipid lowering with simvastatin and ezetimibe in aortic stenosis. N Engl J Med. 2008;359(13):1343-56.

[49] Chan KL, Teo K, Dumesnil JG, Ni A, Tam J; ASTRONOMER Investigators. Effect of Lipid lowering with rosuvastatin on progression of aortic stenosis: results of the aortic stenosis progression observation: measuring effects of rosuvastatin (ASTRONOMER) trial. Circulation. 2010;121(2):306-14.

[50] Helske S, Lindstedt KA, Laine M, Mäyränpää M, Werkkala K, Lommi J, Turto H, Kupari M, Kovanen PT. Induction of local angiotensin II-producing systems in stenotic aortic valves. J Am Coll Cardiol 2004;44:1859–66.

[51] Routledge HC, Townend JN. ACE inhibition in aortic stenosis: dangerous medicine or golden opportunity? J Hum Hypertens. 2001;15(10):659-67.

[52] O'Brien KD, Probstfield JL, Caulfield MT, Nasir K, Takasu J, Shavelle DM, Wu AH, Zhao XQ, Budoff MJ. Angiotensin-converting enzyme inhibitors and change in aortic valve calcium. Arch Intern Med. 2005;165(8):858-62.

[53] Clark BA, Shannon RP, Rosa RM, Epstein FH. Increased susceptibility to thiazide-induced hyponatremia in the elderly. J Am Soc Nephrol. 1994;5(4):1106-11.

[54] Hwang KS, Kim GH. Thiazide-induced hyponatremia. Electrolyte Blood Press. 2010;8(1):51-7.

[55] Moon DG, Jin MH, Lee JG, Kim JJ, Kim MG, Cha DR. Antidiuretic hormone in elderly male patients with severe nocturia: a circadian study. BJU Int. 2004;94(4):571-5.

[56] Cheng JW, Nayar M. A review of heart failure management in the elderly population. Am J Geriatr Pharmacother. 2009;7(5):233-49.

[57] Hunt SA, Abraham WT, Chin MH, Feldman AM, Francis GS, Ganiats TG, Jessup M, Konstam MA, Mancini DM, Michl K, Oates JA, Rahko PS, Silver MA, Stevenson LW, Yancy CW. 2009 focused update incorporated into the ACC/AHA 2005 Guidelines for the Diagnosis and Management of Heart Failure in Adults: a report of the American College of Cardiology Foundation/American Heart Association Task Force on Practice Guidelines: developed in collaboration with the International Society for Heart and Lung Transplantation. Circulation. 2009;119(14):e391-479. Epub 2009 Mar 26. Review. No abstract available. Erratum in: Circulation. 2010 Mar 30;121(12):e258.

[58] American Geriatrics Society 2012 Beers Criteria Update Expert Panel. American Geriatrics Society updated Beers Criteria for potentially inappropriate medication use in older adults. J Am Geriatr Soc. 2012;60(4):616-31.

[59] Hart RG, Pearce LA, Aguilar MI. Meta-analysis: antithrombotic therapy to prevent stroke in patients who have nonvalvular atrial fibrillation. Ann Intern Med. 2007;146(12):857-67.

[60] Iung, B; Baron, G; Butchart, E.G; Delahaye, F; Gohlke-Bärwolf, C; Levang, O.W; Tornos, P;Vanoverschelde, J.L; Vermeer F, Boersma, E; Ravaud P; Vahanian, A. A pro-

spective survey of patients with valvular heart disease in Europe: The Euro Heart Survey on valvular heart disease. Eur Heart J. 2003; 24: 1231 – 1243.

[61] Bach D.S, Nina, C, Deeb G.M. Unoperated Patients With Severe Aortic Stenosis. J Am Coll Cardiol. 2007;50: 2018-2019.

[62] Cribier A, Savin T, Saoudi N, Rocha P, Berland J, Letac B. Percutaneous transluminal valvuloplasty of acquired aortic-stenosis in elderly patients alternative to valve-re-placement. Lancet. 1980;1: 63–7.

[63] Eltchaninoff H, Cribier A, Tron, C; Anselme F, Koning R, Soyer R, Letac B. Balloon aortic valvuloplasty in elderly patients at high-risk for surgery, or inoperable-imme-diate and mid-term results. Balloon aortic valvuloplasty in elderly patients at high-risk for surgery, or inoperable-immediate and mid-term results. Eur Heart J. 1992;16: 1079–84.

[64] Andersen H.R, Knudsen L.L, Hasenkam J.M. Transluminal implantation of artificial heart valves. Description of a new expandable aortic valve and initial results with implantation by catheter technique in closed chest pigs. Eur Heart J. 1992; 13: 704-708.

[65] Cribier A, Eltchaninoff H, Bash A, Borenstein N, Tron C, Bauer F, Derumeaux G, An-selme F, Laborde F, Leon M.B. Percutaneous transcatheter implantation of an aortic valve prosthesis for calcific aortic stenosis: first human case description. Circulation. 2002;106:3006–8.

[66] Buellesfeld L, Gerckens U, Schuler G, Bonan R, Kovac J, Serruys PW, Labinaz M,den Heijer P, Mullen M, Tymchak W, Windecker S, Mueller R, Grube E. 2-year follow-up of patients undergoing transcatheter aortic valve implantation using a self-expand-ing valve prosthesis. J Am Coll Cardiol 2011;57:1650–1657.

[67] Cribier A, Eltchaninoff H, Tron C, Bauer F, Agatiello C, Nercolini D, Tapiero S,Litzler PY, Bessou JP, Babaliaros V. Treatment of calcific aortic stenosis with the percutane-ous heart valve: mid-term follow-up from the initial feasibility studies: the French ex-perience. J Am Coll Cardiol 2006;47:1214–1223.

[68] D'Onofrio A, Rubino P, Fusari M, Salvador L, Musumeci F, Rinaldi M, Vitali EO, Glauber M, Di Bartolomeo R, Alfieri OR, Polesel E, Aiello M, Casabona R, Livi U, Grossi C, Cassese M, Pappalardo A, Gherli T, Stefanelli G, Faggian GG, Gerosa G. Clinical and hemodynamic outcomes of 'all-comers' undergoing transapical aortic valve implantation: results from the Italian Registry of Trans-Apical Aortic Valve Im-plantation (I-TA). J Thorac Cardiovasc Surg 2011;142:768–775

[69] Ambler G, Omar R.Z, Royston P, Kinsman R, Keogh B.E, Taylor K.M. Generic, sim-ple risk stratification model for heart valve surgery. Circulation. 2005;112:224-31

[70] Vahanian A, Otto CM. Risk stratification of patients with aortic stenosis. Eur Heart J, 2010; 31: 416–423

[71] Piazza N, Wenaweser P, van Gameren M et al. Relationship between the logistic Eu-roSCORE and the Society of Thoracic Surgeons Predicted Risk of Mortality score in patients implanted with the CoreValve ReValving System: A Bern-Rotterdam Study. Am Heart J, 2010; 159: 323–329.

[72] Eberhard Grube, Christoph Naber, Alexandre Abizaid, Eduardo Sousa, Oscar Men-diz, Pedro Lemos, Roberto Kalil Filho, Jose Mangione, Lutz Buellesfeld. Feasibility of transcatheter aortic valve implantation without pre-dilation: a pilot study. JACC Car-diovasc. Intervent. 2011; 4:751–757

[73] Leon MB, Smith CR, Mack M, Miller DC, Moses JW, Svensson LG, Tuzcu EM, Webb JG, Fontana GP, Makkar RR, Brown DL, Block PC, Guyton RA, Pichard AD, Bavaria JE, Herrmann HC, Douglas PS, Petersen JL, Akin JJ, Anderson WN, Wang D, Pocock S; PARTNER Trial Investigators. Transcathater aortic valve implantation for aortic stenosis in patients who cannot undergo surgery. N. Engl. J. Med. 2010;363: 1597–607

[74] Smith CR, Leon MB, Mack MJ, Miller DC, Moses JW, Svensson LG, Tuzcu EM, Webb JG, Fontana GP, Makkar RR, Williams M, Dewey T, Kapadia S, Babaliaros V, Thoura-ni VH, Corso P, Pichard AD, Bavaria JE, Herrmann HC, Akin JJ, Anderson WN, Wang D, Pocock SJ; PARTNER Trial Investigators. Transcatheter versus Surgical Aortic-Valve Replacement in High-Risk Patients. N. Engl. J. Med. 2011; 364: 2187–2198

[75] Godino C, Maisano F, Montorfano M, Latib A, Chieffo A, Michev I, Al-Lamee R, Bande M, Mussardo M, Arioli F, Ielasi A, Cioni M, Taramasso M, Arendar I, Grimal-di A, Spagnolo P, Zangrillo A, La Canna G, Alfieri O, Colombo A. Outcomes after transcatheter aortic valve implantation with both Edwards-SAPIEN and CoreValve devices in a single center: the Milan experience. JACC Cardiovasc Interv 2010;3:1110–1121.

[76] Rodés-Cabau J, Webb JG, Cheung A, Ye J, Dumont E, Feindel CM, Osten M, Natara-jan MK, Velianou JL, Martucci G, DeVarennes B, Chisholm R, Peterson MD, Lichten-stein SV, Nietlispach F, Doyle D, DeLarochellière R, Teoh K, Chu V, Dancea A, Lachapelle K, Cheema A, Latter D, Horlick E. Transcatheter aortic valve implantation for the treatment of severe symptomatic aortic stenosis in patients at very high or prohibitive surgical risk. Acute and late outcomes of the multicenter Canadian expe-rience. J. Am. Coll. Cardiol.2010; 55: 1080–1090.

[77] Webb JG, Chandavimol M, Thompson CR, Ricci DR, Carere RG, Munt BI, Buller CE, Pasupati S, Lichtenstein S. Percutaneous aortic valve implantation retrograde from the femoral artery. Circulation. 2006; 113: 842–850

[78] Ge'ne'reux P, Head SJ, Van Mieghem NM, Kodali S, Kirtane AJ, Xu K, Smith CR, Serruys PW, Kappetein AP, Leon MB. Clinical outcomes after transcatheter aortic valve replacement using Valve Academic Research Consortium definitions: a weight-ed meta-analysis of 3519 patients from 16 studies. J Am Coll Cardiol 2012; 59:2317–2326

[79]   Piazza N, Onuma Y, Jesserun E, Kint PP, Maugenest AM, Anderson RH, de Jaegere PP, Serruys PW. Early and persistent intraventricular conduction abnormalities and requirements for pacemaking after percutaneous replacement of the aortic valve. JACC Cardiovasc Interv 2008;1:310–316.

[80]   Godin M, Eltchaninoff H, Furuta A, Tron C, Anselme F, Bejar K, Sanchez-Giron C, Bauer F, Litzler PY, Bessou JP, Cribier A. Frequency of conduction disturbances after transcatheter implantation of an Edwards Sapien aortic valve prosthesis. Am J Cardiol. 2010;106:707–712.

[81]   Gurvitch R, Wood DA, Tay EL, Leipsic J, Ye J, Lichtenstein SV, Thompson CR,Carere RG, Wijesinghe N, Nietlispach F, Boone RH, Lauck S, Cheung A, Webb JG. Transcatheter aortic valve implantation: durability of clinical and hemodynamic outcomes beyond 3 years in a large patient cohort. Circulation. 2010;122: 1319–1327.

[82]   Barbour, J.R. & Ikonimidis, J.S. Aortic Valve Replacement, In: Johns Hopkins Manual of Cardiothoracic Surgery, Yuh, DD; Vricella, L.A. & Baumgartner W.A. 561-606. Mc Graw-Hill Companies, ISBN-13:978-0-07-141652-8, United States of America)

[83]   Heinze, H; Sier, H; Schäfer, U, Heringlake, M. Percutaneous aortic valve replacement: overview and suggestions for anesthestic management. J Clin Anesth, 2010; 22:373-8.

[84]   Connolly HM, Oh JK, Orszulak TA, Osborn SL, Roger VL, Hodge DO, Bailey KR, Seward JB, Tajik AJ.Aortic valve replacement for aortic stenosis with severe left ventricular dysfunction. Prognosticindicators. Circulation. 1997; 20:2395-400.

[85]   Maganti K, Rigolin V.H, Sarano M.E, Bonow O.R. Valvular Heart Disease: Diagnosis and Management. Mayo Clin Proc. 2010; 85(5): 483–500

[86]   Avery, G.J; Ley, S.J; Hill, J.D; Hershon, J.J, Dick S.E. Cardiac surgery in the octogenarian: evaluation of risk, cost, and outcome. Ann Thorac Surg. 2001;71:591-6.

[87]   Aronow, W.S. Valvular aortic stenosis in the elderly. Cardiol Rev. 2007;15:.217-25.

[88]   Taylor KM, Gray SA, Livingstone S, Brannan JJ. The United Kingdom Heart Valve Registry. J Heart Valve Dis. 1992;1(2):152-9

[89]   Bonow, R.O; Carabello, B.A; Chatterjee, K; de Leon, A.C. Jr.; Faxon, D.P; Freed, M.D; Gaasch W.H, Lytle B.W, Nishimura R.A, O'Gara P.T, O'Rourke R.A, Otto C.M, Shah P.M, Shanewise J.S, Smith S.C. Jr; Jacobs, A.K; Adams, C.D; Anderson J.L; Antman, E.M, Fuster, V; Halperin, J.L; Hiratzka, L.F; Hunt, S.A; Lytle, B.W; Nishimura, R; Page, R.L, Riegel B. ACC/AHA 2006 practice guidelines for the management of patients with valvular heart disease: Executive Summary. A Report of the American College of Cardiology/ American Heart Association Task Force on Practice Guidelines (Writing Committee to Revise the 1998 Guidelines for the Management of Patients With Valvular Heart Disease). Developed in collaboration with the Society of Cardiovascular Anesthesiologists. Endorsed by the Society for Cardiovascular An-

giography and Interventions and the Society of Thoracic Surgeons. J Am Coll Cardiol. 2006; 48:1-148

[90] Petersen R.S & Poulsen A. (2010). Quality of life after aortic valve-replacement in patients > or = 75 years. Ugeskr Laeger, Vol.172, No.5, (February, 2010), pp.355-9

[91] Minimally invasive cardiac surgery Daniel J. Goldstein, Mehmet C. Oz. 21 Minimally invasive aortic valve surgery 293-307

[92] Svensson LG. Minimally invasive surgery with a partial sternotomy "J" approach. Semin Thorac Cardiovasc Surg. 2007;19(4):299-303.

[93] GlauberM, MiceliA, BevilacquaS, FarnetiPA.Minimally invasive aortic valve replacement via right anterior minithoracotomy:Early outcomes and midterm follow-up. J Thorac Cardiovasc Surg. 2011;142(6):1577-9.

[94] Olin C.L, Péterffy A. Minimal access aortic valve surgery. Eur J Cardiothorac Surg. 1999; 15:39-43.

[95] Korach A, Shemin R.J, Hunter C.T, Bao Y, Shapira O.M. Minimally invasive versus conventional aortic valve replacement: a 10-year experience. J Cardiovasc Surg. 2010;51: 417-21.

[96] Foghsgaard S, Gazi D, Bach K, Hansen H, Schmidt T.A, Kjaergard H.K. Minimally invasive aortic valve replacement reduces atelectasis in cardiac intensive care. Acute Cardiac Care. 2009;11: 169-72.

[97] Wheatley G.H, Prince S.L, Herbert M.A, Ryan W.H. Port-access aortic valve surgery: a technique in evolution. Heart Surg Forum. 2004;7:628-31

[98] Morita K, Kurosawa H. Indications for and clinical outcome of the Ross procedure: a review]. Nihon Geka Gakkai Zasshi. 2001;102(4):330-6.

[99] Brown JW, Ruzmetov M, Shahriari A, Rodefeld MD, Mahomed Y, Turrentine MW.Midterm results of Ross aortic valve replacement: a single-institution experience. Ann Thorac Surg. 2009 ;88(2):601-7.

[100] Fattouch K, Murana G, Castrovinci S, Nasso G, Mossuto C, Corrado E, Ruvolo G, Speziale G. Outcomes of aortic valve repair according to valve morphology and surgical techniques. Interact Cardiovasc Thorac Surg. 2012;15(4):644-50

Chapter 4

Surgical Valve Replacement (Bioprosthetic vs. Mechanical)

Stamenko Šušak, Lazar Velicki, Dušan Popović and Ivana Burazor

Additional information is available at the end of the chapter

1. Introduction

The aortic valve separates the left ventricular outflow tract from the aorta. It is a tricuspid valve consisting of three semilunar cusps and the aortic valve annulus. The aortic valve annulus is a collagenous structure lying at the level of the junction of the aortic valve and the ventricular septum, which is the nadir of the aortic valve complex. This area is also referred to as the aortic ring and serves to provide structural support to the aortic valve complex. The annulus is shaped like a crown and extends to the level of the aortic sinuses. It attaches to the aortic media distally and the membranous and muscular ventricular septum proximally and anteriorly. There are 3 aortic valve cusps, each half-moon shaped or semilunar in appearance. A small dilatation of the proximal aorta is associated with each cusp; collectively, these are referred to as the sinuses of Valsalva or aortic sinuses, named after the Italian anatomist Antonio Valsalva. Their association with the respective coronary ostia identifies them: left, right, and posterior (or noncoronary).[1]

Aortic stenosis (AS) is one of the most common diseases of the aortic valve. The most common causes of AS are degenerative calcification, bicuspid aortic valve and rheumatic etiology. Age – related degenerative calcific AS is currently the most common cause of AS in adults and most frequent reason for aortic valve replacement (AVR).[2] That atherosclerosis is a cause of AS is derived primarily from five pieces of evidence: 1) that patients with familial homozygous hyperlipidemia usually develop calcific deposits on the aortic aspects of their aortic valve cusps at a very young age, usually by the teenage years (These individuals have serum total cholesterol levels >800 mg/dl from the time of birth.); 2) that progression of AS can be slowed by lowering total and low-density lipoprotein cholesterol levels by statins; 3) that patients >65 years of age with AS involving a three-cuspid aortic valve (unassociated with mitral valve disease) usually have extensive atherosclerosis involving the major epicardial coronary arteries and usually other systemic arterial systems; 4) that serum total cholesterol levels and concomitant coronary bypass grafting tend to be higher in patients with AS involving three-cuspid aortic valves than in patients of similar age and sex without AS or with congenitally bicuspid aortic valves; and 5) that histologic study of three-cuspid stenotic aortic valve demonstrates features similar to those in atherosclerotic plaques.[2] Rare causes of aortic stenosis include obstructive, infective endocarditis, Paget's disease, renal failure, drug induced, familial hypercholesterolemia, systemic lupus erythematosus, irradiation, and ochronosis.[3] As the valves stenosis, valvular abnormality produces turbulent flow, which traumatizes the leaflets and eventually leads to progressive cell proliferation, extracellular matrix production, and calcification of the valve. It is degenerative process that leads to proliferative and inflammatory changes that leading to calcification of the aortic valve. Progressive calcification leads to immobilization of the cusps.[3]

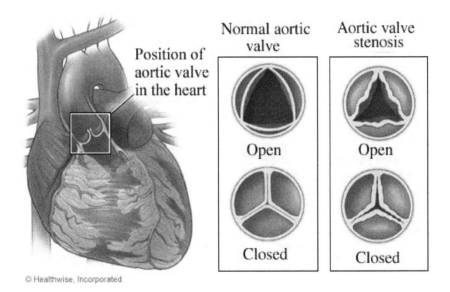

© Healthwise, Incorporated

Figure 1. Normal aortic valve and stenotic aortic valve

The pathophysiology of valvular aortic stenosis is one of progressive obstruction and the resultant compensatory changes. With increasing left ventricular outflow tract obstruction, there is pressure hypertrophy of the left ventricle. Left ventricular cavity size and systolic function is initially maintained, as the increase in left ventricular wall thickness acts as a compensatory mechanism to normalize wall stress. The development of pressure hypertrophy is initially a beneficial adaptation. However, this hypertrophy may result in reduced coronary flow reserve and oxygen supply–demand mismatch. These hypertrophied hearts are also more sensitive to diffuse subendocardial ischemic injury, which may result in both systolic and diastolic dysfunction. As the obstruction progresses to a critical level, the high afterload "overwhelms" the left ventricle and systolic function begins to decrease. With continued severe afterload excess, myocyte degeneration and fibrosis occurs and produces irreversible left ventricular systolic dysfunction. In these patients, both the high afterload and the intrinsic myocardial disease significantly increase wall stress and a vicious cycle of deterioration in ventricular function ensues.[3]

The evaluation of aortic stenosis is based upon the history, the physical examination, and a comprehensive echocardiography. For most patients, two-dimensional echocardiography readily identifies the calcified stenotic aortic valve, and Doppler echocardiography reliably estimates the severity of aortic stenosis in the majority of patients. Many patients with aortic stenosis will remain asymptomatic for decades. The diagnosis of aortic stenosis is usually made in the asymptomatic patient on the basis of a systolic murmur on auscultation and confirmed by echocardiography. Symptoms, when they occur, usually consist of one or more of the classic triad of exertional dyspnea, angina, and syncope. Following symptom onset, there is a high mortality rate with an average survival of 2–3 years. The development of symptoms therefore is a critical point in the natural history of patients with aortic stenosis. Sudden death rarely is the initial manifestation of severe aortic stenosis, occurring at a rate of less than 1% per year in asymptomatic patients.[3] Two-dimensional and Doppler echocardiography is the imaging modality of choice for the diagnosis and quantification of aortic stenosis. Short-axis images from two-dimensional echocardiography demonstrate the number of aortic cusps and the degree of cusp fusion or restricted cusp opening in valvular aortic stenosis. Two dimensional echocardiography is also useful for determining the status of the left ventricle and the degree of hypertrophy. Left atrial enlargement indicates concomitant diastolic dysfunction. The normal area of the adult aortic valve is 3.0 to 4.0 cm². Reduction of the normal area usually does not produce symptoms until the valve reaches one-fourth of its normal dimension.[4] The graduation of AS is given in Table 1.

Severity	Aortic jet velocity (m per second)	Mean gradient (mm Hg)	Aortic valve area (cm²)
Normal	< 2.5	-	3 to 4
Mild	2.5 to 2.9	< 25	1.5 to 2
Moderate	3 to 4	25 to 40	1 to 1.5
Severe	> 4	> 40	< 1

Table 1. Classifications of Aortic Stenosis Severity[4]

There is no effective medical therapy for AS. AVR is the only effective treatment for severe aortic stenosis in adults. Following AVR for AS, one can expect resolution of symptoms, left ventricular hypertrophy (LVH) regression, and improved left ventricular (LV) systolic function secondary to reduced afterload. Importantly, postoperative survival is similar to age-matched controls after AVR for AS when performed prior to the development of LV dysfunction or congestive heart failure (CHF). Similarly, incomplete regression of LVH after AVR has been associated with adverse outcomes such as reduced long-term survival. Contrary to the immediate improvement in systolic performance, diastolic dysfunction may persist for several more years after AVR. In fact, Gjertsson et al. recently evaluated diastolic dysfunction in AS and found that the proportion of patients with moderate-to-severe diastolic dysfunction actually increased with time after AVR despite normalization of LV mass and appropriate adjustments for senile diastolic dysfunction. Finally, AVR is associated with improved quality of life scores, particularly among the elderly, and has been found to be similar to age-matched individuals without heart disease. [3,5,6]

The American College of Cardiology (ACC) and the American Heart Association (ACH) have jointly developed guidelines in which they published indications for AVR:

a. Definite indications:

- Patients who have severe AS and presented with one or more of its classical symptoms (angina, syncope, heart failure, etc.)

- Patients who have severe AS and required coronary artery bypass surgery, surgery on the aorta or other heart valves

- Patients who have severe AS and left ventricle systolic dysfunction (ejection fraction less than 50 %)

b. Possible indications:

- Patients who have moderate AS and required coronary artery bypass surgery, surgery on the aorta or other heart valves

- Asymptomatic patients with severe AS with abnormal exercise test, or an increase in transaortic gradient during exercise, or left ventricle systolic dysfunction (ejection fraction less than 50 %), or left ventricular dilatation, or significantly elevated left ventricular diastolic pressure. [7]

The European Society of Cardiology (ESC) has also developed guidelines in which they published indications for AVR (Table 2).[8] They strongly recommended early AVR in all symptomatic patients with severe AS.

Management of asymptomatic patients requires careful weighing of benefits against risks. Early elective surgery at these patients can only be recommended in selected patients, at low operative risk. This could be the case in:

- The rare asymptomatic patients with depressed LV function not due to another cause

- Those with echocardiographic predictors of poor outcome suggested by the combination of a markedly calcified valve with a rapid increase in peak aortic velocity of ≥ 0.3 m/s per year

- If the exercise test is abnormal, particularly if it shows symptom development, which is a strong indication for surgery in physically active patients.

- However, on the other hand, breathlessness on exercise may be difficult to interpret in patients with only low physical activity, particularly the elderly, making decisionmaking more difficult. There is no strict age limit for performance of exercise testing and it is reasonable to propose it in patients > 70 years old who are still highly active.[8]

Patients with severe AS and any symptoms	IB
Patients with severe AS undergoing coronary artery bypass surgery, surgery of the ascending aorta, or on another valve	IC
Asymptomatic patients with severe AS and systolic LV dysfunction (LVEF < 50%) unless due to other cause	IC
Asymptomatic patients with severe AS and abnormal exercise test showing symptoms on exercise	IC
Asymptomatic patients with severe AS and abnormal exercise test showing fall in blood pressure below baseline	IIaC
Patients with moderate AS undergoing coronary artery bypass surgery, surgery of the ascending aorta or another valve	IIaC
Asymptomatic patients with severe AS and moderate-to-severe valve calcification, and a rate of peak velocity progression ≥ 0.3 m/s per year	IIaC
AS with low gradient (< 40 mmHg) and LV dysfunction with contractile reserve	IIaC
Asymptomatic patients with severe AS and abnormal exercise test showing complex ventricular arrhythmias	IIbC
Asymptomatic patients with severe AS and excessive LV hypertrophy (≥ 15 mm) unless this is due to hypertension	IIbC
AS with low gradient (< 40 mmHg) and LV dysfunction without contractile reserve	IIbC

Table 2. Indications for AVR in AS

In last 50 years, the varieties of prostheses that have become available for use are numerous. An ideal aortic prosthesis would be simple to implant, widely available, possess long-term durability, would have no intrinsic thrombogenicity, would not have a predilection foe endocarditis and would have no residual transvalvular pressure gradient. Such a valve does not currently exist. Currently available options include mechanical valves, stented biological valves, stentless biological valves, allograft valves and pulmonary autograft valves. Commonly in us are mechanical and biological prostheses.[9] When selecting between mechanical and biologic heart valves, the surgeon and patient must balance the risks and benefits of each choice.

2. Mechanical prostheses

Charles Hufnagel in 1952. Used aortic valve ball and cage prosthesis heterotopically in the descending aorta to treat aortic insufficiency. The first aortic valve replacement with an intra cardiac mechanical prosthesis, which led to long terms survivors, was performed in 1960. Mechanical valves are classified according to their structure as caged-ball, single-tilting-disk or bileaflet-tilting-disk valves. The Starr-Edwards caged-ball valve has been available since the 1960's and comprises a silastic ball, which rests on the sewing ring when closed and moves forward into the cage when the valve opens. The single-disk valves, for example, the Bjork-Shiley prosthesis and the Medtronic-Hall prosthesis, contain a disk that tilts between two struts of the orifice housing. The most popular of the mechanical valves at present are the bileaflet valves, of which the St. Jude Medical valve and the Carbomedics valve are widely implanted. Both these devices are implanted within the aortic annulus. The two semi-circular leaflets of the bileaflet valve are connected to the housing by a butterfly hinge mechanism and swing apart during opening of the valve creating three outflow tracts, one central and two peripheral respectively. In contrast to the configuration of the latter, the Carbomedics Top Hat (Sulzer Carbomedics, Austin, TX) bileaflet aortic valve that was introduced in 1993 has a unique supra-annular design with all its components incorporated within the aortic sinuses.[10,11]

Mechanical valves are made from carbon, Teflon, Dacron, titanium and polyester and are very durable. The current designs for the aortic and mitral positions include ball-and-cage valves, single tilting disc prostheses, and bileaflet prostheses. Bileaflet mechanical valves are the standard in current practice, with the St. Jude Medical (St. Jude Medical, Inc., St. Paul, MN) prosthesis the modern prototype, having been first implanted in 1977. Most of these valves are constructed using carbon strengthened with silicon carbide additives. Other examples of bileaflet mechanical valves include those manufactured by CarboMedics (Austin, TX); Advancing the Standard Medical (ATS, Minneapolis, MN); Medtronic, Inc. (Minneapolis, MN); and Medical Carbon Research Institute, LLC (MCRI, Austin, TX). [10,11,12] The On-XR mechanical valve (MCRI) was introduced in Europe in 1996 and differs from other bileaflet mechanical valves in that it is made from pure pyrolytic carbon. The PROACT (Prospective Randomized On-X R Valve Anticoagulation Trial) study is an FDA-approved multicenter trial, sponsored by MCRI, currently enrolling patients to determine whether or not defined patient groups receiving AVR (low versus high risk for TE events) with the On-X R _ valve may be safely maintained on lower doses of warfarin or, for patients in the lowrisk aortic valve arm, on antiplatelet drugs (aspirin plus clopidogrel) alone compared with standard anticoagulation regimens. No single mechanical valve has shown superior patient outcomes, and all demonstrate extremely low rates of structural valve deterioration, the major advantage of mechanical valves.[3]

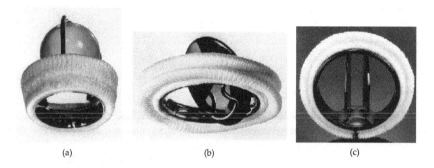

| (a) | (b) | (c) |

Figure 2. Mechanical valves: a) Starr-Edwards cage-ball valve, b) Bjork-Shiley mono-leaflet valve and c) St. Jude Medical bileaflet valve

3. Biological prosthesis

The biological prostheses include a wide variety of devices. Included within this broad category are the bioprostheses, a term which is used for valves with non-viable tissue of biological origin. The bioprostheses include the heterografts, composed of porcine (actual valves of a pig) or bovine tissue (pericardium of a cow) and the allografts, which are preserved human aortic valves. The initial bioprostheses were mounted on stents to which the leaflets and sewing ring were attached but subsequently stentless valves, which are sewn in free hand, have been developed.[13] Stented bioprosthetic valves, which incorporate a semi-rigid external support structure for the valve leaflets, represent the majority of tissue valves implanted in clinical practice. The external support provides accurate valve mounting, improving ease of implantation. Two types of stented bioprosthetic valves are currently available in the United States: porcine aortic valves, which incorporate chemically stabilized porcine valve leaflets mounted on a stented structure or frame, and bovine pericardial valves. The leaflets of the latter valve type are constructed from bovine pericardium and subsequently mounted on a stented frame. Available porcine valves include the Medtronic Mosaic valve (Medtronic Inc., Minneapolis, MN), the St. Jude Medical Biocor and Biocor Supra valves (St. Jude Medical, Inc., St. Paul, MN), and the Carbomedics Mitroflow valve (Carbomedics, Inc., Austin, TX). Bovine pericardial valves include the Carpentier–Edwards (C–E) Perimount (Edward Lifesciences, Irvine, CA) and the CE Perimount Magna valves as well as the Sorin Soprano (Sorin Group, Saluggia, Italy) valves. At present, based on the best available data, no one bioprosthetic valve appears superior with regard to patient outcomes and none requires systemic anticoagulation with warfarin, which is their major advantage. Their major disadvantage is the incidence of structural valve deterioration and subsequent need for reoperation, although the lifespan of the latest generation of tissue valves is unknown. Recent evidence also suggests that stentless biological valves may have better coronary flow reserve compared to stented valves. Additionally, compared with stented bovine pericardial valves, stentless valves have been associated with increased transvalvular EOA and decreased pressure gradients during extended follow-up. However, as seen in other studies, LV mass regression after stentless valve implantation was not different from stented aortic bioprostheses.[3,14]

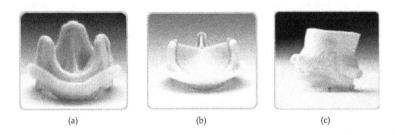

(a)   (b)   (c)

Figure 3. Biological prosthesis: a) stented porcine bioprosthesis, b) pericardial bovine bioprosthesis and c) stentless porcine bioprosthesis

4. Outcomes after aortic valve replacement

The Ad Hoc Liaison Committee for Standardizing Definitions of Prosthetic Heart Valve Morbidity of the American Association of Thoracic Surgery and the Society of Thoracic Surgeons published guidelines during years, which are now widely used in reporting outcomes after valve surgery. They presented a list of developing specific valve-related events during patients remaining lifetime. These valve-related events are:

1. Structural valvular deterioration

2. Nonstructural dysfunction

3. Valve thrombosis

4. Embolism

5. Valvular endocarditis and

6. Bleeding events.[7, 15]

Structural valvular deterioration - Any change in function or deterioration (a decrease of one New York Heart Association functional class or more) of an operated valve due to an intrinsic abnormality, which causes stenosis or regurgitation. Changes intrinsic to the valve include wear, fracture, poppet escape, calcification, leaflet tear stent creep and suture line disruption of the components of the operated valve. The definition excludes changes due to infection or thrombosis. *Mechanical prostheses* are extremely resistant to material fatigue or structural valve deterioration. This is characteristic of mechanical valves

whether they are aortic or mitral valves.[16] Because of the long-term durability of mechanical prostheses a valve replacement rate is less than 2% over 25 years. The most common reasons for reimplantation are pre- and postoperative endocarditis, paravalvular leak
and valve thrombosis.[17] *Bioprosthetic valves* are not as durable, have a shorter lifespan
and are more susceptible to calcification than human and mechanical valves.[13] Bioprostheses have a significantly higher rate of reoperation due to structural valve deterioration.
In large series, freedom from reoperation is > 90% at 10 years, but < 70 % at 15 years.
[17,18,19] There is an important predisposition for premature bioprosthetic structural
valve deterioration in younger patients, especially those under the age of 40 years.[17]

Nonstructural dysfunction - Any abnormality that is not intrinsic to the valve per se, which
causes stenosis or regurgitation. Examples for this include entrapment of pannus, tissue or
suture; paravalvular leak; inappropriate sizing or positioning; residual leak and clinically
important hemolytic anemia. This definition also excludes changes due to infection and
thrombosis. Subvalvular pannus formation is rare with *mechanical bileaflet valves*.[20] Panus
overgrowth and prosthetic structural degeneration interfering with normal valve opening and
closure may cause hemolysis severe enough for reoperation. Paravalvular leak is an operative
complication and it is related to operative technique and to endocarditis.[21]

Valve thrombosis – Any thrombus, in the absence of infection, which is attached to or near an
operated valve that occludes part of the blood flow path or that interferes with function of the
valve. The incidence of prosthesis thrombosis is < 0.2 % per year and it occurs more often in
mechanical prostheses.[22] It is most commonly due to inadequate anticoagulation or noncom-
pliance. Freedom from valve thrombosis at 20 years is > 97 %.[23,24]

Embolism – Any embolic event that occurs, in the absence of infection, after the immediate
peri-operative period. This could be either a neurologic or peripheral embolic event. A
neurologic event includes any new, temporary or permanent focal or global neurologic deficit.
A peripheral embolic event is due to an embolus that produces symptoms from obstruction of
a peripheral (non-cerebral) artery. The incidence of thromboembolic events between bioprostheses and mechanical prostheses are the same.[25] This is a continuous risk factor that is
present through the life of patients with *mechanical valve prosthesis*, so they must maintain
therapeutic anticoagulant levels. The embolic risk is highest in the first few months, before the
ring and valve components have fully endothelialized.[26] Acceptable thromboembolic rates
range between 0.8 and 2.3 % per patient-year.[21,22,25] 50 % of these events are neurologic, 40
% are transient and 10 % are peripheral.[21]

Valvular endocarditis – Any infection involving an operated valve diagnosed by customary
clinical criteria. It is rare case with prophylactic antibiotics. Around 60 % of events occur early
and are associated with staphylococci. The mortality for this event is high. Freedom from
endocarditis with mechanical prosthesis is 97 to 98 % at 20 to 25 years. A number of studies
have reported a higher incidence of valvular endocarditis after *mechanical valve* replacement
in comparison with the biologic valve replacement during the initial few months after
implantation. *Bioprostheses* are less susceptible to early infection, which is often restricted to
the leaflets, making cure with antibiotics more likely but increasing the chances of late failure
due to degeneration of the cusps.[27,28,29]

Bleeding event – Formerly classified as anti-coagulant hemorrhage, a bleeding event is an episode of major internal or external bleeding that causes death, hospitalization, and permanent injury or requires transfusion. This definition applies to all patients, irrespective of anti-coagulation status. *Mechanical valves* are durability but anticoagulation is key of long-term success. International Normalized Ratio (INR) is the standard to which anticoagulation levels should be targeted. Level of INR should be individual for each person. Complications occur during fluctuations in the INR and less during steady-state levels, be they high or low.[30,31] When levels of INR increase, bleeding episodes become more common, and when levels of INR decrease thromboembolic episodes become more common. Some studies showed that around 40 % of the bleeding episodes occurred in the first year after surgery, when levels of INR are more likely to fluctuate. Many studies suggested that in the early postoperative period slowly raise the level of INR to therapeutic levels is needed, to prevent bleeding events. [21,32,33] According to ACC and ACH after mechanical AVR, the goal of antithrombotic therapy is usually to achieve an INR of 2.5 to 3.5 for the first 3 months after surgery and 2.0 to 3.0 beyond that time. At that level of anticoagulation, the risk of significant hemorrhage appears to be 1% to 2% per year.[7] Low-dose aspirin is also indicated in addition to warfarin to result in a lower incidence of thromboembolic event, with a low possibility for bleeding.[34] Older patients are at higher risk for thromboembolic event because of the greater number of risk factors that accumulate with aging.[30] Anticoagulation-related hemorrhage (ARH) is the most common valve-related event. More often it will occur during fluctuations in INR, which happens most often early after valve replacement.[21,22] The most common places for ARH are gastrointestinal tract and central nervous system.[21] Acceptable ARH rates range from 1.0 to 2.5% per patient-year in long term reports.[21,22,25,35] It is very dangerous complication, because mortality more often occurs in relation to bleeding events than in relation to thromboembolic events.[21]

Operative mortality – Operative mortality is defined as all-cause mortality within 30 days of operation. According to the Society of Thoracic Surgeons mortality for isolated AVR is 4.3% and for AVR with concomitant coronary artery disease is 8%.[36] Many factors have been associated with an increased risk of operative mortality in isolated AVR. Some of these risk factors are age, female gender, diabetes, renal failure, and emergency status, previous operation, advanced preoperative NYHA class, lower cardiac index, concomitant coronary artery bypass grafting and longer aortic crossclamp and cardiopulmonary bypass time respectively.[37] In the absence of major comorbidities and preserved ejection fraction, isolated AVR can be performed with an expected mortality of less than 2%.[38]

Several studies have evaluated independent risk factors for operative mortality after AVR. Five variables predictive of increased mortality risk after AVR are common to each of these analyses: preoperative renal failure, urgency of AVR, preoperative heart failure, presence of CAD or recent MI, and redo cardiac operation. Other factors independently associated with operative mortality from the individual studies include preoperative atrial fibrillation, active endocarditis, preoperative stroke, advanced age, lower body surface area, multiple valve procedures, and hypertension. [39, 40]

5. Factors affecting long-term outcome after AVR

- Demographic
  - Older age
  - Male sex
- Clinical
  - Higher pre-operative NYHA functional class
  - Pre-operative atrial fibrillation and non-sinus rhythm
  - Pure aortic regurgitation
  - Hypertension
  - Diabetes mellitus
  - Renal failure
- Surgery-related
  - Longer cardiopulmonary bypass time
- Morphological
  - Previous myocardial infarction
  - Left ventricular structure and functional abnormality
  - Previous aortic valve surgery
  - Coronary artery disease (CAD)

Older patients have a lot of comorbiditis and they are at higher risk for valve-related events. Atrial fibrillation is one of the risk factor for thromboembolism, because of that INR levels must be higher (INR 2.5 to 3.5) than regular.[30,34] The majority of patients undergoing AVR have other cardiac lesions, most commonly CAD, and more complex pathology has been associated with increased risk. Combined myocardial revascularization and AVR increases cross-clamp time and has the potential to increase perioperative myocardial infarction and early postoperative mortality compared with patients undergoing isolated AVR.[7] In addition to severity of CAD and AS, the multivariate factors for late postoperative mortality include low ejection fraction, severity of LV dysfunction, age greater than 70 years (especially in women), and presence of NYHA functional class IV symptoms.[36]

6. Patient selection

Propter selection of patients for valve replacement can bring us excellent long-term results, long-term survival and low incidence of valve-related complications.

In some studies of patients followed over longer time frames, freedom from all valve-related events and freedom from reoperation were improved in patients with mechanical valve prostheses as compared to patients with biological prostheses. [9,16,25] Key of long-term success of mechanical valve prostheses is anticoagulation. Patients that are inconsistent, noncompliant or incapable of managing medications are not good candidates for long-term chronic anticoagulation.[39,41] Also patients with higher levels of education and those from geographic areas with a good medical infrastructure have better compliance with necessary medications and anticoagulant monitoring.[31]

Many centers used bioprosthetic valves for patients who are older than 70 year, based on data by Akins.[42] In patients younger than 60 years of age, the best solution would be implantation of mechanical valves, based on prosthesis durability and they have low-risk for valve-related events.[21] In decade between 60 and 70 years of age, other factors have to be taken into account.[7] According to some studies, patients over 65 years at the time of surgery should receive a biologic valve. Patients under the age of 60 should have a mechanical prosthesis to minimize the risk of structural failure requiring repeat AVR in an octogenarian. Patients between 60 and 65 represent the group in whom there is still considerable debate regarding prosthesis selection. Those patients who have comorbidities such as severe CAD may be less likely to outlive their prosthesis and should receive a biologic valve. A detailed discussion of these risks and benefits of prosthesis selection should occur with all patients and their families prior to entering the operating room. [3,7,22,24,25,37,38]

In the early follow-up period, anticoagulation – related hemorrhage is the most common unwanted event for mechanical valve prostheses. Over the first 10 years of follow-up there is a higher incidence of valve-related events in patients with mechanical prostheses as opposed to those with biologic valves.[32] However, in the next 10 to 20 years after AVR, the incidence of valve failure and valve-related complications are much higher at biologic prostheses than those with mechanical valve prostheses. Some series showed that the time to biologic valve failure was only 7.6 years.[43] This failure rate will increase over time. However, freedom from valve-related events is more strongly influenced by pre-existing comorbidities than the presence of mechanical prostheses.[21], [22, 25, 31]

The elderly patient with severe aortic stenosis poses a therapeutic challenge. In considering elderly patients for aortic valve replacement, important factors include the presence of symptoms, physiologic age, patient expectations, anticipated future activities, and comorbidity. The operation itself carries a higher risk than in younger patients. Extensive calcification of the aorta and annulus as well as fragile tissue presents significant technical difficulties for the surgeon. In addition, particularly in women, the aortic root and annulus may be small and require concomitant enlargement to accommodate the valve prosthesis. Furthermore, protruding arch atheroma occurs in one-fifth of patients > 65 years of age and significantly increases the risk of stroke and mortality during cardiac surgery. Major postoperative complications, nevertheless, remain high, with the incidence of permanent stroke between 4 and 6%. Rehabilitation can also be a problem, as elderly patients take longer to recover from surgery. Survival has clearly improved in these elderly patients with severe symptomatic aortic stenosis who undergo aortic valve replacement. Survival is 80–85% at 1 year and 60–

70% at 5 years, which is similar to an age- and sex-matched population without aortic valve disease. Most patients report improved functional capacity and quality of life, with more than 90% of patients feeling better after surgery.[3]

A major deterrent to mechanical valve replacement in the younger patient is the impact of long-term anticoagulation. Mechanical valves are, however, more ideal for younger patients due to their excellent durability characteristics. Most importantly, younger patients (i.e., patients under the age of 50 years) are a low-risk subset for valve related events. These individuals have very few risk factors for TE, and thus anticoagulation can be run at the lower end of the therapeutic target range, decreasing the incidence of anticoagulant-related hemorrhage without altering the incidence of TE. In fact, many infants and children have been managed with only aspirin with quite good long term results. While this is not recommended in patients older than infancy, it is a feasible alternative. A recent study in patients under 50 years of age followed 254 patients for up to 20 years and found an exceedingly low rate of valve related events, an exceptional long-term overall survival of nearly 88%, and event-free survival probability of 92% at 19 years.[3,44,45]

Patients with an absolute requirement for long-term anticoagulation such as atrial fibrillation, previous thromboembolic events, hypercoagulable state, severe LVD, another mechanical heart valve in place, or intracardiac thrombus, should receive a mechanical valve regardless of age. Patients in whom anticoagulation with warfarin is contraindicated, such as women of child-bearing age wishing to become pregnant, patients with other bleeding disorders, or those who refuse anticoagulation should receive a bioprosthesis. There is growing interest in using mechanical prostheses in women of child-bearing age and providing anticoagulation with subcutaneous low-molecular weight heparin injections. Patients with end-stage renal failure were previously believed to have significantly elevated risk for early bioprosthetic structural valve deterioration. However, increased anticoagulation- related complications are also more likely in this group, and the current ACC/AHA guidelines do not recommend routine use of mechanical prostheses in these patients.[3,7,8,9,10]

The decision between bioprosthetic and mechanical valve should be made by the patient with educated input regarding the pros and cons of each option from the patient's physicians. Today surgeons implant bioprosthetic valves in younger patients who wish to avoid anticoagulation due to lifestyle concerns (e.g. young, active individual, desire to become pregnant, etc.), although surgeons generally will guide patients toward a mechanical option at the time of redo-AVR if their life expectancy exceeds 10–15 years at that time.[3]

7. Operative technique

Aortic valve replacement is most frequently done through a median sternotomy, meaning the incision is made by cutting through the sternum. Once the pericardium has been opened, the patient is put on a cardiopulmonary bypass machine. This machine takes over the task of breathing for the patient and pumping their blood around while the surgeon replaces the heart valve.

Once the patient is on bypass, a cut is made in the aorta and a crossclamp applied. The surgeon then removes the patient's diseased aortic valve and a mechanical or biological valve is put in its place. Once the valve is in place and aorta has been closed, the patient is taken off the heart-lung machine. Transesophageal echocardiogram can be used to verify that the new valve is functioning property. Pacing wires are usually put in place, so that the heart can be manually paced should any complications arise after surgery. Drainage tubes are also inserted to drain fluids from the chest and pericardium following surgery. These are usually removed within 36-48 hours while the pacing wires are generally left in place until right before the patient is discharged from the hospital.

8. Patient-prosthesis mismatch

Prosthesis-patient mismatch (PPM) is that a smaller than expected effective orifice area (IEOA) in relation to the patient's body surface area (BSA) will result in higher transvalvar gradients. It is condition that occurs when the valve area of a prosthetic valve is less than the area of that patient's normal valve.[46] Several authors suggest that prosthesis-patient mismatch occurs at an IEOA of 0.85 cm^2/m^2.[46,47] Transvalvular gradients begin to rise substantially at IEOAs below this value, and these elevated gradients potentially cause increased left ventricular work that prevents adequate regression of left ventricular hypertrophy. Several factors including age, body mass index (BMI), and pre-operative status of left ventricular function may potentially influence the effect of PPM on post-operative outcomes.[46] PPM is associated with a significant reduction in cardiac index during the postoperative course. The incidence of congestive heart failure was significantly higher in patients with PPM.[48] Several studies reported that early mortality is significantly increased in patients with PPM.[47, 48, 49, 50]

The projected indexed EOA should be systematically calculated at the time of the operation to estimate the risk of PPM. PPM can be avoided by using a simple strategy at the time of operation. Pibarot suggested that surgeon first calculate the patient's BSA from his or her weight and height. Than multiply BSA by 0.85 cm^2/m^2, the result being the minimum EOA that the prosthesis to be implanted should have to avoid PPM, and than choose the prosthesis and the reference values for the different types and sizes of prosthesis.[46, 47]

Due to concerns over PPM, stentless bioprosthetic valves, which generally have a larger EOA sizefor- size compared with mechanical or stented bioprosthetic valves, have been increasingly utilized for AVR. In initial evaluation, stentless valves had better hemodynamics and improved survival rates relative to stented biological or mechanical valves and were more durable than stented biological valves. Stentless valves may be preferred in patients with a small aortic root, and arguments have been made that wider utilization of stentless valves may minimize PPM. Stentless valves also appear to have better hemodynamic profiles than stented valves during exercise testing. Technical reasons for not implanting stentless valves include extensive aortic root calcification, coronary ostia opposed by 180, presence of the two coronary ostia in close proximity, or unusual disproportion between the sinotubular junction and the aortic annulus. Whereas stented valves allow perfect valve mounting within the aortic annulus, thus reducing the risk of implanting an incompetent valve, postoperative AR and limited durability remain a concern with the free-hand stentless valve insertion technique. This issue may be circumvented with full aortic root replacement using a stentless porcine root.[3.49,50]

Author details

Stamenko Šušak[1]*, Lazar Velicki[1], Dušan Popović[1] and Ivana Burazor[2]

*Address all correspondence to: drsusak@gmail.com

1 Institute of Cardiovascular Diseases Vojvodina, Sremska Kamenica, Serbia

2 Clinical Centers, Nis, Serbia

References

[1] Malouf, J. F, Edwards, W. D, Tajik, A. J, & Seward, J. Functional anatomy of the heart. In: Fuster V, O'Rourke RA, Walsh RA, Poole-Wilson P, eds. Hurst's The Heart. 12th ed. New York, NY: McGraw-Hill Companies, Inc; (2008).

[2] Otto, C. M, Lind, B. K, Kitzman, D. W, et al. Association of aortic valve sclerosis with cardiovascular mortality and morbidity in the elderly. N Eng J Med (1999).

[3] Andrew WangThomas S. Bashore. Valvular Heart Disease. Humana Press, a part of Springer Science Business Media, LLC (2009).

[4] Gjertsson, P, Caidahl, K, Farasati, M, et al. Preopeartive moderate to severe diastolic dysfunction: A novel Doppler echocardiographic long-term prognosis factor in patients with severe aortic stenosis. J Thorac Cardiovasc Surg (2005).

[5] Connolly, H. M, Oh, J. K, Orszulak, T. A, et al. Aortic valve replacement for aortic stenosis with severe left ventricular dysfunction: prognostic indicators. Circulation (1997). , 95, 2395-400.

[6] Gjertsson, P, Caidahl, K, & Bech-hanssen, O. Left ventricular diastolic dysfunction late after aortic valve replacement in patients with aortic stenosis. Am J Cardiol (2005). , 96, 722-7.

[7] Bonow, R. O, Carabello, B. A, & Chatterjee, K. de Leon AC Jr, Faxon DP, Freed MD, Gaasch WH, Lytle BW, Nishimura RA, O'Gara PT, O'Rourke RA, Otto CM, Shah PM, Shanewise JS. ACC/AHA 2006 guidelines for the management of patients with valvular heart disease: a report of the American College of Cardiology/American Heart Association Task Force on Practice Guidelines (Writing Committee to Develop

Guidelines for the Management of Patients With Valvular Heart Disease). Circulation. (2006). ee231. DOI:CIRCULATIONAHA.106.176857, 84.

[8] The European Society of Cardiology Guidelines on the management of valvular heart disease European Heart Journal (2007.

[9] Gott, V. L. Alejo DE: Mechanical heart valves: 50 years of evolution. Ann Thorac Surg (2003). S2230

[10] Bloomfield, P. Choice of heart valve prosthesis. Heart. (2002). , 87, 583-9.

[11] Dewall, R. A, Qasim, N, & Carr, L. Evolution of Mechanical Heart valves. Ann Thorac Surg. (2000). , 69, 1612-21.

[12] Bonow, R. O, Carabello, B. A, Chatterjee, K. C, De Leon, J. R, Faxon, A. C, Freed, D. P, Shah, M. D, & Acc, P. M. AHA 2006 guidelines for the management of patients with valvular heart disease. Journal of the American College of Cardiology, 48(3), 1-148.doi:10.1016/j.jacc.2006.05.021

[13] YangThang, "Mechanical Versus Bioprosthetic Valve Replacement in Valvular Heart Disease: A Systematic Review" ((2011). School of Physician Assistant Studies. Paper 240.http://commons.pacificu.edu/pa/240

[14] Tsialtas, D, Bolognesi, R, Beghi, C, et al. Stented versus stentless bioprostheses in aortic valve stenosis: effect on left ventricular remodeling. Heart Surg Forum (2007). E, 205-10.

[15] Golubovic, M, Mihajlovic, B, Kovacevic, P, Cemerlic-adjic, N, Pavlovic, K, Velicki, L, & Susak, S. Postoperativne neletalne komplikacije posle operacije na otvorenom srcu. Vojnosanitetski pregled (2012). , 69(1), 27-31.

[16] Stamenko, S. Susak. Mitralna regurgitacija- kardiohirurski aspekti dijagnostike i terapije. Mediterran Publishing, Biblioteka Academica, knjiga 15, Novi Sad (2010).

[17] Emery, R. W, Arom, K. V, Krogh, C. C, et al. Reoperative valve replacement with the St.Jude Medical valve prosthesis: long-term follow up. J Am Coll Cardiol (2004). A

[18] Desai, N. D, Merin, O, Cohen, G. N, et al. Long-term results of aortic valve replacement with the St.Jude Toronto stentless porcine valve. Ann Thorac Surg (2004).

[19] Grunkemeier, G. L, Jamieson, W. R, & Miller, D. C. Starr A: Actuarial versus actual risk of porcine structural valve deterioration. J Thorac Cardiovasc Surg (1994).

[20] Vongpatanasin, W, & Hills, L. D. Lange RA: Prosthetic heart valve. N Eng J Med (1996).

[21] Emery, R. W, Krogh, C. C, Arom, D. V, et al. The ST. Jude Medical cardiac valve prosthesis: A year experience with single valve replacement. Ann Thorac Surg (2005). , 25.

[22] Ikonomidis, J. S, Kratz, J. M, Crumbley, A. J, et al. Twenty-year experience with the St.Jude Medical mechanical valve prosthesis. J Thorac Cardiovasc Surg (2003).

[23] Lengyel, M. Vandor L: The role of thrombolysis in the management of left-sided prosthetic valve thrombosis: a study of 85 cases diagnosed by transesophageal echocardiography. J Heart Valve Dis (2001).

[24] Durrleman, N, Pellerin, M, Bouchard, D, et al. Prosthetic valve thrombosis: twenty-year experience at the Montreal Heart Institute. J Thorac Cardiovasc Surg (2004).

[25] Khan, S. S, Trento, A, Derobertis, M, et al. Twenty-year comparison of tissue and mechanical valve replacement. J Thorac Cardiovasc Surg (2001).

[26] Heras, M, Chesebro, J. H, Fuster, V, et al. High risk of thromboemboli early after bioprosthetic cardiac valve replacement. J Am Coll Cardiol (1995).

[27] Mahesh, B, Angelini, G, Caputo, M, Jin, X. Y, & Bryan, A. (2005). Prosthetic valve endocarditis. Ann. Thorac. Surg., 0003-4975, 80(3), 1151-1158.

[28] Velicki, L, Susak, S, Cemerlic-adjic, N, & Redzek, A. Aortic valve endocarditis, Chapter in: Ying-Fu Chen and Chwan-Yau Luo- Aortic valve, InTech Publishing (2011).

[29] Velicki, L, Susak, S, & Srdanovic, I. Kovacevic M; Infective endocarditis of native aortic valve: destruction of leaflet with an aorto-cavitary fistula to the right ventricle, Chirurgia (2010). , 23(6), 261-266.

[30] Koertke, H, Minami, K, Boethig, D, et al. INR self-management permits lower anticoagulation levels after mechanical heart valve replacement. Circulation (2003). Suppl II):II-75.

[31] Butchart, E. G, Ionescu, A, Payne, N, et al. A new scoring system to determine thromboembolic risk after heart valve replacement. Circulation (2003). Suppl II):II-68.

[32] Kumar, D, & Elefteriades, J. Ezekowitz MD: Anticoagulation in patients with prosthetic heart valves. Cardiac Surg Today (2004).

[33] Koo, S, Kucher, N, Nguyen, P. L, et al. The effect of excessive anticoagulation on mortality and morbidity in hospitalized patients with anticoagulant-related major hemorrhage. Arch Intern Med (2004).

[34] Massel, D. Little SH: Risk and benefits of adding antiplatelet therapy to warfarin among patients with prosthetic heart valves: a metaanalysis. J Am Coll Cardiol (2001).

[35] Lund, O, Nielsen, S. L, Arildsen, H, et al. Standard aortic St. Jude valve at 18 years: performance, profile and determinants of outcome. Ann Thorac Surg (2000).

[36] Society of Thoracic Surgeons National Cardiac Surgery DatabaseAvailable at: http://www.sts.org/documents/pdf/STS-ExecutiveSummaryFall2005.pdf. November (2005).

[37]　Edwards, F. H, Peterson, E. D, Coombs, L. P, et al. Prediction of operative mortality after valve replacement surgery. J Am Coll Cardiol (2001).

[38]　David TE: Surgery of the aortic valve. (1999). *Curr Probl Surg.*

[39]　Rankin, J. S, Hammill, B. G, Ferguson, T. B, et al. Determinants of operative mortality in valvular heart surgery. J Thorac Cardiovasc Surg (2006). , 131, 547-57.

[40]　Kuduvalli, M, Grayson, A. D, Au, J, et al. A multi-centre additive and logistic risk model for in-hospital mortality following aortic valve replacement. Eur J Cardiothorac Surg (2007). , 31, 607-13.

[41]　Butchart, E. G, Payne, N, Li, H, et al. Better anticoagulation control improves survival after valve replacement. J Thorac Cardiovasc Surg (2002).

[42]　Akins, C. W, Buckley, M. J, Daggett, W. M, et al. Risk of reoperative valve replacement for failed mitral and aortic bioprostheses. Ann Thorac Surg (1998).

[43]　Potter, D. D, & Sundt, T. M. rd, Zehr KJ, et al: Operative risk of reoperative aortic valve replacement. J Thorac Cardiovasc Surg (2005).

[44]　Cabalka, A. K, & Emery, R. W. Petersen RJ: Long-term follow-up of the St. Jude Medical prosthesis in pediatric patients. Ann Thorac Surg (1995). S618

[45]　Emery, R. W, Erickson, C. A, Arom, K. V, et al. Replacement of the aortic valve in patients under 50 years old with the St. Jude Medical prosthesis. Ann Thorac Surg (2003).

[46]　Dumesnil, J. G. Pibarot P: Prosthesis-patient mismatch and clinical outcomes: the evidence continues to accumulate. J Thorac Cardiovasc Surg (2006).

[47]　Pibarot, P, & Dumesnil, J. G. Prosthesis-patient mismatch: definition, clinical impact, and prevention. Heart. (2006). , 92, 1022-9.

[48]　Milano, A D, De Carlo, M, Mecozzi, G, et al. Clinical outcome in patients with 19-mm and 21-mm St. Jude aortic prostheses: comparison at long-term follow-up, Ann Thorac Surg (2002). , 7337-43.

[49]　Rao, V, Jamieson, W, & Ivanov, E. J. et al Prosthesis-patient mismatch affects survival following aortic valve replacement. Circulation (2000). IIIIII9.III9, 5.

[50]　Blais, C, Dumesnil, J G, Baillot, R, et al. Impact of prosthesis-patient mismatch on short-term mortality after aortic valve replacement. Circulation (2003). , 108983-988.

Chapter 5

New Therapeutic Approaches to Conventional Surgery for Aortic Stenosis in High-Risk Patients

Omer Leal, Juan Bustamante, Sergio Cánovas and Ángel G. Pinto

Additional information is available at the end of the chapter

1. Introduction

Aortic stenosis (AS) is the most frequent type of valvular heart disease in Europe and North America. It mainly presents as calcified aortic stenosis in older adults (2-7% of the population> 65 years), which is the most common cause of valve replacement in the western world. Its incidence increases with age [1]. With the increasing age and life expectancy of the population, an increase in the prevalence of aortic stenosis had been observed. Furthermore, the elderly patient usually presents multiple comorbidities associated with increased surgical risk. Aortic valve replacement (AVR) is currently the treatment of choice in patients with symptomatic aortic stenosis and/or left ventricular systolic dysfunction (see Indications for surgery), even though some cases present high or extremely high surgical risk.

Our goal is to update the treatment of severe aortic stenosis in high-risk patients, mainly the elderly and those cases where risk assessment scales indicate a high- or very high-risk patient. Here we analyse the role of new therapeutic approaches in the treatment of these patients and their short and long-term results, as well as the use of new devices and prosthesis.

2. Etiology

AS without accompanying mitral valve disease is more common in men than in women [2] and rheumatic etiology is currently rare. Age-related degenerative calcific AS is currently the most common cause of AS in adults and the most frequent reason for aortic valve replacement (AVR) in patients with AS. Sclerosis of the aortic valve is observed in up to 30%

of elderly people: 25% of people aged 65 to 74, and 48% of people older than 84 years [3,4]. This calcific disease progresses from the base of the cusps to the leaflets, eventually causing a reduction in leaflet motion and effective valve area without commissural fusion. Calcific AS is an active disease process characterized by lipid accumulation, inflammation, and calcification, with many similarities to atherosclerosis. In approximately half of cases there is a bicuspid aortic valve basis. Bicuspid aortic valve valvulopathy affects 2% of the population, making it the most frequent congenital anomaly, representing the more common cause among young adults [5].

3. Evaluation and grading the degree of stenosis

Patient history and physical examination remain essential. Careful exploration for the presence of symptoms (shortness of breath on exertion, angina, dizziness, or syncope) is critical for proper patient management. It is important to be aware that patients may not notice symptoms but they significantly reduce their activities. The characteristic systolic murmur draws attention and guides further diagnostic work in the right direction. However, on occasion the murmur may, be faint and the primary presentation may be heart failure of unknown cause. The disappearance of the second aortic sound is specific to severe AS, however, it is not a sensitive sign.

Several studies [6-9] reports that biomarkers such as B-type natriuretic peptide (BNP) has been shown to be related to functional class and prognosis, particularly in AS and MR. In fact, Lancellotti et al. [9] reports in their study that a left atrial area index of > or = 12.4 cm2/m2, systolic annular velocity of < or = 4.5 cm/s, E/Ea ratio >13.8, late diastolic annular velocity of < or = 9 cm/s, and BNP of > or = 61 pg/ml were identified as the best cutoff values to predict events (death, symptoms, or surgery). They found, in asymptomatic AS, tissue Doppler imaging and BNP measurements provide prognostic information beyond that from clinical and conventional echocardiographic parameters. However, Natriuretic peptides have been shown to predict symptom free survival and outcome in normal- and low-flow severe AS and may be useful in asymptomatic patients, helping to discriminates those patients who can benefits from an early intervention [7-9]. Nevertheless, evidence regarding its incremental value in risk stratification remains limited so far.

Echocardiography is indicated when there is a systolic murmur of grade III/VI or higher, a single S2, or symptoms that might be due to AS [10]. A 2-dimensional (2D) echocardiogram is valuable for assessing valve anatomy and function and determining the LV response to pressure overload. In nearly all patients, the severity of the stenotic lesion can be defined with Doppler echocardiographic measurements. Echocardiography is also used to assess LV size and function, degree of hypertrophy, and presence of other associated valvular disease. Transoesophageal echocardiography (TOE) is rarely helpful for the quantification of AS, as valve area planimetry becomes difficult in calcified valves [11] however, it is useful when transthoracic visualization is poor and leaflets only moderately calcified [12]. TOE may, however, provide additional evaluation of mitral valve abnormalities and has gained importance in assessing annulus diameter before TAVI and in guiding the procedure. Intraprocedural TOE enables us to monitor the results of percutaneous procedures [11]. Three-dimensional TOE offers a more detailed examination of valve anatomy than two-dimensional echocardiography and is useful for the assessment of complex valve problems or for monitoring surgery and percutaneous intervention [11]. Three-dimensional echocardiography (3DE) is useful for assessing anatomical features which may have an impact on the type of intervention chosen, if it is needed. AS severity could be graded on the basis of a variety of hemodynamic and natural history data, using definitions of aortic jet velocity, mean pressure gradient, valve area and velocity ratio as shown in Table 1.

	Aortic Stenosis		
Indicator	*Mild*	*Moderate*	*Severe*
Aortic jet velocity (m/s)	2.6-3	3-4	≥4
Mean gradient (mmHg)	≤30(25)	30-50(25-40)	≥50(40)
Indexed AVA (cm²/m²)	≥0.9	0.6-0.9	≤0.6
AVA (cm²)	≥1.5	1-1.5	≤1
Velocity ratio	≥0.50	0.25-0.50	≤0.25

Table 1. Classification of the Severity of Aortic Valve Disease in Adults

Based on the European Society of Cardiology (ESC) Guidelines on the management of valvular heart disease [12], American College of Cardiology/American Heart Association (ACC/AHA) Guidelines for the Management of Patients With valvular heart disease [10] and ASE/EAE Recommendations for Quantitation of Stenosis Severity, [13] ACC/AHA guidelines use lower mean gradient cutoffs as indicated in parentheses. The ESC definitions apply only in the presence of normal flow conditions. The velocity ratio is included in the ASE/EAE guidelines only.

Multi-slice computed tomography (MSCT) and cardiac magnetic resonance (CMR) provide additional information on the assessment of the ascending aorta when it is enlarged. MSCT may be useful in quantifying the valve area and coronary calcification, which aids in assessing prognosis. MSCT may contribute to the evaluation of the severity of valve disease, particularly in AS, either indirectly by quantifying valvular calcification, or directly through the measurement of valve planimetry. Also, MSCT has become an important diagnostic tool for evaluation of the aortic root, the distribution of calcium, the number of leaflets, the ascending aorta, and peripheral artery pathology and dimensions before undertaking TAVI [11]. In patients with inadequate echocardiographic quality or discrepant results, CMR should be used to assess the severity of valvular lesions—particularly regurgitant lesions—and to assess ventricular volumes and systolic function, as CMR assesses these parameters with higher reproducibility than echocardiography [11]. In practice, the routine use of CMR is limited because of its limited availability, compared with echocardiography. Due to its high negative predictive value, MSCT may be useful in excluding CAD in patients who are at low risk of atherosclerosis [11]. MSCT plays an important role in the work-up of high-risk patients with AS considered for TAVI. The risk of radiation exposure—and of renal failure due to contrast injection—should, however, be taken into consideration.

There are contraindications for exercise testing in symptomatic patients with AS, however it is useful for unmasking symptoms and in the risk stratification of asymptomatic patients with severe AS [12]. Stress tests are currently under-used in patients with asymptomatic AS. In some patients, it may be necessary to proceed with cardiac catheterisation and coronary angiography at the time of initial evaluation [10]. This could be appropriate if there is a discrepancy between clinical and echocardiographic examinations or if symptoms might be due to coronary artery disease (CAD).

4. Indications for surgery

Early valve replacement should be strongly recommended in all symptomatic patients with severe AS, because it is the only effective treatment. Thus, the development of symptoms identifies a critical point in the natural history of AS. The interval from the onset of symptoms to the time of death is approximately 2 years in patients with heart failure, 3 years in those with syncope, and 5 years in those with angina, with a high risk of sudden death (Figure 1).

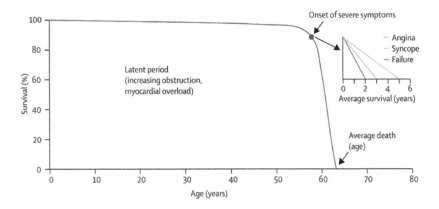

Figure 1. Natural History. Ross J Jr. & Braunwald E, 1968 [14]

There is some disagreement about the optimal timing of surgery in asymptomatic patients, and the decision to operate on this kind of patient requires careful weighing of the benefits against the risks. Early elective surgery, at the asymptomatic stage, can only be recommended in selected patients, with low operative risk [12]. A proposed management strategy for patients with severe AS based on the ESC Guidelines on the management of valvular heart disease [12] and ACC/ AHA Guidelines for the Management of Patients with valvular heart disease [10] is shown in Figure 2.

Although there are no prospective randomized trials, data from retrospective analysis indicates that patients with moderate AS (mean gradient in the presence of normal flow 30–50 mmHg, valve area 1.0–1.5 cm^2) will generally benefit from valve replacement at the time of coronary surgery. However, individual judgement must be recommended [12], based on the evolution of the echocardiography severity parameters and the patient's clinical evaluation.

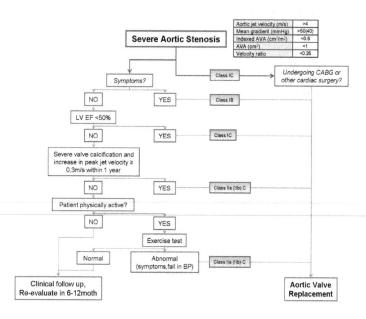

Figure 2. Management of Severe Aortic Stenosis.

Based on the ESC Guidelines on the management of valvular heart disease [12] and ACC/ AHA Guidelines for the Management of Patients with valvular heart diseaseb [10]. ACC/AHA recommendations has been shown in parentheses.

5. Risk stratification

Patient selection for AVR for AS is well outlined by ACCF/AHA and ESC guidelines. Problems arise when the patients present significant symptoms and significant structural disease, complicated by the presence of significant comorbidity. A number of risk algorithms for cardiac surgery have been developed. Experience accrued since the development of the Parsonnet scale reveals that this scale assigns too much weight to age. Nowadays the STS score and logistic EuroSCORE are the most commonly used. These provide information concerning short term operative risks, however, they are not able to predict symptom resolution, quality-of-life improvement, or return to independent living.

As discussed above (see also Evaluation and Grading the Degree of Stenosis), several studies have reported the usefulness of BNP in risk stratification of asymptomatic or mildly symptomatic patients, which could help to discriminate which patients would benefit from an early surgical management. However, there is not enough evidence to recommend the routine use of these biomarkers.

Although both are accurate in low-risk patients, accuracy is reduced in higher-risk subsets [15]. The logistic EuroSCORE is based on 12 covariates derived from 14,799 patients undergoing all types of cardiac operations in 8 European countries in 1995. On the other hand, the STS risk predictor is based on 24 covariates derived from 67,292 patients undergoing isolated AVR only in the United States between 2002 and 2006. Both use an algorithm based on the presence of coexisting illnesses in order to estimate 30-day operative mortality. There is a much simpler variation of the EuroSCORE logistic model, which can be calculated at the patient's bedside, adding points manually. This model is called the additive EuroSCORE. It assigns a specific value to each risk factor, and the points are simply added to obtain the estimated operative mortality rate.

With improved outcomes after cardiac surgery in more recent years, EuroSCORE has become less well calibrated. EuroSCORE II has been developed using data from 22.381 patients who underwent cardiac surgery during 2010, and represents a necessary and timely update of the original EuroSCORE models. EuroSCORE II improves on the original logistic EuroSCORE, though mainly for combined AVR and CABG cases. However, concerns still exist, about its use for isolated AVR procedures, aortic surgery and miscellaneous procedures. There is still room for improvement in risk modelling and several studies are currently being carried out to validate EuroScore II. Nevertheless, Grant et al [16] report that EuroSCORE II performs well overall in contemporary UK adult cardiac surgery, with good discrimination for all kinds of cardiac surgery; in fact, they report that the logistic EuroSCORE is now obsolete and their study demonstrates that it is appropriate to use EuroSCORE II as a generic risk model for contemporary UK cardiac surgery.

There is growing debate about the definition of high-risk patients and the validity of risk assessment using different risk-scoring systems for prediction of mortality (see also **High-Risk Patient**). Current models do not include some risk factors that may be particularly important in the prediction of outcomes for high- or very high-risk populations including frailty, pulmonary hypertension (PH), porcelain aorta, and the presence of hepatic dysfunction, although all these have been included in EuroSCORE II.

Nevertheless, the sample of elderly patients considered for the design of these scales represents a small proportion of the population, resulting in less accurate risk assessment, and interpretation should be made with caution. In this regard, a recent study which included 1245 elderly patients (mean age 77.2 years) who underwent AVR with or without CABG reports that only STS-PROM correlated with mortality rates [17]. Thielmann et al [18] also report that the logistic EuroSCORE and the Parsonnet score clearly overestimated the risk of mortality, whereas the STS score and the additive EuroSCORE were much more accurate in predicting the risk of mortality.

Certain authors, such as Rosenhek [19] and others, suggest the need to include other variables such as cognitive function and functional capacity in surgical risk stratification, mainly in the elderly group. There are physiological characteristics inherent to elderly patients that make them different in risk estimation; an example of this is the amount of creatinine considered in the EuroSCORE scale as a predictor of mortality. This scale assigned a particular score (2 points) to patients with creatinine levels greater than 2.26 mg / dl, which through a logistic regression analysis could estimate risk in percentage terms. However creatinine is not the best parameter to define renal function and its value can be influenced by various factors such as age, race, muscle mass and metabolic state, as has been demonstrated in several studies, hence glomerular filtration rate provides a much more accurate estimation [20]. Obviously in the elderly there is a physiological involution of organs and systems that should be taken into account since surgery represents a stressful situation that can reveal or tip the balance for certain pathologies. However, numerous reports have demonstrated excellent results in terms of morbidity and mortality in most patients. Hospital mortality is significantly related to the preoperative presence of depressed left ventricular systolic function, pulmonary hypertension, symptoms of heart failure, kidney failure, long-standing mitral valve disease, and nutritional deficiencies. When these risk factors are absent in the preoperative period, mortality is similar to that of the youngest patients. It should be emphasized that risk models serve as one aspect of patient selection, but need to be considered alongside clinical judgement and other methods of risk assessment.

6. High risk and elderly patients, are they the same?

6.1. Elderly patient

The ageing of the population is an important social and sanitary phenomenon. Consensus about allowing access to health care unconstrained by age limits, together with increased life expectancy and advances in highly specialised medicine have brought us to the point where surgical treatment is indicated in progressively older sectors of the population [21]. The diagnosis and management of valvular heart disease in the elderly has been affected by the dramatic increase in life expectancy that began in the last half of the 20th century. In the United States, for example, the number of persons aged 80 years or older is expected to increase from 6.9 million in 1990 to approximately 25 million by the year 2050. As a result, degenerative valve disease is likely to become an increasing problem. In the Helsinki Ageing Study [22], 501 randomly selected men and women aged 75 to 86 underwent imaging and Doppler echocardiography. The prevalence of at least moderate aortic stenosis, defined as an aortic valve area (AVA) ≤1.2 cm^2 and velocity ratio ≤0.35, was 5 percent; the prevalence of critical aortic stenosis (AVA ≤0.8 cm^2, and velocity ratio ≤0.35) increased with age from 1 to 2 percent in persons aged 75 to 76 up to almost 6 percent in those aged 86. With the rapidly increasing geriatric population, it is common in current practice to have elderly patients referred for surgical treatment of AS. In 2006, in the United States, approximately 40% of patients undergoing AVR were at least 75 years old Nevertheless, even though valve replacement is the procedure of choice in this population, currently a large percentage of suitable candidates are, unfortunately, not referred for surgery, mostly because of their age.

As in [21], increased risk in these patients is related to:

• Ageing, which causes structural changes in the heart and reduces the physiological reserves of most organs, thus impairing the capacity to recover from surgical aggression;

• An increase in associated diseases, as studied by Rodríguez et al [23], especially diabetes, kidney failure, arterial hypertension, chronic obstructive pulmonary disease, and cerebrovascular disease;

• The advanced phase of heart disease, as indicated by the greater incidence of heart failure, depressed left ventricular function, and preoperative pulmonary hypertension;

• Reduction of the inflammatory response to surgical aggression,

• Undernourishment, measured by anthropometric and biochemical parameters, which is a frequent preoperative finding before cardiac surgery; its incidence is even greater in older persons and is associated with an increment in postoperative complications due to an impaired response to surgical aggression.

• The increased complexity of surgical techniques for these patients, due to the presence of severe calcification of the aortic ring and the greater incidence of associated coronary and valvular surgery, which require longer aortic clamping times.

Age has been considered an independent predictive factor for mortality, but the way to estimate its influence on the calculation of the risk of surgery has evolved since the introduction of the Parsonnet risk scale, which gave excessive weight to age. Currently the most accepted risk assessment tools are the STS-PROM score and EuroSCORE (with the EuroSCORE II currently being validated).Although they are widely used, there is a possibility of overestimating the operative mortality rates by using these risk-prediction models, and an inescapable discrepancy between the estimated and observed mortality rate has been acknowledged. In a study published in Ann Thorac Surg in 2009 Thielmann et al [18] report that the logistic EuroSCORE clearly overestimates the risk of mortality, whereas the STS score seems to be more accurate in predicting the risk of mortality. Moat et al. [24] also report the relative lack of utility of EuroSCORE in risk/outcome prediction for their group of patients and confirm the need for more sophisticated and procedure-specific (rather than generic) scoring systems. There is no perfect method for weighing all of the relevant factors and identifying specifically high- and low-risk elderly patients, but this risk can be estimated well in individual patients, and the decision to proceed with surgery should depend on many factors, including the patient's wishes and expectations.

Although the proportion of elderly patients with multiple comorbidities is increasing, operative outcomes following AVR have improved over the past decade. Likosky et al [25] published the outcomes of the very elderly undergoing aortic valve surgery in a study comprising 7584 patients, including 815 over the age of 80. They found that short- and long-term survival was favourable across all age groups. Specifically, more than half of the patients undergoing aortic valve procedures were alive 6 years after surgery. Among patients under 80 years of age, survival favoured those undergoing isolated AVR procedures, but among octogenarians, concomitant CABG surgery did not result in reduced survival. Yamane K et al [26] published the outcome of a single-centre study of conventional AVR in patients aged 70 or older. In their analysis, patients aged 80–92 who underwent isolated AVR or AVR with CABG showed an acceptable mortality rate of 4.0%, comparable to the 3.8% mortality rate in patients aged 70–79. Brown et al [27] published the outcomes of isolated AVR in North America by analysing the STS National Database, comprising 108,687 patients, and compared the mortality rates in 1997 with those in 2006. In their analysis, patients aged 70–75 had a mortality rate of 3.2% in 1997 and 2.9% in 2006; for patients aged 80–85, the mortality rate was 6.3% in 1997 and 4.9% in 2006. These improvements in operative outcome over the past decade could be related to multiple factors, including patient selection and perioperative management. A better understanding of the role of preoperative respiratory preparation, improved myocardial protection of otherwise severely hypertrophic myocardium, as well as normothermic cardiopulmonary bypass may have contributed to the improved early postoperative results in recent studies as compared to those several decades ago. Yamane K et al [26] propose that with the elderly, especially those aged 80 years or older, goal-oriented strategies such as early extubation, judicious sedation management, medication dosage based on renal or liver function, early involvement of physical or occupational therapists, and speech/swallow specialists are all indispensable.

From a patient's perspective, functionality after surgery may be more important than simple survival. Using the Seattle Angina Questionnaire, Huber et al [28] interviewed 136 patients who were 80 years of age at the time of cardiac surgery (isolated CABG, AVR, or AVR +CABG). They found that 95% lived in their own homes, and 93% reported that they had experienced no reduction in their quality of life. Kolh et al [29] interviewed 61 long-term survivors of AVR and found that 92% of patients believed that having heart surgery at age 80 was a "good choice," with 88% of patients feeling "as good or better" than they had before surgery. Also, Maillet et al [30] reported results from 84 octogenarians undergoing either AVR or AVR+CABG between 1998 and 2001. The majority (91.1%) lived in their own homes (compared with 75% of the general French population aged 80 years), whereas 26.7% of patients required help with activities of daily living (compared with 35% to 40% of the general population). Sundt et al [31] reported functional status and survivorship up to 5 years among 133 patients undergoing AVR with or without CABG. Patient-reported functional status was comparable to the general population.

Because there is no effective medical therapy and balloon valvotomy is not an acceptable alternative to surgery, AVR is the gold standard for the treatment of severe stenosis and must be considered in all elderly patients who have symptoms caused by AS [10]. Age, per se, should not be considered a contraindication for surgery. Decisions should be made on an individual basis, taking into account patients' wishes and cardiac and non-cardiac factors

[12]. In this population, the need for an emergency operation, or, at the other end of the clinical spectrum, very early intervention at an asymptomatic stage, should be avoided.

The surgical community worked vigorously over the past two decades to reduce the trauma of the conventional aortic valve operation. Ongoing studies of transcatheter aortic valve implantation (TAVI) have demonstrated feasible short- and mid-term results in patients who were not considered suitable candidates for conventional AVR. Minimally invasive approaches like partial upper sternotomy have replaced the conventional complete median sternotomy when performing AVR in many centres. By aiming for smaller incisions, without compromising the quality of the operation and the effectiveness of myocardial protection, improved early outcomes have been achieved.

In a prospective randomised trial, Dogan et al [32] show that minimally invasive AVR can be performed with only slightly longer operative times, good cosmetic results and improved rib cage stability as well as significantly less blood loss. Furthermore, limited surgical access had no negative effects on the patients' neurological outcome nor the efficacy of myocardial protection. More recently, the implantation technique for AVR has also been modified, without compromising the hemodynamic performance of the valve substitute, all in order to reduce implantation times, and therefore reduce ischemia in the myocardium and cardiopulmonary bypass times. In 2009 Martens et al [33] reported on initial clinical experiences with the sutureless, nitinol-stented Enable (Medtronic Inc., Minnesota, USA) aortic valve prosthesis in 32 patients. Implantation time could be significantly reduced, down to 9±5 minutes, the first report of multi-centre experience with this particular valve substitute and implantation technique in 140 patients was published in the European Journal of Cardiothoracic Surgery in 2011. Reproducibility as well as feasibility and safety were demonstrated with the ATS 3f Enable® Bioprosthesis. Valve implantation resulted in excellent hemodynamics and significant clinical improvement. Further comparative studies are under way to prove the clinical benefit using this less-time-consuming implantation technique versus the conventional one.

6.2. High risk patient

How could we define a cardiac high-risk patient? Which parameters must we consider in order to assess risk? Which is the most accurate assessment tool to calculate a patient's risk?

We could define high risk cardiac patients as those who present several factors that significantly affect their outcome after surgery and could compromise their survival. Multiple series have documented that patients were deemed to have a high risk of operative complications or death on the basis of coexisting conditions such as advanced age, diabetes mellitus, existence of preoperative shock, LVEF ≤40%(≤30%), preoperative NYHA class III or IV, concomitant CAD, concomitant surgical procedure (CABG, valve surgery or surgery on thoracic aorta), renal failure and chronic obstructive pulmonary disease (COPD). Although attempts have been made to identify the high-risk population for AVR, there is currently no ideal model for precisely identifying high-risk patients. STS-PROM score and the European System for Cardiac Operative Risk Evaluation (EuroSCORE) have been used as part of the inclusion/exclusion criteria for the TAVI trials and to quantify the operative risk of conventional AVR. Nevertheless, several previous reports on TAVI defined high-risk patients as patients with a logistic EuroSCORE between 10% and 30% [18]. Smith et al [34] in a TAVI versus AVR paper published in the New England Journal of Medicine in 2011 used as a guideline a score of at least 10% on the risk model developed by the STS to define high-risk patients. However, there are multiple additional risk factors, which are not currently considered by existing risk scoring systems; for example the presence of a porcelain aorta and considerations such as social integration, mobility, frailty, and the individual's overall health status must be taken into account, as well as the patient's wishes and expectations. A further definition that must be taken into account for evaluation of those patients who underwent TAVI is that very or extremely high-risk patients are those with a logistic EuroSCORE above 30% or STS score higher than 15% (see Table 2). The 2012 ACCF/AATS/SCAI/STS Expert Consensus Document on Transcatheter Aortic Valve Replacement [15] used the term *prohibitive risk*. This includes some patients for whom surgery might be deemed unsuitable based on the physician's assessment of the patient's risk for surgery; whereas in others, the surgeon may decide that the operation cannot be performed successfully because of technical considerations.

	Risk assessment tool	
	EuroSCORE	**STS score**
High risk	10-30%	"/>10%
Very or extremely high risk	"/>30%	"/>15%

Based on the 2012 ACCF/AATS/SCAI/STS Expert Consensus Document on Transcatheter Aortic Valve Replacement [15].

Table 2. Risk Assessment

In the absence of evidence in the literature and recommended guidelines, the determination of inoperability in any given patient depends on the judgement of the Heart team. It is generally agreed that patients with limited life expectancy due to concurrent conditions such as malignant tumours, dementia, primary liver disease or COPD, among others, are not appropriate for AVR. Frailty and poor physical condition are known to result in an inability to recover from major heart surgery such as AVR. These conditions can potentially contribute to increased surgical mortality and morbidity in the elderly. The surgeon may judge a patient inoperable as a result of technical considerations that preclude safe performance of AVR, such as prior mediastinal irradiation, porcelain aorta or severe periannular calcification, severe atheromatous disease, prior cardiac operations, and other conditions such as the internal mammary artery crossing the midline. In summary, a substantial percentage of patients with AS are judged to be inoperable for surgery based primarily on the physician's or surgeon's determination of operative risk and probability of survival [15]. Although some patients may be found to be inoperable for technical and surgical reasons, most inoperable patients are considered to be too ill due to associated comorbid conditions. In conclusion, the decision to proceed with AVR or TAVI requires careful weighing of the potential for improved symptoms and survival and the morbidity and mortality of surgery.

7. Surgical approach

7.1. Conventional AVR

Aortic valve replacement has permitted thousands of lives to be saved since it was first successfully carried out by Harken and Starr in 1960 [35, 36]. Since then, advances in prosthetic technology including improved hemodynamics, durability and thromboresistance, and techniques in cardiac surgery such as cardioplegia, management of the small aortic root, and replacement of associated aortic aneurysm have resulted in improvements in both operative and long-term results.

The conventional approach to AVR is the following: A mid-line incision and sternotomy is made and a pericardial well created. The patient is cannulated via the aorta and a single atrial venous cannula. After cross-clamping of the aorta, a transverse aortotomy is made approximately 1 cm above the take-off of the right coronary artery, slightly above the level of the sinotubular ridge (Figure. 3).

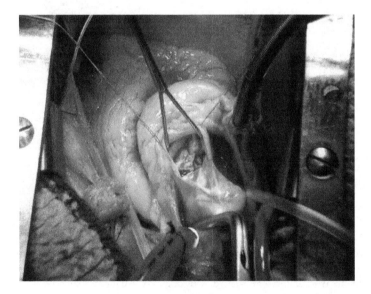

Figure 3. Transverse aortotomy

The incision is extended three-quarters of the way around the aorta, leaving the posterior one-quarter of the aorta intact allowing excellent visualization of the native aortic valve and annulus. The leaflets of the aortic valve are excised to the level of the annulus and the annulus is thoroughly debrided of any calcium. Braided 2-0 sutures with pledgets are applied. Beginning at the non-coronary commissure, the annulus is encircled with interrupted mattress sutures (Figure 4) extending from the ventricular to the aortic surface.

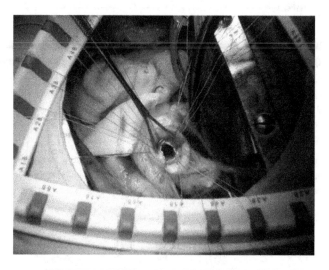

Figure 4. Aortic annulus encircled with interrupted mattress sutures

Next, each half of the suture bundles are implanted in the sewing ring and the prosthesis seated. The sutures are tied first at the left coronary cusp extending to the mid-portion of the right coronary cusp. Lastly, the sutures of the non-coronary cusp are secured, seating the valve appropriately. In case of mechanical valve prosthesis leaflet motion should always be checked and the surgeon must be assured that the coronary arteries are not obstructed. The aortotomy is closed with a double layer of polypropylene suture consisting of an underlying mattress suture and a more superficial over-and-over suture.

7.1.1. Conventional AVR results

Regardless of surgical approach, elected AVR is the gold standard for the treatment of severe AS. Several studies have shown acceptable short- and long-term outcomes, as well as improved quality of life in elderly patients. Although the proportion of elderly patients with multiple comorbidities is expanding, operative outcomes following AVR were still improving in the past decade. Recent series such as Likosky et al [25], report 30-day mortality among patients who underwent isolated AVR of 3.7% for patients <80, 6.7% in the 80 to 84 age group, and 11.7% in those ages >85 (P<0.001). Among patients undergoing AVR+CABG, 6.2% of patients <80 years died within 30 days, 9.4% among those 80 to 84, and 8.5% of patients ≥85 years (P=0.01). Also M. Di Eusanio et al [37] published a multi-centre study including 638 octogenarians who underwent AVR from an Italian regional cardiac surgery registry (2003-2009), They report hospital mortality of 4.5%, which favourably compares with those reported in other series (ranging from 4.3% to 13.7%). Recent surgical series [3, 38] report operative mortality rates for aortic valve replacement as low as 1%, increasing to 9% in higher-risk patients. Long-term survival after valve replacement is 80% at 3 years, with an age-corrected postoperative survival that is nearly normalized. Significant postoperative morbidity, such as thromboembolism, haemorrhagic complications from anticoagulation, prosthetic valve dysfunction, and endocarditis, are rare and occur at a rate of 2% to 3% per year [38]. These improvements in operative outcome could be related to multiple factors, including patient selection and perioperative management.

A number of studies have also examined outcomes of AVR conducted with concomitant CABG surgery. With few exceptions, concomitant CABG surgery does not increase a patient's operative risk. Considering the mounting evidence for the acceptable perioperative outcomes after AVR with or without concomitant CABG in the elderly, perhaps the fact that as many as one-third of patients >80 years of age with severe aortic stenosis are still denied surgery because of their age is due at least in part to the lack of evidence for long-term outcomes. Likosky et al [25] published the outcome of the very elderly undergoing aortic valve surgery comprising 7584 patients, including 815 over the age of 80. They have demonstrated that aortic valve replacement with or without concomitant CABG is a safe and effective option for elderly patients with severe aortic stenosis. Specifically, more than half of the patients undergoing aortic valve procedures were alive 6 years after surgery. Although concomitant CABG adds a slight mortality risk in the immediate postoperative period, it does not appreciably affect long-term survival among patients older than 80 years.

Survival has been also improved in elderly patients who underwent AVR. Asimakopoulos et al [39] reviewed United Kingdom Heart Valve Registry data from 1100 patients >80 years of age who underwent AVR from January 1986 to December 1995. They reported 30-day mortality as 6.6% with actuarial survival of 89%, 79.3%, 68.7%, and 45.8% at 1, 3, 5, and 8 years, respectively. Likosky et al [25] report a 6-year survival of 54.7% in patients aged 80 to 84 following AVR and 53.3% in patients aged 80 to 84 following AVR+CABG. Yamane et al [26] published their single centre study in 2011, reporting Survival at 1, 3, 5, and 10 years in patients aged 70–79 as 91.6%, 85.1%, 77.2%, and 38.0%, respectively, as compared with 84.1%, 75.7%, 63.0%, and 21.7% in patients aged 80– 92 (P=0.002). More recently M. Di Eusanio et al [37] report a 1, 3 and 6 year survival of 91.3%, 80.6% and 67.5% respectively in octogenarian patients who underwent isolated AVR.

In several studies, estimates of quality of life, as measured by NYHA functional class improvement, autonomy or satisfaction after receiving surgery have shown excellent functional recovery after AVR in patients >80 years (also see Elderly patient). Wu et al [40] in a recent study, determining the economic value of the additional life given to patients undergoing AVR, concluded that AVR is cost-effective for all ages, and still worthwhile in octogenarian and nonagenarian patients.

In conclusion, conventional AVR in selected octogenarians has similar outcomes to those in "younger" elderly patients, with good mid-term survival and excellent functional recovery with a marked improvement in quality of life; in fact, their level of function and quality of life are the same as a general population of age-matched subjects.

7.2. Minimally Invasive Surgical (MIS) approaches

MIS approaches appear to improve the results observed in conventional surgery. The latter shows good results with acceptable morbidity and mortality rates in most cases, including in patients with aortic valve disease, however, in some subgroups of patients these outcomes tend to be worse. Minimally invasive surgery aims to minimise the degree of surgical intrusiveness. Currently there are several surgical approaches. A partial upper sternotomy is the most frequently used incision for a minimally invasive approach to the aortic valve and this is usually carried out via a parasternal incision over the second and third intercostal space, depending on the patient's anatomy as observed in preoperative imaging studies such as CT. The partial sternotomy is also frequently used, and there are several possible approaches. The table below summarises the various possible techniques (Table 3).

Partial sternotomy
Para-sternal incision [41,42]
Trans-sternal incision [41]
Upper sternotomy (Byrne et al., 2000) [38]
T mini-sternotomy [44]
V-shaped incision [45]
Inverted L incision [44]
Reversed L incision [46]
J incision [41,47]
Reversed C incision
Inverted T incision [48]
Thoracotomy
Right anterior thoracotomy 2° or 3° inter-costal space [49]
Right anterior thoracotomy 4° or 5° inter-costal space [50]
Video-assisted vision
Port access [51]
Video-direct vision
AESOP 3000 (Computer Motion, Goleta, CA) [52]
Da Vinci System (Intuitive Surgical, Sunnyvale, CA) [53]
Zeus (Computer Motion, Goleta, CA) [41]
Bustamante et al., 2012 [54]

Table 3. Minimally Invasive Approaches.

The "J" incision is the most widely used approach among the partial sternotomy approaches (Figure 5 & 6).

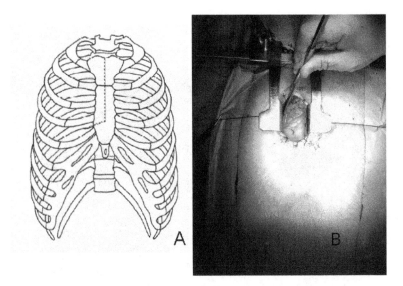

Figure 5. A & B: Reversed L incision.

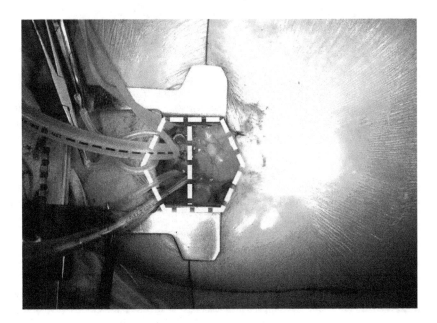

Figure 6. Operative field distribution from surgeon view.

However there are other approaches that are gaining popularity and some groups are beginning to use it quite often, so is the case of the right anterior thoracotomy through 2º or 3º inter-costal space (Figure 7).

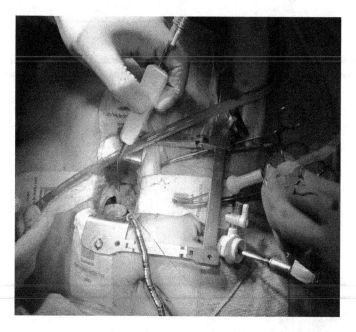

Figure 7. Right anterior thoracotomy through 2º or 3º inter-costal space.

Some controversy exists as to the benefits of these approaches. There are currently very few randomized studies able to answer this question and those that do exist have certain limitations [55, 56]. However, in the medical literature we do find numerous articles that report broad series of patients in which the effects can be observed and several aspects of these approaches can be compared to conventional approaches.

A series of advantages traditionally exist in the application of MIS for aortic valve replacement. There is no methodological uniformity across the studies that have been carried out, which sometimes complicates comparison between studies and makes it difficult to draw conclusions about the impact of these approaches on patient treatment. This is due to the fact that the aspects considered by the different studies differ in some cases. For example, some focus on length of hospitalization and specific complications and others give more relevance to surgical aspects such time spent with extracorporeal circulation or clamping. In summary, we can say that there is a group of patients about which there is a certain consensus as to the benefits of the MIS approaches. This group includes the elderly [50], and patients who have previously undergone interventions involving myocardial revascularisation [43]. In the first case the benefit fundamentally lies in the reduction of surgical aggression in cases where patients are more susceptible to developing post-operative complications, leading to a much faster functional recovery time compared to patients subjected to conventional interventions. In the second case the benefit lies in the fact that it is not necessary to dissect the mediastinal structures, thus avoiding the risk of damaging coronary implants, and the complications that would entail [57, 58].

7.2.1. Advantages and disadvantages of MIS approaches in aortic stenosis

In other patients there are arguments in favour of MIS. Benefits have been observed in certain aspects such as:

- Reduction in bleeding in surgery and therefore in the use of hemoderivatives. There are also discrepancies in this aspect, as while some studies indicate the benefit [55, 59-61], others, such as Stamou et al [44] do not observe this effect. A possible explanation for this disparity of results is that in the assessment of reduced post-operative bleeding, no prior adjustments for risk factors for post-operative bleeding were made. The debate is further complicated by the fact that Dogan et al [32], observed differences in the reduction of post-surgical bleeding in a randomised study. In our group we did observe a statistically significant reduction in blood loss during surgery and in the need for hemoderivatives.

- Reduction in the pain perceived by the patient. Numerous studies indicate this benefit [55, 62, 63] which is based on a reduction in the distension of costovertebral ligaments and traction of the brachial plexus. This results in reduced consumption of analgesic pharmaceuticals by the patient.

- Less reduction in tidal lung volume, thus reducing the appearance of respiratory complications such as atelectasis by maintaining the integrity of the thorax [56].

- Better aesthetic results. This is one of the clear benefits of the technique, due to the reduced size of the surgical incisions and their relocation to less visible areas.

- There are other benefits, such as the reduction in complications in the surgical wound/ infections. Grossi et al [64] observe an incidence of infection of 0.9% for minimally invasive approaches as against 5.7% in cases of patients with the approach by sternotomy, p=0.05. It has been observed that this difference increases in elderly patients (1.8 and 7.7% respectively). Other authors observe that in comparison with the classical approach there is a lesser incidence of infectious complications [65, 66].

A certain consensus exists around the benefits mentioned above. There is also the question of the impact of MIS on duration of surgery. There is disparity in the results found in the literature. Along with other research groups, we observed that, once the learning curve has been overcome, these times tend to equal out and there is no significant difference to be observed between the different approaches. Studies that support an increase in the time for cardiopulmonary bypass and aortic clamping are Farhat et al, Detter et al, de Vaumas et al, and Stamou et al. [44, 46, 48, 67]; contradictory results can be found in Corbi et al., Sharony et al or the randomised study by Bonachi et al. [45, 50, 55]. Another aspect that is highly valued in MIS surgery is the impact it has on the duration of hospitalisation and time spent in intensive care units. This has been taken into consideration in reducing the cost of the process, in a context of increased life expectancy and rising healthcare costs. In terms of patient treatment it is relevant in that the reduction of both is accompanied by a lesser incidence of other complications, basically infections, particularly respiratory infections, surgical wound infections and urinary tract infections.

7.3. Transcatheter Aortic Valve Replacement (TAVR)

Transcatheter aortic valve implantation (TAVI) was developed as an alternative to AVR in the very or extremely high-risk patient population. The first implant in man was performed by Cribier [68] in 2002, using a balloon expandable frame and equine valve. Since the introduction of minimally invasive and catheter-based therapies, patients want less invasive options for all types of medical procedures including general surgical, orthopaedic, spinal, and urological operations with the goal of decreasing morbidity and mortality and shortening recovery time. Other issues with traditional aortic and mitral valve surgery include the fact that patients may not even be offered operation; in multiple series from different centres and in different countries, up to 40% of patients with severe aortic stenosis are treated medically [69, 70]. Some of these patients may be deemed to be too sick for surgery because of associated medical comorbidities, and some may be considered too old. Finally, some who may benefit the most from an operation may decline surgery even though they develop irreversible damage from the valve lesion that could have been treated. These factors have led to the continuous development of less invasive strategies with lower mortality, lower morbidity, and less invasiveness [71]. Transcatheter aortic valve replacement seems to offer a new window of treatment for those patients with severe aortic valve stenosis that are either extremely high-risk or inoperable for conventional aortic valve replacement. Today around 40000 patients have received a transcatheter aortic valve implantation (TAVI) worldwide. Multiple single- and multi-centre registries, and a single randomized trial, the PARTNER trial (Placement of AoRTic TraNscathetER Valve Trial), have documented favourable outcomes using a wide spectrum of endpoints, including survival, symptom status, quality of life, and need for repeat hospitalization.

7.3.1. Implantation techniques

TAVI is currently carried out using two main approaches (retrograde transfemoral and antegrade transapical), which share the same main principles. Trans-axillary artery or transaortic are other approaches that are gaining popularity when the transfemoral approach is not feasible. Specific anatomic issues must be considered in device design. These include the rigid structure and pattern of the valvular calcification and the aortic annulus, and the need for as full an apposition as possible to the annulus in an attempt to minimize periprosthetic leaks. In the case of eccentric, bulky calcifications, this may be difficult. The close proximity to the coronary ostia, the width and height of the sinuses, the membranous ventricular septum with the His bundle and the anterior leaflet of the mitral valve are also important anatomical considerations. In addition, the size and degree of severity of peripheral arterial disease are all factors that could limit catheter size [15]. It is therefore highly recommended to perform an adequate preoperative assessment of the degree of peripheral arterial disease through imaging studies such as CT (Figure 8).

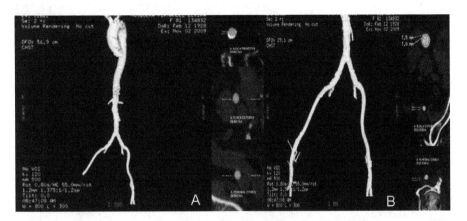

Figure 8. (A) CT reconstruction of the aorta. (B) CT reconstruction of iliofemoral arteries

Most teams perform the procedure under general anaesthesia, although sedation and analgesia may suffice for the transfemoral approach. Peri-procedural transoesophageal echocardiography (TEE) monitoring is desirable to correctly position the valve as well as to detect complications. After crossing the aortic valve, Balloon aortic valvuloplasty is performed to pre-dilate the native valve and serve as a rehearsal for TAVI. Simultaneous rapid pacing decreases cardiac output, stabilizing the balloon during inflation. Normal blood pressure must be completely recovered between sequences of rapid pacing. In order to position the prosthesis at the level of the aortic valve annulus different methods can be used, such as fluoroscopy to assess the level of valve calcification (Figure 9); aortography, using different views, performed at the beginning of the procedure and repeated with the undeployed prosthesis in place, to determine the position of the valve and the plane of alignment of the aortic cusps; and echocardiography. TEE is particularly helpful in cases with moderate calcification.

Three dimensional real-time TEE seems to provide extra information to the teams that use it. When positioning is considered correct, the prosthesis is released. Rapid pacing is used at this stage for balloon-expandable devices but not for self-expanding ones. Immediately after TAVI, aortography and, whenever available, TEE or, in the absence of TEE, Transthoracic echocardiogram(TTE) are performed to assess the location and degree of aortic regurgitation and the patency of the coronary arteries, and to rule out complications such as haemopericardium, and aortic dissection. The hemodynamic results are assessed using pressure recordings and/or echocardiography. After the procedure, the patients should stay in intensive care for at least 24 hours and be closely monitored for several days, particularly as regards hemodynamics, vascular access, rhythm disturbances (especially late atrioventricular block), and renal function.

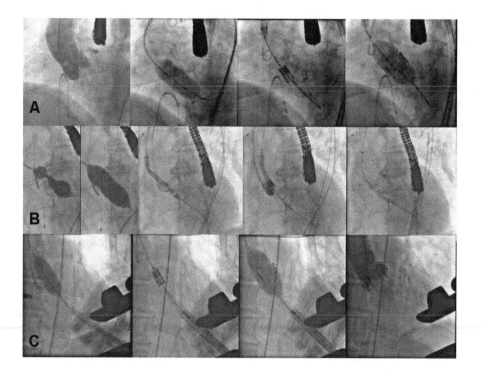

Figure 9. First row (A). Edwards Sapiens transfemoral implantation. Second row (B). Transfemoral Corevalve implantation. Third row (C). Edwards Sapiens transapical implantation.

The specific issues related to the different approaches include the following: In the transfemoral approach, close attention should be paid to the vascular access. The common femoral artery can be either prepared surgically or approached percutaneously. Echo-guided femoral access could be useful. Manipulation of the introductory sheaths should be careful and fluoroscopically guided. Depending on the size of the device, closure of the vascular access can be effected surgically or using a percutaneous closure device. Femoral access and cardiopulmonary bypass should be on standby for patients for whom surgical conversion is an option in case of complications.

The transapical approach requires an antero-lateral mini-thoracotomy (Figure 10), pericardiotomy, identification of the apex, and then puncture of the left ventricle using a needle through purse-string sutures. Subsequently, an introductory sheath is positioned in the LV, and the prosthesis is implanted using the antegrade route.

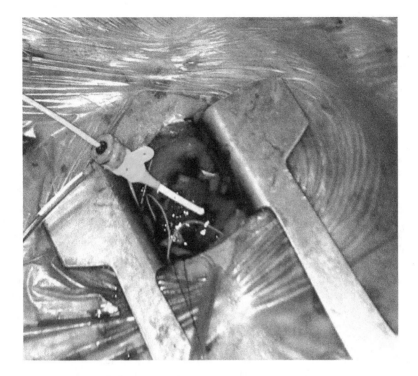

Figure 10. Anterior minitoracotomy for transapical approach of a TAVI procedure.

7.3.2. TAVR results

The PARTNER trial has been followed with great interest. The PARTNER trial was basically 2 parallel trials: 1) PARTNER Cohort A, which randomized high-risk surgical patients to either traditional aortic valve replacement or to TAVI by either a transfemoral or transapical approach; and 2) PARTNER Cohort B in which patients who were inoperable were randomized to either a TAVR by a transfemoral approach or to conventional medical therapy, which typically consisted of balloon aortic valvuloplasty.

Screening required evaluation by 2 experienced cardiac surgeons to agree on the surgical risk using the STS Predicted Risk of Mortality score and was rigorous, with approximately one-quarter to one-third of screened patients subsequently enrolled. The primary endpoint was death from any cause at 1 year. The results of PARTNER Cohort B included 358 patients deemed unsuitable for conventional aortic valve replacement because of predicted probability of≥ 50% mortality or the risk of a serious irreversible complication within 30 days. At 1 year, all-cause mortality with TAVR was 30.7% versus 50.7% with medical therapy (hazard ratio: 0.55, 95% confidence interval: 0.40 to 0.74). Despite the marked improvement in survival and event-free survival, there were some significant safety hazards, particularly a higher incidence of major strokes (5.0% versus 1.1%) as well as increased major vascular complications (16.2% versus 1.1%) with TAVR, both of which may adversely impact early and longer-term outcome. Longer-term outcomes will be required. These results were received enthusiastically; however, they have important limitations. Firstly, they can be applied only in patients similar to those in the study (i.e., those patients deemed to be inoperable). Secondly, they are the result of treatment by very experienced operators working as a heart team in a hybrid operating room or similar facility with a specific device and do not necessarily apply to other devices.

The results of the PARTNER Cohort A trial also have important implications. The primary endpoint of the trial was met, with TAVR found not to be inferior to aortic valve replacement for all-cause mortality at 1 year (TAVR versus aortic valve replacement, 24.2% versus 26.8%, respectively, p=0.001 for non-inferiority). Death at 30 days was lower than expected in both arms of the trial: TAVR mortality (3.4%) was the lowest reported in any series, despite an early generation device and limited previous operator experience. Aortic valve replacement mortality (6.5%) was lower than the expected operative mortality (11.8%). Furthermore, both TAVR and aortic valve replacement were associated with important but different peri-procedural hazards: major strokes at 30 days (3.8% versus 2.1%, p=0.20) and 1 year (5.1% versus 2.4%, p=0.07), and major vascular complications were more frequent with TAVR (11.0% versus 3.2%, p<0.001). Major bleeding (9.3% versus 19.5%, p<0.001) and new onset atrial fibrillation (8.6% versus 16.0%, p<0.001) were more frequent with aortic valve replacement.

Rates of stroke were similar whether the access was transfemoral or transapical. Bioprosthetic-valve gradients and orifice areas were slightly better after transcatheter replacement than after surgical replacement, probably because of the less bulky support frame with transcatheter replacement [34]. However, transcatheter replacement resulted in much more frequent paravalvular aortic regurgitation. Although this condition was stable at 1 year, repeat intervention was required in some cases. A reduction in the incidence and severity of paravalvular AR represents an obvious target for technical improvements in the design of transcatheter valves and of implantation techniques [24]. Clinical benefits of transcatheter replacement included significantly shorter stays in the intensive care unit and in hospital. In addition, the NYHA functional class and 6-minute walk distance were strikingly improved at 1 year [34]. Transcatheter aortic valve implantation by means of either the transfemoral or the transapical approach is a reasonable and promising treatment option for patients who are at high risk or had been refused for conventional AVR. Recommendations made to individual patients must balance the appeal of avoiding the known risks of open-heart surgery against the less invasive transcatheter approach, which has different and less well understood risks, particularly with respect to stroke and paravalvular aortic regurgitation.

8. New prostheses in mini-invasive approaches

These prostheses were designed by industry with a view to facilitating the implantation of the prosthesis through conventional surgery; that is to say, using a cardio-pulmonary bypass and aortic clamping. The gold standard for the use of these prostheses is in association with MIS approaches, providing a reduction in surgical aggression in addition to the reduction in ECC and aortic clamping time, the consequences of which we have already examined. These designs have the common feature of being expandable, anchoring themselves to the aortic ring in a similar way to the devices used in TAVI.

To date there are three commercially available models: 3f Enable ® (Medtronic Inc, Minneapolis, MN), Perceval S (Sorin Group Cardio Srl, Sallugia, Italy) and Intuity (Edwards Lifesciences, Irvine, California). These differ from each other in a few characteristics.

3f Enable ® aortic bioprosthesis (Figure 11): This prosthesis is especially indicated in patients with small aortic annulus where the possibility of having a severe mismatch is high with the use of conventional prosthesis. Several studies report an acceptable hemodynamic behavior with this type of prosthesis. Furthermore, there is no need to match the measure between the annulus and the sinotubular junction, because the prosthesis is anchored only to the annulus. Of the three prostheses this is the oldest and different models have been developed since its initial commercialisation with a view to improving hemodynamics, durability and facilitating surgeons in its implantation [72-74]

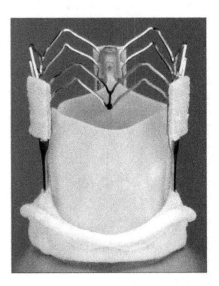

Figure 11. Enable ® (Medtronic Inc, Minneapolis, MN)

Perceval S (Sorin Biomedica Cardio Srl, Sallugia, Italy) (Figure 12): Prosthesis aimed at patients with a high surgical risk in which a reduction in surgery time may have a significant impact, for patients where it is necessary to carry out mixed procedures, and patients undergoing re-intervention, and patients with a small aortic ring, because of the hemodynamic characteristics of the prosthesis [75, 76]

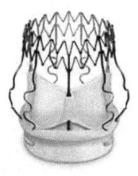

Figure 12. Perceval S (Sorin Biomedica Cardio Srl, Sallugia, Italy)

Intuity (Edwards Lifesciences, Irvine, California) (Figure 13): Of these three prostheses this is the most recently commercialised and results as to its hemodynamic profile and durability in clinical practice are not available. Arguments in its favour, as put forward by the company, are the conjunction between the Edwards Perimount bioprosthesis, the clinical and hemodynamic results of which are widely known, and the experience in the development of new prostheses such as the Sapien transcatheter. The mode of implantation for this prosthesis allows the aortic clamping and extracorporeal circulation times to be reduced. For a number of reasons, one of the most important being ischemic reperfusion, these two variables are known to be directly related to the surgical morbidity and mortality of procedures, which is why this model may be attractive, in addition to the comfort of implantation, as it does not require stitches in the aortic ring.

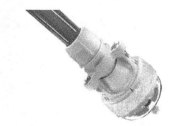

Figure 13. Intuity (Edwards Lifesciences, Irvine, California)

The disadvantage of these prostheses is their cost, as they ultimately increase resource consumption. Results for hemodynamics and durability are becoming better understood as preliminary studies are published. From the beginning we find data in the literature relating to safety and effectiveness in the implantation of aortic valve replacements. Some of the complications associated with their use, such as perivalvular leaks are understood to be intimately related to the decalcification of the ring; in some cases, it has been possible to correct other complications, such as bad positioning, with new designs being applied to the already existing prosthetics [77]

9. Conclusions

Medical science is progressing faster than ever and the field of cardiovascular disease is one of its greatest exponents. Patient care and treatment must adapt to changing patient characteristics as well as to new technologies and treatment options. In the case of aortic valve disease, whose prevalence is booming in the western world, we must be capable of a comprehensive approach to ensure optimal results and efficient use of resources. Currently, age, *per se*, is not a contraindication for the treatment of aortic valve disease; hence a thorough assessment should be undertaken to design the best therapeutic approach for high-risk patients. Understanding of treatment options of this disease has increased. New devices have been developed and advances have been made in perioperative management of cardiac surgical patients. Nevertheless, there is still room for improvement in this interesting field of cardiac surgery.

Author details

Omer Leal[1], Juan Bustamante[1*], Sergio Cánovas[2] and Ángel G. Pinto[3]

*Address all correspondence to: jbustamantemunguira@gmail.com

1 Department of Cardiovascular Surgery, Hospital Universitario La Princesa, Madrid, Spain

2 Department of Cardiac Surgery, Hospital General Universitario de Valencia, Valencia, Spain

3 Department of Cardiac Surgery, Hospital Universitario Gragorio Marañon, Madrid, Spain

References

[1] Schmitto J.D., Mohr F.W., Cohn L.H. Minimally invasive aortic valve replacement: how does this perform in high-risk patients? Curr Opin Cardiol. 2011; 26(2):118-122.

[2] Chambers J.B. Aortic stenosis. Eur J Echocardiogr. 2009; 10(1):i11-9.

[3] Freeman RV, Otto CM. Spectrum of calcific aortic valve disease: pathogenesis, disease progression, and treatment strategies. Circulation. 2005 Jun 21;111(24): 3316-3326.

[4]   Otto CM, Lind BK, Kitzman DW, Gersh BJ, Siscovick DS. Association of aortic-valve sclerosis with cardiovascular mortality and morbidity in the elderly. N Engl J Med. 1999 15;341(3):142-147.

[5]   Kurtz CE, Otto CM. Aortic stenosis: clinical aspects of diagnosis and management, with 10 illustrative case reports from a 25-year experience. Medicine (Baltimore). 2010;89(6):349-379.

[6]   Steadman CD, Ray S, Ng LL, McCann GP. Natriuretic peptides in common valvular heart disease. J Am Coll Cardiol 2010;55:2034-2048.

[7]   Bergler-Klein J, Klaar U, Heger M, Rosenhek R, Mundigler G, Gabriel H, et al. Natriuretic peptides predict symptom-free survival and postoperative outcome in severe aortic stenosis. Circulation 2004; 109:2302-2308.

[8]   Monin JL, Lancellotti P, Monchi M, Lim P, Weiss E, Pie'rard L, et al., Risk score for predicting outcome in patients with asymptomatic aortic stenosis. Circulation 2009;120:69-75.

[9]   Lancellotti P, Moonen M, Magne J, O'Connor K, Cosyns B, Attena E, et al., Prognostic effect of long-axis left ventricular dysfunction and B-type natriuretic peptide levels in asymptomatic aortic stenosis. Am J Cardiol 2010; 105:383-388.

[10] Bonow RO, Carabello BA, Chatterjee K, de Leon AC Jr, Faxon DP, Freed MD, et al. 2008 focused update incorporated into the ACC/AHA 2006 guidelines for the management of patients with valvular heart disease: a report of the American College of Cardiology/American Heart Association Task Force on Practice Guidelines (Writing Committee to revise the 1998 guidelines for the management of patients with valvular heart disease). Endorsed by the Society of Cardiovascular Anesthesiologists, Society for Cardiovascular Angiography and Interventions, and Society of Thoracic Surgeons. J Am Coll Cardiol. 2008 23;52(13):e1-142.

[11] Vahanian A, Alfieri O, Andreotti F, Antunes MJ, Barón-Esquivias G, Baumgartner H, et al. Guidelines on the management of valvular heart disease (version 2012): The Joint Task Force on the Management of Valvular Heart Disease of the European Society of Cardiology (ESC) and the European Association for Cardio-Thoracic Surgery (EACTS). Eur J Cardiothorac Surg. 2012 27. doi:10.1093/eurheartj/ehs109.

[12] Vahanian A, Baumgartner H, Bax J, Butchart E, Dion R, Filippatos G, et al. Guidelines on the management of valvular heart disease: The Task Force on the Management of Valvular Heart Disease of the European Society of Cardiology. Eur Heart J. 2007;28(2):230-268.

[13] Baumgartner H, Hung J, Bermejo J, Chambers JB, Evangelista A, Griffin BP, et al. American Society of Echocardiography; European Association of Echocardiography. Echocardiographic assessment of valve stenosis: EAE/ASE recommendations for practice. J Am Soc Echocardiogr. 2009;22(1):1-23.

[14] Ross J Jr, Braunwald E. Aortic stenosis. Circulation. 1968;38(1 Suppl):61-67.

[15] Holmes DR Jr, Mack MJ, Kaul S, Agnihotri A, Alexander KP, Bailey SR, et al. 2012 ACCF/AATS/SCAI/STS expert consensus document on transcatheter aortic valve replacement: developed in collaboration with the American Heart Association, American Society of Echocardiography, European Association for Cardio Thoracic Surgery, Heart Failure Society of America, Mended Hearts, Society of Cardiovascular Anesthesiologists, Society of Cardiovascular Computed Tomography, and Society for Cardiovascular Magnetic Resonance. Ann Thorac Surg. 2012;93(4):1340-1395.

[16] Grant SW, Hickey GL, Dimarakis I, Trivedi U, Bryan A, Treasure T, et al. How does EuroSCORE II perform in UK cardiac surgery; an analysis of 23 740 patients from the Society for Cardiothoracic Surgery in Great Britain and Ireland National Database. Heart. 2012 Aug 21. doi:10.1136/heartjnl-2012-302483.

[17] Frilling B, von Renteln Kruse W, Riess FC. Evaluation of operative risk in elderly patients undergoing aortic valve replacement: the predictive value of operative risk scores. Cardiology. 2010;116(3):213-218.

[18] Thielmann M, Wendt D, Eggebrecht H, Kahlert P, Massoudy P, Kamler M, et al. Transcatheter aortic valve implantation in patients with very high risk for conventional aortic valve replacement. Ann Thorac Surg. 2009;88(5):1468-1474.

[19] Rosenhek R, Iung B, Tornos P, Antunes MJ, Prendergast BD, Otto CM, et al. ESC Working Group on Valvular Heart Disease Position Paper: assessing the risk of interventions in patients with valvular heart disease. Eur Heart J. 2012;33(7):822-828.

[20] Bustamante J, Gómez-Martínez ML, Bustamante E, Tamayo E. Occult chronic kidney disease in the ederly with coronary heart disease. Med Clin (Barc). 2009;133(13):524.

[21] Herreros JM. Cardiac surgery in elderly patients. Rev Esp Cardiol. 2002;55(11):1114-1116.

[22] Lindroos M, Kupari M, Heikkilä J, Tilvis R. Prevalence of aortic valve abnormalities in the elderly: an echocardiographic study of a random population sample. J Am Coll Cardiol. 1993;21(5):1220-1225.

[23] Rodríguez R, Torrents A, García P, Ribera A, Permanyer G, Moradi M, et al. Cardiac surgery in elderly patients. Rev Esp Cardiol. 2002;55(11):1159-1168.

[24] Moat NE, Ludman P, de Belder MA, Bridgewater B, Cunningham AD, Young CP, et al. Long-term outcomes after transcatheter aortic valve implantation in high-risk patients with severe aortic stenosis: the U.K. TAVI (United Kingdom Transcatheter Aortic Valve Implantation) Registry. J Am Coll Cardiol. 2011;58(20):2130-2138.

[25] Likosky DS, Sorensen MJ, Dacey LJ, Baribeau YR, Leavitt BJ, DiScipio AW, et al. Long-term survival of the very elderly undergoing aortic valve surgery. Circulation. 2009;120(11 Suppl):S127-133.

[26] Yamane K, Hirose H, Youdelman BA, Bogar LJ, Diehl JT. Conventional aortic valve replacement for elderly patients in the current era. Circ J. 2011;75(11):2692-2698.

[27] Brown JM, O'Brien SM, Wu C, Sikora JA, Griffith BP, Gammie JS. Isolated aortic valve replacement in North America comprising 108,687 patients in 10 years: changes in risks, valve types, and outcomes in the Society of Thoracic Surgeons National Database. J Thorac Cardiovasc Surg. 2009;137(1):82-90.

[28] Huber CH, Goeber V, Berdat P, Carrel T, Eckstein F. Benefits of cardiac surgery in octogenarians a postoperative quality of life assessment. Eur J Cardiothorac Surg. 2007;31(6):1099-1105.

[29] Kolh P, Lahaye L, Gerard P, Limet R. Aortic valve replacement in the octogenarians: perioperative outcome and clinical follow-up. Eur J Cardiothorac Surg. 1999;16(1): 68-73.

[30] Maillet JM, Somme D, Hennel E, Lessana A, Saint-Jean O, Brodaty D. Frailty after aortic valve replacement (AVR) in octogenarians. Arch Gerontol Geriatr. 2009;48(3): 391-396.

[31] Sundt TM, Bailey MS, Moon MR, Mendeloff EN, Huddleston CB, Pasque MK, et al. Quality of life after aortic valve replacement at the age of >80 years. Circulation. 2000;102(19 Suppl 3):III70-74.

[32] Dogan S, Dzemali O, Wimmer-Greinecker G, Derra P, Doss M, Khan MF, et al. Minimally invasive versus conventional aortic valve replacement: a prospective randomized trial. J Heart Valve Dis. 2003;12(1):76-80.

[33] Martens S, Sadowski J, Eckstein FS, Bartus K, Kapelak B, Sievers HH, et al. Clinical experience with the ATS 3f Enable® Sutureless Bioprosthesis. Eur J Cardiothorac Surg. 2011;40(3):749-755.

[34] Smith CR, Leon MB, Mack MJ, Miller DC, Moses JW, Svensson LG, et al. Transcatheter versus surgical aortic-valve replacement in high-risk patients. N Engl J Med. 2011;364(23):2187-2198.

[35] Harken, D.E., Soroff, H.S., Taylor, W.H. Aortic valve replacement, in Merendino KA (ed): Prosthetic Valves for Cardiac Surgery. Springfield, IL, Thomas; 1961, p 508-526

[36] Starr A, Edwards ML. Mitral replacement: clinical experience with a ball-valve prosthesis. Ann Surg. 1961; 154:726-740.

[37] Di Eusanio M, Fortuna D, Cristell D, Pugliese P, Nicolini F, Pacini D, et al. Contemporary outcomes of conventional aortic valve replacement in 638 octogenarians: insights from an Italian Regional Cardiac Surgery Registry (RERIC). Eur J Cardiothorac Surg. 2012;41(6):1247-1252.

[38] Rahimtoola SH. Choice of prosthetic heart valve in adults an update. J Am Coll Cardiol. 2010;55(22):2413-2426.

[39] Asimakopoulos G, Edwards MB, Taylor KM. Aortic valve replacement in patients 80 years of age and older: survival and cause of death based on 1100 cases: collective results from the UK Heart Valve Registry. Circulation. 1997;96(10):3403-3408.

[40] Wu Y, Jin R, Gao G, Grunkemeier GL, Starr A. Cost-effectiveness of aortic valve replacement in the elderly: an introductory study. J Thorac Cardiovasc Surg. 2007;133(3):608-613.

[41] Cohn LH, Adams DH, Couper GS, Bichell DP, Rosborough DM, Sears SP, Aranki SF. Minimally invasive cardiac valve surgery improves patient satisfaction while reducing costs of cardiac valve replacement and repair. Ann Surg. 1997;226(4):421-426.

[42] Navia JL, Cosgrove DM 3rd. Minimally invasive mitral valve operations. Ann Thorac Surg. 1996;62(5):1542-1544

[43] Byrne JG, Karavas AN, Adams DH, Aklog L, Aranki SF, Couper GS, Rizzo RJ, Cohn LH, et al. Partial upper re-sternotomy for aortic valve replacement or re-replacement after previous cardiac surgery. Eur J Cardiothorac Surg. 2000;18(3):282-286.

[44] Stamou SC, Kapetanakis EI, Lowery R, Jablonski KA, Frankel TL, Corso PJ. Allogeneic blood transfusion requirements after minimally invasive versus conventional aortic valve replacement: a risk-adjusted analysis. Ann Thorac Surg. 2003;76(4): 1101-1106.

[45] Corbi P, Rahmati M, Donal E, Lanquetot H, Jayle C, Menu P, et al. Prospective comparison of minimally invasive and standard techniques for aortic valve replacement: initial experience in the first hundred patients. J Card Surg. 2003;18(2):133-139.

[46] Detter C, Deuse T, Boehm DH, Reichenspurner H, Reichart B. Midterm results and quality of life after minimally invasive vs. conventional aortic valve replacement. Thorac Cardiovasc Surg. 2002;50(6):337-341.

[47] Doll N, Borger MA, Hain J, Bucerius J, Walther T, Gummert JF, et al. Minimal access aortic valve replacement: effects on morbidity and resource utilization. Ann Thorac Surg. 2002;74(4):S1318-1322.

[48] Farhat F, Lu Z, Lefevre M, Montagna P, Mikaeloff P, Jegaden O. Prospective comparison between total sternotomy and ministernotomy for aortic valve replacement. J Card Surg. 2003;18(5):396-401.

[49] Burfeind WR, Glower DD, Davis RD, Landolfo KP, Lowe JE, Wolfe WG. Mitral surgery after prior cardiac operation: port-access versus sternotomy or thoracotomy. Ann Thorac Surg. 2002;74(4):S1323-1325.

[50] Sharony R, Grossi EA, Saunders PC, Schwartz CF, Ribakove GH, Culliford AT, et al. Minimally invasive aortic valve surgery in the elderly: a case control study. Circulation. 2003;108 Suppl 1:II43-47.

[51] Galloway AC, Shemin RJ, Glower DD, Boyer JH Jr, Groh MA, Kuntz RE, et al. First report of the Port Access International Registry. Ann Thorac Surg. 1999;67(1):51-56.

[52] Falk V, Walther T, Autschbach R, Diegeler A, Battellini R, Mohr FW. Robot-assisted minimally invasive solo mitral valve operation. J Thorac Cardiovasc Surg. 1998;115(2):470-471.

[53] Carpentier A, Loulmet D, Aupècle B, Kieffer JP, Tournay D, Guibourt P, et al. Computer assisted open heart surgery. First case operated on with success. C R Acad Sci III. 1998;321(5):437-442.

[54] Bustamante J, Cánovas S, Fernández AL, Minimally Invasive Aortic Valve Surgery - New Solutions to Old Problems In Hirota M (Ed) Aortic Stenosis - Etiology, Pathophysiology and Treatment. Rijeka: InTech; 2012. p 91-114.

[55] Bonacchi M, Prifti E, Giunti G, Frati G, Sani G. Does ministernotomy improve postoperative outcome in aortic valve operation? A prospective randomized study. Ann Thorac Surg. 2002;73(2):460-465.

[56] Moustafa MA, Abdelsamad AA, Zakaria G, Omarah MM. Minimal vs median sternotomy for aortic valve replacement. Asian Cardiovasc Thorac Ann. 2007;15(6): 472-475.

[57] Yap CH, Sposato L, Akowuah E, Theodore S, Dinh DT, Shardey GC, et al. Contemporary results show repeat coronary artery bypass grafting remains a risk factor for operative mortality. Ann Thorac Surg. 2009;87(5):1386-1391.

[58] Yau TM, Borger MA, Weisel RD, Ivanov J. The changing pattern of reoperative coronary surgery: trends in 1230 consecutive reoperations. J Thorac Cardiovasc Surg. 2000;120(1):156-163.

[59] Cosgrove DM 3rd, Sabik JF, Navia JL. Minimally invasive valve operations. Ann Thorac Surg. 1998;65(6):1535-1538.

[60] Tam RK, Almeida AA. Minimally invasive aortic valve replacement via partial sternotomy. Ann Thorac Surg. 1998;65(1):275-276.

[61] Mächler HE, Bergmann P, Anelli-Monti M, Dacar D, Rehak P, Knez I, et al. Minimally invasive versus conventional aortic valve operations: a prospective study in 120 patients. Ann Thorac Surg. 1999;67(4):1001-1005.

[62] Candaele S, Herijgers P, Demeyere R, Flameng W, Evers G. Chest pain after partial upper versus complete sternotomy for aortic valve surgery. Acta Cardiol. 2003;58(1): 17-21.

[63] Liu J, Sidiropoulos A, Konertz W. Minimally invasive aortic valve replacement (AVR) compared to standard AVR. Eur J Cardiothorac Surg. 1999;16 Suppl 2:S80-83.

[64] Grossi EA, Galloway AC, Ribakove GH, Zakow PK, Derivaux CC, Baumann FG,et al. Impact of minimally invasive valvular heart surgery: a case control study. Ann Thorac Surg. 2001;71(3):807-810.

[65] Lee JW, Lee SK, Choo SJ, Song H, Song MG. Routine minimally invasive aortic valve procedures. Cardiovasc Surg. 2000;8(6):484-490.

[66] Tabata M, Umakanthan R, Cohn LH, Bolman RM 3rd, Shekar PS, Chen FY, et al. Early and late outcomes of 1000 minimally invasive aortic valve operations. Eur J Cardiothorac Surg. 2008;33(4):537-541.

[67] de Vaumas C, Philip I, Daccache G, Depoix JP, Lecharny JB, Enguerand D, et al. Comparison of minithoracotomy and conventional sternotomy approaches for valve surgery. J Cardiothorac Vasc Anesth. 2003;17(3):325-328.

[68] Cribier A, Eltchaninoff H, Bash A, Borenstein N, Tron C, Bauer F, et al. Percutaneous transcatheter implantation of an aortic valve prosthesis for calcific aortic stenosis: first human case description. Circulation. 2002;106(24):3006-3008.

[69] Charlson E, Legedza AT, Hamel MB. Decision-making and outcomes in severe symptomatic aortic stenosis. J Heart Valve Dis. 2006;15(3):312-321.

[70] Pellikka PA, Sarano ME, Nishimura RA, Malouf JF, Bailey KR, Scott CG, et al. Outcome of 622 adults with asymptomatic, hemodynamically significant aortic stenosis during prolonged follow-up. Circulation. 2005;111(24):3290-3295.

[71] Holmes DR Jr, Mack MJ. Transcatheter valve therapy a professional society overview from the American college of cardiology foundation and the society of thoracic surgeons. J Am Coll Cardiol. 2011;58(4):445-455.

[72] Cox JL, Ad N, Myers K, Gharib M, Quijano RC. Tubular heart valves: a new tissue prosthesis design- preclinical evaluation of the 3F aortic bioprosthesis. J Thorac Cardiovasc Surg. 2005;130(2):520-527.

[73] Pillai R, Ratnatunga C, Soon JL, Kattach H, Khalil A, Jin XY. 3f prosthesis aortic cusp replacement: implantation technique and early results. Asian Cardiovasc Thorac Ann. 2010;18(1):13-16.

[74] Wendt D, Thielmann M, Buck T, Jánosi RA, Bossert T, Pizanis N, et al. First clinical experience and 1-year follow-up with the sutureless 3F-Enable aortic valve prosthesis. Eur J Cardiothorac Surg. 2008;33(4):542-547.

[75] Flameng W, Herregods MC, Hermans H, Van der Mieren G, Vercalsteren M, Poortmans G, et al. Effect of sutureless implantation of the Perceval S aortic valve bioprosthesis on intraoperative and early postoperative outcomes. J Thorac Cardiovasc Surg. 2011;142(6):1453-1457.

[76] Shrestha M, Folliguet T, Meuris B, Dibie A, Bara C, Herregods MC, et al. Sutureless Perceval S aortic valve replacement: a multicenter, prospective pilot trial. J Heart Valve Dis. 2009;18(6):698-702.

[77] Aymard T, Kadner A, Walpoth N, Göber V, Englberger L, Stalder M, et al. Clinical experience with the second-generation 3f Enable sutureless aortic valve prosthesis. J Thorac Cardiovasc Surg. 2010;140(2):313-316.

Chapter 6

Stentless Bioprostheses for Aortic Valve Replacement in Calcific Aortic Stenosis

Kaan Kirali

Additional information is available at the end of the chapter

1. Introduction

The classic case of aortic stenosis is a healthy middle-aged patient with/without symptoms, but in practical life, patients with severe calcific aortic valve come with several and severe comorbidities such as advanced age, coronary artery disease, atherosclerotic aorta, significant left ventricular dysfunction. Aortic valve replacement (AVR) is the only options in these patients, and it requires patient-by-patient analysis of clinical, echocardiograhic, and hemo-dynamic data with associated pathologies. The curative treatment of calcific aortic valve stenosis is the replacement of the aortic valve with a prosthetic valve, and selection of a perfect prosthetic valve is the main goal to get a successful treatment. But, there is no any perfect heart valve prosthesis which may mimic the characteristics of the normal native aortic valve: excellent hemodynamics, life-long durability, thromboresistance, and excellent implantability. That means that native valve disease will be traded for prosthetic valve disease and the outcome of AVR is affected by the type of prosthetic valve. Mechanical valves are non-limited durable, but have a substantial risk of hematologic complications (thromboemboli, thrombotic obstruction, hemorrhage related life-long anticoagulation therapy) with/without hemolysis potential. In contract, bioprosthetic valves have a low risk of thromboembolism without anticoagulation, but their durability is limited by calcific or noncalcific tissue deterioration. Biological prostheses, especially homografts, are often believed to be the substitute of choice in AVR, but the limited availability of homografts prevents their more broadly usage. To overcome this problem and all possible complications of mechanical valves, xenogenic biological prostheses have been developed. The design of bioprosthetic valves purports to mimic the anatomy of the native aortic valve and their flow characteristics are better than mechanical valves, whereas stentless bioprostheses have hemodynamic performance similar to the healthy native aortic valve. Although stented bioprostheses can be implanted easier, they decrease the effective orifice area due to the rigid stent and result turbulent flow through the valve. Stented valves also increase stress at the attachment of the stent which cause earlier primary tissue failure. Stentless biologic valves have been introduced into clinical practice to solve all these problems and to reproduce the anatomy and function of the native aortic valve, but their clinical use has still not exceeded the number of stented aortic bioprostheses because of more demanding technique of implantation. To gain more widespread clinical use and general recommendation of stentless bioprostheses, their advantages and simple implantation techniques must be popularized.

It is believed that the aortic root is probably the best stent for the native or prosthetic aortic valve. The anatomy and function of the aortic root may dampen the mechanical stress to which the leaflets are subjected during diastole. The ideal stentless prosthesis should have no synthetic materials, preserve the aortic root dynamics, restore flexibility and distensibility of the native valve annulus after decalcification, and have minimal xenograft aortic wall, short implantation time, and excellent hemodynamic performance to facilitate the recovery of left ventricular function.

1.1. Historical background

Homografts were the first biological prostheses used in clinical practice to treat aortic valve stenosis in early 1960s, and they were the first stentless valves, too [1,2]. The authors used the aortic root of the patient to secure the homograft aortic valve in the subcoronary position. The most complicated implantation technique and the restricted availability of homografts prevented their widespread usage. First stentless pig and calf xenografts were used in limited patients, but the valves were abandoned because of poor tissue fixation [3]. Stented bioprostheses were considered as the gold standard for several years, but abnormal stress on the leaflets was believed to decrease durability. To overcome this problem with a rigid stent on the aortic position, stentless bioprostheses were re-introduced in the middle of 80's [4], whereas new designed stentless xenografts were proposed and popularized in daily use at the beginning of 1990s [5]. The main problem (early failure of bioprostheses) was solved with new bioengineering improvement (antimineralization, zero-pressure fixation) [6]. The other problem was partial dehiscence when the heterograft contained muscular bar resulting paravalvular leakage in the area corresponding to the muscular bar, and this problem was abolished with a fine Dacron cloth covered the outside wall of the stentless porcine aortic valve along its inflow [7]. Recognizing the range of aortic root variability and disease of the root itself, the concept of stentless valve replacement was expanded to replacement of the entire aortic root. Full root replacement with a bioprosthesis brought the challenges of homeostasis and coronary reimplantation. In spite of hemodynamic advantages proven for the root replacement technique, acceptance was slowed by risk/benefit ratio concerns. The whole aortic root could be prepared and implanted with modified root inclusion or subcoronary implant techniques.

Biological stentless valve can be prepared by pulmonary autograft, homograft, xenograft, autologous or xenogenic pericardium. Pulmonary autograft has limited durability beyond the first decade [8]. The same problem has been observed with homografts in the aortic position, especially in younger patients, which are less durable than commercially available stentless bioprostheses and cannot be recommended as the ideal device [9]. The use of the patients own pericardium for constructing a heart valve prosthesis is biologically more appealing than the use of animal tissue or heterologous material. The feasibility of autologous pericardial stentless aortic valve was shown in an animal study [10]. The feasibility and durability of truly stentless autologous pericardial AVR sutured directly onto the aortic wall has been also performed in human recently [11]. Stentless porcine or pericardial xenogenic bioprostheses have been introduced to get better long-term durability and become a routine device when a stentless biologic valve is implanted.

There are a lot of stentless bioprostheses with/without the aortic root in the market, but some of them are not used widespread and implantation of a few xenografts is stopped (Table 1). The first modern (first generation) stentless valves were glutaraldehyde-fixed porcine prostheses with a fully scalloped shape or a complete aortic root (Figure 1). The most preferred approach was root replacement technique because subcoronary approach needed more suture line. The second generation of stentless valves improved the technical difficulties related to free-hand implantation with two rows of sutures for subcoronary implantation of porcine bioprostheses (Figure 2). The third generation of stentless prostheses are made by xenogenic pericardium, because the pericardial valve is free from the compromises of the porcine aortic root, it is flexible, and easy to implant either with an interrupted or running suture technique (Figure 3). There are different xenogenic pericardial valves (bovine or equine), and horse pericardium is thinner, however, stronger than the bovine pericardium and also much more pliable. The fourth generation of stentless valves are produced by a proprietary process and the unique conditioning technology paves the way for autologous repopularization of the valve in patients. The durability of current bioprosthetic heart valves is diminished by glutaraldehyde-associated leaflet calcification or by the host immune reaction. As a novel tissue engineering approach to improving replacement heart valve durability, a new acellular (nonglutaraldehyde-fixed) tissue heart valve for autologous recellularization is developed to limit xenograft antigenicity. As no glutaraldehyde is used in the whole process lack of calcification and also lack of toxicity, and the method delivers a very pliable valve with very low gradients. To use of autologous pericardium fixed with glutaraldehyde avoids any immune reaction between the host and the implanted heart valve and so minimizes tissue calcification and pannus formation. The last generation of stentless valves provides avoidance of suture lines during AVR: closed [transcatheter (transfemoral or transapical)] or open (transaortic = sutureless) techniques (Figure 4).

2. Hemodynamic recovery

Every effort should be made to avoid moderate prosthesis-patient mismatch during AVR. Stentless valves enable to select the largest bioprosthesis to the patient's annulus and provide better aortic root and valve behavior, larger effective orifice area (EOA), reduced transprosthetic gradient and greater left ventricular mass regression.

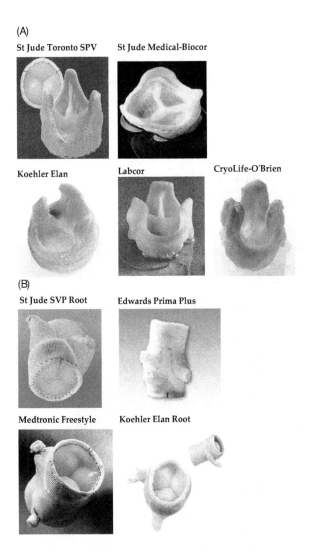

Figure 1. First generation bioprostheses (Porcine Stentless Xenografts) A) Scalloped stentless porcine bioprostheses B) Root stentless porcine bioprostheses.

To prevent early or late prosthetic failure, maintenance of the aortic root with physiological anatomy must be the primary goal during AVR with a stentless prosthesis. Any kind of bioprosthetic valve will deviate from native aortic valve in terms of leaflet dynamics. Stiffening of the aortic root either by glutaraldehyde or by stent degenerates the opening (wrinkles and blurry edges of leaflets) and closing (asynchronism) behavior of native aortic valve leaflets.

Shelhigh Suprestentless

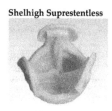

Figure 2. Second generation bioprostheses.

Sorin Pericarbon Freedom   Sorin Pericarbon Freedom SOLO   3F Therapeutics

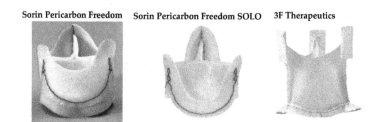

Figure 3. Third generation bioprostheses (Pericardial Stentless Xenografts)

3F Enable model 6000   Perceval S

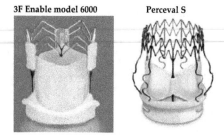

Figure 4. Sutureless Pericardial Stentless Xenografts

Stented valves fixe the native commissures and do not allow cyclic change of the commissural dimension as it normally occurs. This cyclic expansion of the commissural area serves reduction of stress on the leaflets, which is preserved by stentless bioprostheses. Second, the intrinsically obstructive nature of the stented bioprostheses increases pressure gradient and creates turbulent flow patterns, however, normal laminar flow patterns can be restored after AVR with stentless tissue valves. The opening and closing of the stentless biologic valve constitute a passive mechanism responding to pressure difference between the left ventricle and the aorta. Like the native aortic valve, a stress created by this difference heads toward the central coaptation area of the bioprosthesis during diastole. The negative pressure difference during diastole helps prosthetic valve to be closed. The valve opens rapidly at the beginning of ejection because of rising of pressure difference and persists to remain open as a tunnel

A. Autograft	
B. Homograft	
C. Xenografts	
I. First generation (Stentless Porcine Bioprosthesis)	
Dacron reinforced inflow tract	
Toronto SPV (stentless porcine valve)	St Jude Medical, Inc., St Paul, MN, USA
St Jude Medical-Biocor	St Jude, Belo Horizonte, MG, Brazil
CryoLife-O'Brien Model 3000	CryoLife International Inc, Atlanta, GA, USA
Toronto SPV Root	St Jude Medical, Inc., St Paul, MN, USA
Edwards Prima Plus	Edwards Lifesciences, Inc., Irvine, CA,USA
Medtronic Freestyle	Medtronic, Inc., Minneapolis, MN, USA
pericardial reinforced inflow tract	
Koehler Elan	Koehler, Bellshill, Scotland
Koehler Elan Root	
tri-composite design (three noncoronary leaflets)	
Labcor	Labcor, Inc., Belo Horizonte, MG, Brazil
II. Second generation (porcine with single suture line, No-react treatment)	
Shelhigh Suprestentless	Shelhigh, Inc, Millburn, NJ, USA
III. Third generation (Stentless Pericardial Bioprosthesis)	
porcine pericardium	
Sorin Pericarbon Freedom	Sorin Biomedica Cardio SpA, Saluggia, Italy
Sorin Pericarbon Freedom SOLO	
horse (equine) pericardium	
3F Therapeutics	3F Therapeutics, Inc., Lake Forest, CA, USA
IV. Fourth generation (non-gluteraldayhde fixed + decellularized)	
Matrix A	
V. Sutureless generation (Sutureless + Stentless Pericardial Bioprosthesis)	
3F Enable model 6000	3F Therapeutics, Inc., Lake Forest, CA, USA
Perceval S	Sorin Biomedica Cardio SpA, Saluggia, Italy
D. Autologous pericardium	

Table 1. Stentless Bioprostheses.

during systole, and the aortic root may also expanse at the late diastole to help opening of the leaflets (in native aortic valve, expansion of the aortic root is about 12% and that starts opening the leaflets to about 20%). At the end of systole, the backward blood flow into the sinuses of Valsalva (behind prosthetic leaflets) and initialization of pressure difference help prosthetic leaflets to revert to their original closed position. An in-vivo-study has showed that there is no difference in opening velocities among native, stented and subcoronary stentless valves in a porcine model [12]. However, the closing velocities are significantly higher in the pericardial valves. The bending deformation increases when implanting a glutaraldehyde-treated valve subcoronary. Porcine stentless valves display a distinct folding pattern during opening resulting in an altered stress distribution and also tend to fold during opening causing increased leaflet bending stress [13].

One of the key parameters for stentless xenograft performance is the EOA. In spite of the EOA is significantly higher in stentless bioprostheses it is also dependent on the design and the implantation technique of the prostheses. The EOA will increase especially during the first year and the transvalvular gradient drops dramatically in the first 3 to 6 months after surgery, but some further drop may be seen more later [14]. The reason may be remodeling of the left ventricular outflow tract, diminished aortic root edema, and slight dilatation of the aortic root. Transvalvular gradient is closely related to the EOA: the larger orifice area the lower is the transvalvular gradient. The second reason to increase transvalvular gradient is usage of a rigid stent. Avoidance of a stent enlarges inner diameter of prosthetic valve and eliminates intraluminal obstruction which increases the EOA. Several studies have shown transvalvular gradient across stentless valves is always lower than for their stented valves, especially mean and/or peek gradients [15-1617]. The third possible reason can be excessive tissue of a bioprosthesis: the lesser tissue implanted within the recipient aortic root the lesser obstruction. The full root prostheses reduce the intraluminar obstruction because nothing is implanted inside, and they have larger EOA than subcoronary prostheses. The main differences of stentless biologic tissue valves are the specific gravity of the leaflets which is not equal to that of blood like native human aortic leaflets and the specific thickness of the leaflets which is thinner in pericardial tissue valves. Both parameters cause transvalvular gradient during ejection which is lesser in fully pericardial stentless valves than porcine. The other reasons may be small aortic annulus and physically active patients. The change in gradients during exercise is interesting: when cardiac output increases it also increases the transvalvular flow and raises transprosthetic gradient, but these gradients under exercise are lower with stentless valves than stented bioprostheses, which provide better opening-closing behavior [18].

Left ventricular output is maintained by the development of the left ventricular hypertrophy which results in a large pressure gradient across the stenotic valve. The left ventricle mass increases and becomes less compliant. Left ventricular hypertrophy and increased mass can be correlated with sudden death, congestive heart failure, and other cardiovascular events. Left ventricular hypertrophy will regress after AVR regardless of the type of prostheses, and an improved hemodynamic performance of prostheses should result in a faster regression, especially in patients with severe calcific aortic stenosis and left ventricular hypertrophy, because incomplete regression after AVR is related to poor long-term outcome [19]. This regression is related to EOA and transvalvular gradient constituted by the prosthetic valve. A significant improvement will occur in all type of valves in the first year, but this improvement is greater and faster with the stentless bioprostheses [20]. A lasting benefit beyond the first year is possible, especially in severely enlarged ventricles [21]. These improvements include mass regression, wall thickening, fractional shortening, and diastolic relaxation. Patients with small aortic annuli or with compromised left ventricular function (EF < 50%) might benefit more from stentless prostheses [22,23].

3. Structural and nonstructural durability

One of the foremost concern of any tissue valve is its long-term patency, because the limited durability represents the main disadvantage of these devices. Tissue valve degeneration causing stenosis or regurgitation is the primer indication for reoperation.

Durability of any kind of stentless bioprosthesis can be affected adversely by internal (structural) or external (nonstructural) factors.

Structural valve deterioration (SVD) is a primary tissue failure after biological valve implantation. A major cause of SVD is cusp tear with consequent aortic regurgitation where urgent or emergent reoperation is necessary due to congestive heart failure and hemolytic anemia. The other major reason is prosthetic valve sclerosis and calcification which could permit an elective reoperation in stable condition. An in vivo animal study has shown that native aortic valves are significantly more distensible at the level of the sinotubular junction, commissures and ascending aorta when compared with all-valve prosthesis [24]. There is no any study to evaluate how the late scar with/without calcification tissue formation spread and effect this distensibility. We can argue that annular calcification developed during follow-up acts similar in native and stentless valves and fixes the aortic annulus. The zero-pressure fixation and antimineralization techniques have improved durability of tissue valves. To avoid from well known limited durability of xenogenic bioprostheses owing to structural degeneration and calcification, the use of autologous pericardium may be an attractive alternative with several advantages: no immune reaction, minimum tissue calcification and pannus formation, excellent hemodynamics and dynamics of the aortic root, no complicated reoperation [11].

Nonstructural valve deterioration (NSVD) is independent on the xenograft's tissue. In spite of leaflets of xenografts work very well, stentless bioprosthesis shows incompetence. There are several reasons causing prosthetic stenosis or regurgitation (Table 2).

Technical inadequacy during stentless valve implantation cause hemodynamic problems like regurgitation, turbulent flow, uncoaptation or stretching of leaflets which aggregate tissue degeneration. Any increase in mechanical stress causing by surgical implantation techniques has a negative impact on durability. Description of all implantation techniques with their tips is not adequate to avoid iatrogenic valve degeneration, all details of these techniques should be well known. The best way to avoid mechanical stress may be to use the full root replacement technique, but most surgeon do not like to replace the aortic root without any pathology

A. Endocarditis
B. Technically implantation errors
C. Aortic root enlargement
I. Sinotubular junction dilatation
II. Sinus of Valsalva aneurysm (± rupture)
III. Aortic dissection
IV. Left ventricular dilatation
D. Partial dehiscence after preserved non-coronary sinus
E. Insufficiently decalcification
I. Poor decalcification (intra-operatively)
II. Suture rupture or loosening (post-operatively)
III. Calcification on the native aorta (follow-up)
F. Subvalvular fibrous band
G. Hematologic problems (hemolysis, thrombocytopenia)

Table 2. Non-structural Deterioration (regurgitation or stenosis).

(dilatation, calcification) because of higher operative risk. Subcoronary implantation technique is more acceptable approach for isolated AVR with stentless bioprostheses. Technical errors relating to xenograft sizing and failure to achieve appropriate geometry of the xenograft within the aortic root are 2 major reasons for early valve failure. The learning curve associated with subcoronary implantation is the main reason for these technical errors. Suboptimal implantation resulting in distortion of the valve or bulking of valve tissue into the outflow tract may be involved in the evolution of higher gradients. Undersizing of xenograft results regurgitation due to handicapping leaflet coaptation, whereas oversizing may cause higher transvalvular gradient due to making leaflet opening difficult. The other error is to decide and apply the wrong implantation technique, especially in small or dilated aortic root, and subcoronary technique might be associated with higher gradient or regurgitation [25].

On the other hand, improvement of the long term patency of an aortic prosthetic valve is dependent on avoidance of paravalvular complications which can be very serious and cause reoperation. Paravalvular regurgitation is a dangerous long-term result of insufficient decalcification, which causes incompetence suturing or suture rupture during follow-up.

Partial dehiscence of the stentless xenograft indeed occurs and that it has a strong predilection for the preserved non-coronary sinus after modified subcoronary technique. Supposedly, proteolytic enzymes from captured blood cells in the dead space between native and donor aortas or the potential usefulness of biologic glues might prevent adequate fusion of the walls and healing of the anastomosis [26].

Subvalvular fibrous band is a rare complication resulting significant left ventricular outflow tract obstruction, which can be a derivative of the pannus discovered on the sewing ring of stented valves. The etiology is unknown, but it may result from thrombus formation or inflammation related to host factors. A chronic inflammatory infiltrate composed of lymphocytes and macrophages occurs in equine or porcine stentless valves, which suggests equal immunogenicity among different various biologic graft materials [27].

4.1. Aortic valve surgery

4.1.1. Cardiopulmonary bypass

Aortic valve surgery can be performed through a median full sternotomy or upper ministernotomy with conventional or minimal skin incision. The distal ascending aorta cannulation is usually the standard approach in most patients, but the arcus aorta or axiller artery can be also cannulated when the ascending aorta should be replaced [28]. A single dual-stage venous cannula is inserted through the right atrium appendage. After cardiopulmonary bypass is initiated the aorta is clamped and cardiac arrest is be achieved with antegrade isothermic blood cardioplegia administered into the aortic root. Myocardial protection is continued due to retrograde cardioplegic cannula during whole procedure, and retrograde cardioplegia is continuously infused whenever clear visulation of the aortic root is not required [29]. Rarely the retrograde cannula cannot be introduced safely into the coronary sinus, in this situation intermittent antegrade isothermic blood cardioplegia is performed using selective coronary ostial cannulation after transverse aortotomy incision. If both approaches are unsuccessful, bicaval cannulation is performed and the retrograde cannula is placed in the coronary sinus under direct vision. A vent cannula is inserted into the left atrium through the right upper pulmonary vein after cross clamp to prevent the left ventricle distention. Mild-moderate hypothermia (30-32°C) is achieved and continued during extracorporeal circulation, and rewarming of patients is started before the closure of the aortotomy.

4.1.2. Aortotomy

A small transverse aortotomy incision is made initially at least 15 to 20 mm above the origin of the right coronary ostium or the sinotubular junction. The calcific aortic valve and whole aortic root should be investigated under direct vision and decided which approach will be preferred. If the aortic root will not be replaced then the transverse aortotomy incision is extended on both sides until 3D view of the aortic root appears. That helps surgeons for excision of the severe calcific aortic valve, selection of an appropriate stentless bioprosthesis and insertion simple and/or continuous sutures easily and correctly. A transverse aortotomy is also required to image 3D shape of the aortic root which is the main condition for resuspention of the prosthetic commissures and to hold a stentless tissue valve in corrected position for prevention of the iatrogenic valve degeneration. An oblique or hockey-stick incision is preferred very seldom, but it could be useful in patients with small aortic root. If the aortic root is replaced it is excised completely and aortic root implantation technique is performed. Reoperation for severe calcific aortic stenosis is not rare in patients with previously coronary artery bypass surgery, and patent proximal anastomoses on the ascending aorta can be a serious problem during aortotomy. I have offered a simple aortotomy incision "Reverse U aortotomy" to save proximal anastomoses and if it is necessary to apply direct antegrade cardioplegia through proximal anastomoses [30].

4.1.3. Excision of the calcific aortic valve

Aortic valve stenosis appears with fusion of one or both commissures, thickening and retraction of the cusps, and restriction of effective orifice area. Calcific involvement of native aortic valve is the last step which can be widespread very aggressively: aortic annulus, mitral annulus, aortic root, coronary ostia. The typically pathologic findings of calcific aortic stenosis are discrete, focal lesions on the aortic side of the leaflets. The severe form is characterized by diffuse calcification of the aortic root and the deposits involve the sinuses of Valsalva and the ascending aorta (porcelain aorta). The calcification presents as a cauliflower-like mass within the leaflets and often extends deep into the annulus and surrounding tissues. All these contiguous anatomical structures can have adverse affects on the surgical techniques.

A surgically complete decalcification of the aortic annulus is an important point. The flexible continuity of the aortic annulus with sub- and supra-annular tissues is indispensable condition to get better durability and hemodynamics with stentless xenografts, and to avoid from a whole aortic root replacement technique, which hinders surgeons to perform AVR with a stentless xenograft. Surgeons must care 1) not to leave any calcific tissue around the aortic annulus, 2) not to allow fragments of calcium to fall into the left ventricle, 3) not to disrupt the annulus as possible, 4) not to detach the anterior mitral leaflet from the annulus (non-coronary sinus), 5) not to rupture subannular muscular septum (right coronary sinus), 6) not to perforate outside the heart (left coronary sinus).

The calcific aortic valve is excised and trimmed with a scissor leaving a 2-3 mm margin at the annulus if the annular margin of the leaflets are healthy. The frequent scenario is conversely that and extensive calcific involvement of the whole aortic annulus is observed very often. First of all, complete resection of the calcific aortic valve should be performed without any complication listed above. Excision of the calcific leaflets with a scissor is usually unsuccessful and dangerous because of breaking of calcification and falling calcium debris into the left ventricle. The best alternative to remove the diseased tissue is excision all of them with a lancet (number 15). A folded segment of sponge or tampon is not necessary to place in the left ventricle and it hinders to see the cavity and to remove any calcium particle. The easiest excision with the lancet is to perforate the healthy leaflet near the annulus in partial calcified aortic valve or to begin excision at the commissure between the non-coronary and right coronary leaflets in en-bloc calcific aortic valve. Cutting of the calcification is begun at the nearest end and the lancet incises the calcified valve from the healthy annular tissue. The sharp edge of the lancet should be headed toward the calcified valve, and cutting is performed just below of calcification. The whole calcified valve must be incised as en-block, without fragmentation. If calcification is very heavy or invaded into the annulus it can be cut with the scissor and then the residual calcifications will be gently crushed and removed with a rounger. After completion of the aortic valve excision, all residual diseased and/or calcified tissue or particles should be removed from around the annulus. Before sizing the prosthesis, the left ventricular cavity is flushed and irrigated with saline solution.

4.1.4. Sizing the stentless aortic bioprosthesis

The stented prostheses must fit snugly in the annulus, because a very loose or tight fit indicates inadequate effective orifice area (patient-prosthesis mismatch) or oversizing the prosthesis. For the truly measurement of a stented valve, the seizer should be inserted through the aortic annulus and the same (supra-annular) or one number smaller (intra-annular) stented prosthesis must be chosen.

Sizing a stentless bioprosthesis is different from stented valves. The most important phase is the choice of an appropriate stentless bioprosthesis, and measurement of the aortic annulus must be done with the seizer that corresponds to the specific bioprosthesis. The true seizer should be chosen to implant the appropriate tissue valve with the optimum size. If the prosthetic valve is too small, the inflow end obstructs the EOA which increases transvalvular gradient and the outflow end is stretched out with decreased leaflet coaptation which causes more regurgitation. On the other hand, oversizing to fit a larger sinotubular junction leads to buckling of the inflow end which can produce both relative stenosis and regurgitation as well as harmful turbulent flow. How the stentless valves sized and implanted will influence its function and durability in future. The larger surface area of the cusps allows greater coaptation area which reduces the risk of bioprosthesis regurgitation. This relatively larger bioprosthesis can simplify replacement, especially the running sutures for all sinuses. But, it is imperative to avoid over-sizing of stentless valves with the tubular structure achieved by three tabs on the commissures, and if sizing is uncertainty the smaller prosthesis should be implanted.

In normal aortic root, the diameter of the aortic annulus is 10-15% larger than those of the sinotubular junction and measurement of the aortic annulus is the correct way to choice an appropriate sized stentless valve. However, most patients with calcific aortic stenosis have an abnormal aortic root and the relationship between both diameters is usually altered. In this situation, the diameter of the sinotubular junction is more important because the three commissures of stentless valves are secured at approximately the level of the sinotubular junction if not the full-root replacement technique will be used.

A cylindrical silicon seizer is more practical to measure the true valve size when both the annulus and the sinotubular junction are measured. The rule is that the sinotubular junction should be dominate during measuring and if there is a major difference (> 3 mm) subcoronary implantation technique can be not used because the commissures of stentless valves are pulled outward and cause valvular insufficiency and an alternative technique (root replacement) or stented bioprosthesis must be used. Supra-annular sizing is the best measurement method to choice an appropriate stentless bioprosthesis, especially during single suture line technique. I prefer this more practical way and put the appropriate seizer into the aortic root in supra-annular position (not into the annulus) where I put continuous proximal suture line, so I can choice an acceptable size that is equal to the sinotubular junction size or one number larger stentless prosthesis can be chosen if the seizer fits aortic orifice tightly in patients with aortic root enlargement. Trans-annular measurement is adequate to get a fit stentless valve for subcoronary implantation in patients with normal aortic root, but preferring one size larger prosthesis is better if full-root replacement technique will be performed or a small aortic root is present. I never suggest to play some traction sutures at the commissures or in the nadir of the annulus to open the aortic orifice. It can be useful during the replacement of a stented valve, but it will be better to release the aortic root in its original shape during sizing stentless valves.

5. Implantation techniques

Stentless aortic biologic prostheses can be different in origin: autogenous, homogenous, heterogeneous. Procuring of aortic auto- or homograft is not easy, but production of xenografts is a sufficiently technical supply of the industry for the treatment of aortic valve diseases. All stentless biologic valves can be implanted using different techniques: the subcoronary method, the full root implantation technique, and the root inclusion alternative.

The subcoronary technique is the simplest method for implantation, and either a porcine root can be adapted intra-operatively or a prefabricated tissue valve can be utilized. The main advantages are to avoid the manipulation of coronary ostia and bleeding from suture lines. The disadvantages could be difficulties occurring in the small aortic annulus and calcified aortic root, and possibilities of valve insufficiency by changing the shape of the stentless valve in a diseased aortic root [31]. Subcoronary implantation technique can be performed in two methods: double suture lines (classic) or single suture line (simple) approach.

In classical subcoronary implantation technique, stentless valves are fixed into the host aortic root using double suture lines. The first suture line attaches the inflow site of the stentless bioprosthesis in the left ventricular outflow tract: annular suture line. The second suture line, which is constructed using 1 or 3 continuous sutures, connects the outflow site of the prosthesis with the aortic wall below the coronary ostia: supra-annular suture line. The first suture line consists usually of interrupted sutures, but to reduce cross-clamp and cardiopulmonary times a continuous suture can be preferred [32]. Because the conventional continuous inflow suture line can increase the postoperative heart block risk, an alternative subcoronary technique has been reported in which the inflow suture line is raised at the level of right-non-coronary commissure [33].

The single suture line technique is a simple, quick, safe and reliable method to replace the native aortic valve with a stentless valve. This approach is used for implantation of scalloped new generation tissue valves in supra-annular position and placement of the sutures below or through the annulus should be avoided. Running sutures avoid any prosthetic dead space between prosthetic valve and native aortic wall, and selecting a prosthesis a size larger than the host annulus minimizes the stress on the suture lines. These new generation pericardial valve can have manufactured scalloped design [34] or it can be prepared by trimming away all the extra tissue of the valve inflow side ond scalloping the outflow side [35]. If stentless prostheses are designed with a tubular structure, the tabs on the commissures should be attached to the aortic wall [36].

The total root technique requires reimplantation of coronary arteries using the button technique. The main advantages are normal physiological shape of the aortic root and choice of a larger valve in small aortic annulus, and both avoid any patient-prosthesis mismatch. The total root technique also prevents torsions of the commissures which avoiding postoperative prosthetic dysfunction. The main disadvantages are implantation difficulties, requirement of interposition a vascular tubular graft between xenograft and native ascending aorta, and xenograft aortic wall calcification making reoperation difficulty. The learning curve seems to be more pronounced when using the total root technique, whereas single suture line technique may be also performed by young surgeons without any problem. Surgeons decide on their experience and the patient's anatomy pre- and intra-operatively which approach with appropriate stentless bioprosthesis type they will use for AVR. Isolated AVR using the subcoronary technique is the best and easiest way in calcific aortic stenosis and using single suture line technique increases the success of implantation a stentless xenograft.

The direct suture of autologous pericardium to the aortic wall creating a new aortic valve does not need any supporting stent, sewing ring or cuff, allowing to rebuilt 3 symmetrical aortic cusps independent of the geometry of the native aortic valve. Harvesting a circular pericardium about 8-10 cm in diameter, treating with glutaraldehyde, sizing-cutting-shaping (a trefoil) with a specially designed instrument, and suturing the cut pericardium mounted on a tissue holder are the steps of this technique which does not take more time. The important goal is to reconstruct a newly geometrically symmetric valve and to ensure adequate coaptation with no prolapse. the suture technique is similar to the single suture line technique and running sutures are placed onto supra-annular aortic wall.

5.1. Subcoronary implantation technique

This approach is a simple method to implant a stentless bioprosthesis. In spite of the only handicap is the inexperience in this field, geometric thinking is the key point to perform a successful stentless AVR using this approach. A transverse aortotomy helps to image 3D shape of the aortic root which simplifies sizing and implanting a stentless valve. The proximal suture line is performed with the simple interrupted suture technique. This technique requires 18-24 sutures (4/0 Ticron or Polypropylene) which are placed in a circular plane coursing through the aortic annulus (annular suture line) and passed through the inflow end of the stentless valve (subannular suture line). All sutures are passed through the Dacron skirt of the bioprosthesis just below the lowest aspect of the cusps, but the sutures at the native commissures must be passed through the same level of prosthetic commissures to create a geometrical shape without any distortion. It is also important not to injury or perforate the prosthetic cusps when the needles are passed through the skirt of the stentless valve. If the aortic annulus is weakened or destroyed pledgeted sutures (4/0 Ticron) should be placed in subannular position to hold suture securely, which provides satisfactory buttressing effect and repairs annular ruptures. Because xenografts are not as pliable as homografts and its inversion into the left ventricle followed by being pulled up into the aorta may damage the device, I never use this maneuver. The prosthesis is lowered into the aortic root and sutured with its annulus to the aortic annulus as the baseline line, and all sutures are tied on the skirt. If the prosthesis has three own sinuses, at least the two sinuses facing the native left and right coronary ostia are scalloped out below the level of those recipient coronaries, leaving a 4-5 mm rim of prosthetic tissue behind. To suture sinuses of bioprosthesis to the native aortic sinuses, three continuous suture lines (5/0 polypropylene) are started in the nadir of each sinus below the native coronary ostia and in the nadir of the non-coronary sinus and progress upward to the top of three commissures (supra-annular suture line), taking care not to buckle the stentless tissue or distort the positions of the commissural posts. The sutures are taken outside the aorta, buttressed with a pledget and tied together. The deep bites of continuous sutures on the aortic sinuses can be transverse or horizontal, but they must be full-thickness at the host aortic wall. The broad bites must be taken on the aortic sinuses of bioprosthesis to avoid any space under device. It is also important to pass the needle well away from the margin of the stentless cusp attachment and not to injury the cusps. If the non-coronary sinus of the stentless valve is kept intact (modified subcoronary technique), it is not necessary to use the third suture, and the distal suture line is completed by running along the top to join the first two sutures. A stay suture (pledgeted 2/0 Ticron) may be placed at the top of each commissure to achieve 3D geometric shape of the device. If it is necessary the tops are trimmed down to the level of the native aorta. The aortotomy is closed with double continuous pledgeted sutures (4/0 polypropylene) beginning from each edge.

5.2. Single suture line technique

It is a simple modification of the subcoronary technique and it can be performed according to the design of stentless valve.

Classical subcoronary stentless valves could be implanted with only supra-annular running suture line that places the stentless annulus above and along the native annulus up and around each commissure (Sorin Freedom Solo, CryoLife O'Brien). In this approach, the device should fit the supra-annular area because the aortic trimmed wall of stentless valves is sutured and attached only with proximal supra-annular suture line directly to native aortic sinuses in supra-annular position. Three polypropylene sutures are started at the nadir of each sinus and brought progressively up to each commissural tip with the ends brought outside the aorta for tying (as described above). Because the stentless valve will be placed supra-annular we can choice a 1 or 2 number larger size than the true annular-size and that prevents any transvalvular gradient.

An alternative approach must be preferred in some stentless prostheses designed as having a tubular structure. The outflow orifice is supported by 3 commissural tabs at the distal junction of the leaflets. Inflow implantation is performed with the same running suture line, but the tops of three commissures are equipped at an appropriate location with stay sutures (pledgetless 2/0 Ticron) tied on the outside of the aorta (3f ATS, Shelhigh Superstentless). These tabs are sewn onto the patient's aortic wall, thereby maintaining the tubular integrity of the prosthesis. It is imperative to achieve true-sizing. Should uncertainty arise, the smaller prosthesis should be implanted because larger prosthesis can block a rapid and unobstructed opening, whereas to small prosthesis restricts of fully leaflet-opening. The same problem can also occur with an excessive or insufficient distal traction on the tabs.

5.3. Root inclusion technique

If the original cylindrical shape of the bioprosthetic root devices wants to be preserved without replacement of the native aortic root to avoid bleeding complication, the root inclusion technique can be chosen. A glutaraldehyde-treated porcine aortic root is implanted inside the patient's aortic root. But this technique is more difficult because both native coronary ostia should be anastomosed to the prosthesis like in classic Bentall procedure. After transverse aortotomy a proximal suture line is performed like the subcoronary technique in a circular plane coursing below the commissures. Appropriate opening for coronary ostia are made by excising the sinuses facing the right and left main coronary ostia and then both are sutured continuously (5/0 polypropylene). The only difference between the root inclusion and subcoronary techniques is that the complete sinotubular junction of the stentless valve is preserved. This method is not used nowadays, and if this technique is preferred it should not be used unless the root is large enough to place 23-mm or larger prosthetic root.

5.4. Root replacement technique

Complete replacement of the native aortic root is last preference for those devices. This technique is used mostly during auto- or homograft replacement. A part of the patient's ascending aorta with total aortic root is excised and a new glutaraldehyde-treated porcine aorta with total aortic root is inserted using a single proximal and distal suture lines. Only indication to prefer this approach is an extended pathology through aortic root (endocarditis, annular abscess, porcelain aorta, dissection) if a stentless valve is used. Since the tubular 3D geometry is not altered, its factory-tested performance is not affected by the implantation. All aortic root is excised and both coronary ostia are separated from the root. The valve seizer should fit in the aortic annulus and 1 or 2 number bigger stentless bioprosthesis is chosen. Depending on the anatomical details of the native right coronary artery, the device may be implanted anatomically or rotated to put the porcine left in the patient's right sinus. The proximal suture line is constructed with continuous polypropylene suture or interrupted sutures (4/0). The coronary buttons are re-implanted as the standard fashion (5/0 polypropylene). The distal end of the bioprosthesis is usually smaller than the distal native aorta, but it can be not a problem during distal anastomosis (4/0 polypropylene).

5.5. Direct suture technique of autologous pericardium

Truly stentless AVR using autologous pericardium sutured directly onto the aortic wall without supporting stents is a safe and feasible alternative with excellent hemodynamics of the aortic root [11]. With the use of specially designed instruments, the sinotubular junction is sized, the pericardium is placed on a base, and a cutting blade of the matching size is placed on top of the pericardium, which cuts it to the required size and shape (a trefoil). The cut pericardium is then mounted on a tissue holder to facilitate suturing it to the aortic wall. The prepared autologous pericardium is then sutured directly onto the aortic wall close to the marked annulus using 4–0 polypropylene sutures. Each running suture starting from the base of the leaflet cusp ends at each commissure where it passes through to the outside of the aorta, at which point the knot is tied. The commissures are then securely fixed by passing another mattress suture from inside the commissure to outside the aorta where it is tied. Leaflet symmetry and coaptation are assessed directly at the end of the procedure before closing the aortotomy.

5.6. Sutureless implantation technique

Aortic valve replacement with prosthetic heart valves is the treatment of choice for calcific aortic valve stenosis. Stentless valves are the best option with larger EOA and lower trans-valvular gradient, but technically the implantations of these valves are more demanding resulting in longer operation times. However, important comorbid conditions in elderly patients referred for aortic valve replacement require alternative treatment options with possible reductions of the extracorporeal bypass and cross-clamp times and reliable hemody-namic features. In order to comply with these requirements, transcatheter (transfemoral or transapical) valves and sutureless surgical valves have been developed. The transcatheter techniques have the advantage of being performed without circulatory bypass but leaving the aortic calcifications in place, thereby resulting in a high degree of paravalvular insufficiency, atrioventricular block and strokes [37]. The surgical approach has the advantage of removing all calcifications and the valves can be optimally implanted, resulting in minimal paravalvular leak with a low incidence of atrioventricular block and strokes; however, it requires cardio-pulmonary bypass. The design of sutureless bioprosthesis stems from the intention to offer an alternative to traditional flexible stentless prostheses using conventional open-heart surgery. Sutureless new designed bioprosthesis is a trileaflet bovine or equine pericardial valve mounted on an expandable metal frame in nitinol (equiatomic alloy of nickel and titanium). New designed stentless bioprostheses have several advantages: reducing cross-clamp and cardiopulmonary bypass times, reducing related risk by placing of proximal sutures, less risk of tearing the aortic annulus and wall, avoiding damage of the bundle of His, preventing foreign particle embolization. The primary benefit of this aortic bioprosthesis is the potential for surgeons to provide the same gold standard outcomes of traditional surgical AVR but without the need for sutures, thereby facilitating less invasive or minimally invasive proce-dures.

The transverse aortic incision is performed 1 cm above the sinotubular junction to preserve a segment of the ascending aorta above the prosthetic valve. Severe calcific aortic valve is removed and aortic annulus should be decalcified for implantation (it is not necessary a complete decalcification). To ensure the correct positioning and orientation of the prosthesis guide-suture(s) can be used. Avoidance of proximal suture lines makes the procedure easier. The architectural design of this new kind of bioprosthesis allows perfect function after it adapts itself to the aortic root. They have two cylindrical ring segments: 'outflow ring' comprises straight posts designed to support the valve and 'inflow ring' allows the prosthesis to be anchored to the aortic root in the Valsalva sinuses and reaches a final diameter compatible with the aortic root. The configuration of the stentless valve is perfect which allows higher hemodynamic performance. There are two types of sutureless aortic bioprostheses in the market.

The Perceval S Aortic Bioprosthesis (Sorin Biomedia Cardio Srl, Sallugia, Italy) has been introduced for minithoracotomy incision [38]. After the device is introduced and parachuted down into aortic annulus and checking corrected position, a balloon dilatation of the inflow ring is performed in the Perceval S valve. If the device is in malpositioning the valve can be quickly removed using the 'χ movement' and repositioned [39]. Because there are only three number valves (21, 23, 25), paravalvular leakage can be observed in higher incidence (4.4% postoperatively and 4% during follow-up) which can be a result of either inadequate sizing or due to inappropriate decalcification of the annulus [40]. For an enlarged aorta with a ratio greater than 1.3, the predicted diameter according to body surface area represents a contraindication for this device. Early mortality (total 2.4%) and late death (total 2.5%) is acceptable with lower transvalvular gradient (10.8 mmHg) at the first postoperative year [41].

The 3f Enable Aortic Bioprothesis (Model 6000; Medtronic Inc, Minneapolis, USA) is more different and the implantation is more easier: after insertion the device into aortic root in the corrected position, only pour warmer saline (> 30°) onto the device to fully deploy the Nitinol frame into its original shape [42]. If malpositioning occurs after complete deployment, rinsing with chilled saline makes the nitinol stent flexible and enhances repositioning until the valve is correctly placed. Early clinical and hemodynamic performances of the 3f aortic bioprosthesis are similar to those of the regular stentless aortic valves, but both parameters could be inconsistent with the established stentless valves during mid-term follow-up: unfavorable mean gradient especially with smaller number (≤ 23 mm), incomplete left ventricular regression, higher incidence of neurologic complications [43]. However, a multi-center study has shown better early and mid-term results: major paravalvular leakage 2.1%, neurologic events 0.7%, lower mean gradient (10.2 mmHg), lower valve-related early mortality rate (1.4%; total 3.6%); lower late mortality rate (1.5%; total 9.6%), excellent freedom from valve-related mortality at 1-year (96.5%; hazard ratio 1.6%/year), lower paravalvular leakage (0.8%/year) [44].

The analysis of the current outcome of the use of sutureless aortic bioprostheses must take into consideration the preliminary nature of these devices and the relevant implantation learning curve. There are no comparative study analyzing the outcomes of sutureless and stentless bioprostheses, but it can be said that sutureless bioprostheses have better outcome (mortality, neurologic deficit, renal failure, bleeding) than conventional stentless valves in high-risk patients with aortic stenosis (such as older, female, left ventricular dysfunction, calcification in the ascending aorta, previously cardiac operation, pulmonary or renal disease? [45].

5.7. Transcatheter (transfemoral or transapical) aortic valve implantation

The approval of transcatheter aortic valve implantation (AVI) represents a fundamental change in the management of calcific aortic stenosis by offering an alternative to traditional surgical AVR in carefully selected patients. Patient-selection is very strict nowadays, and AVI is a reasonable alternative to surgical AVR in adults with severe symptomatic calcific aortic stenosis if they have suitable aortic and vascular anatomy for transcatheter AVI and a predicted survival > 12 months [46]. Transcatheter AVI can be prefer in patients with severe calcific aortic stenosis if their aortic valve is trileaflet. There are some exclusion criteria in calcific aortic stenosis: en-block calcification (like unicusp), bicuspid aortic valve, severe massive calcification closely coronary ostia, small aortic annulus (< 18 mm) or large aortic orifice (> 25 mm), thoraco-abdominal aortic or peripheral arterial pathologies. Transapical AVI is the another alternative in patients with calcific aortic stenosis associated thoraco-abdominal aortic or peripheral arterial pathologies.

As experience is gained and technology evolves, new areas will be met with this approaches. The most optional area is bioprosthesis dysfunction requiring reoperation and an attractive option is to use a AVI procedure in which the device is deployed within the previously placed bioprosthesis: valve-in-valve. Valve-in-valve procedures require a large enough bioprosthetic valve inserted at the index operation to prevent patient-prosthetic mismatch with the AVI valve.

6. Special situations

Calcific aortic stenosis is a long-term disease and usually associated with other cardiovascular pathologies. Before AVR, all these situations must be reassessmended and case-specific operation procedure and its alternatives must be planned. If we do not think preoperatively that any specific situation needs an intervention intra-operatively, spontaneously home-made resolutions can be also very helpful in the theater when we decide to correct this pathology.

6.1. Proximal ascending aorta aneurysm

Severe aortic stenosis is usually combined with proximal ascending aorta aneurysm causing by turbulent flow. The gold standard treatment is composite aortic valve and root replacement. Several surgical teams have devised strategies to construct their homemade composite conduits intra-operatively. It can be a mechanical valved conduit with excellent long-term results [47]. If any contra-indication for anticoagulation therapy, a composite bioprosthetic valved conduit will be the best alternative. Because severe calcific aortic stenosis is often an elderly disease, improved durability of bioprostheses stimulates also their use in the setting of ascending aorta replacement if proximal ascending aorta requires replacement in this population. The concept of composite bioprosthetic valved conduits has also been taken up by the industry and these conduits are already commercially available in different sizes. There are several technical options to allow replacement of the aortic root and ascending aorta using either stented or stentless bioprosthesis [48]. There are basically two alternatives to built a composite graft with a stentless bioprosthesis: the subcoronary technique and the full-root technique.

The subcoronary implantation technique requires a tubular graft and double suture lines for device implantation is necessary. A stentless valve is placed inside a Dacron tube graft leaving a proximal free margin (3-5 mm) and the proximal suture line of the stentless bioprosthesis is fixed to the graft with a running mattress suture [49]. The free end of the tube graft is then sutured to the native annulus with pledgeted interrupted mattress sutures, and following this, the upper circumference of the stentless valve is reimplanted within the tube graft using a second running mattress suture. To avoid the potential drawbacks of a straight cylindrical tube an aortic graft with pseudo-sinuses can be used [50] or David-V procedure using a stentless bioprosthesis can be applied to build new sinuses [51]. I implant firstly tubular synthetic graft using pledgeted interrupted mattress sutures subannularly, and then a stentless valve is implanted using the single suture line technique as described above. The ready-to-use composite biological valved graft is also available in practice currently [The BioValsalva composite grafts (Sulzer Vascutek, Renfrewshire, Scotland, UK)] [52].

The full-root technique is preferred in order to reduce distortion risk leading valve regurgitation or deterioration, but the commercially available stentless porcine aortic root devices are usually too short to replace the host ascending aorta. There are also four alternatives to suture a stentless conduit directly to the distal ascending aorta with extended tubular devices: extended version of stentless porcine aortic root bioprosthesis, direct anastomosis after extensive mobilization of the host aorta, interposition of a Dacron tube graft, and total xenopericardial valved conduit. The availability of extended root xenograft is extremely limited, but this approach can achieve an anastomosis between xenograft and the distal ascending aorta [53]. Primary end-to-end anastomosis might prevent the need for graft interposition, but extensive mobilization of the aortic arch and its branches can be dangerous and some tension might be left at the distal anastomosis with a risk of late dehiscence and false aneurysm development [54]. The most practical technique appears to be the insertion of a Dacron tube graft between the xenograft root and the native distal ascending aorta [55]. There is a new bioprosthetic conduit, constructed using individual non-coronary porcine cusps, which are fitted on a scalloped shaped tubular bovine pericardium [56]. The 15 cm long pericardial cuff is long enough to facilitate the anastomosis between the conduit and the remaining distal aorta. If mid- or long-term results will confirm excellent results, this option will be an attractive alternative to the others techniques.

6.2. Small aortic annulus

Aortic valve replacement with a small stented prosthetic valve is technically straightforward and frequently performed, but it may result in patient-prosthesis mismatch and a high residual outflow gradient, which is significant risk factor for early mortality [57]. Patient-prosthesis mismatch is associated with an increase in all-cause and cardiac-related mortality over long-term follow-up, and current efforts to prevent prosthesis-patient mismatch should receive more emphasis and a widespread acceptance to improve long-term survival after AVR [58]. When the aortic annulus diameter is less than 20 mm, a relatively high transvalvular velocity has to be expected after valve replacement. In these cases, a stentless bioprosthesis with/ without aortic root enlargement would provide better hemodynamic results than stented valves.

For severe small aortic root with small aortic annulus, a xenograft root replacement can be the first alternative and this technique avoids the aortic annulus enlargement, but it can be problematic because of reimplantation of the coronary arteries, calcified aorta and/or coronary ostia, or prolonged operation times. The full-root replacement technique is technically more demanding, but it prevents residual gradient postoperatively, and if one number larger conduit is selected the possible largest orifice area will be gained. Subcoronary techniques with/without intact non-coronary sinus can be also used in these patients with excellent hemodynamics in smaller valve sizes and appropriate device can be implanted safely and easily [59].

Another alternative technique is aortic annulus enlargement to prevent patient-prosthesis mismatch and a two-size-larger prosthesis could be inserted. The most commonly used technique is enlargement of the aortic annulus with a biologic or synthetic patch which can be performed in different approach [60]. A modification of the Manouguian technique has been introduced for aortic annulus enlargement without using a patch [61]. A tubular aortic bioprosthesis of one or two sizes larger than the size of the native annulus is prepared for modified subcoronary implantation technique and non-coronary sinus wall be kept intact. The prosthesis is sutured directly on the enlarged annulus after the aortic incision is extended through the commissure, and the aorta is closed directly with the mural wall of the tubular xenograft.

6.3. Porcelain aorta

The scope of porcelain aorta ranges from isolated plaques to the circumferential calcification of the ascending aorta. Typically, a heavily calcified ascending aorta with calcific aortic stenosis involves aortic annulus, aortic valve, aortic root and ascending aorta (± distal aortic segments). This scenario is associated with higher operative mortality and morbidity than isolated severe calcific aortic stenosis. A more recent study have been demonstrated a link between arteriosclerotic changes in aortic valve and ascending aorta [62]. This study compared healthy patients with severe aortic stenosis patients shows that the prevalence of aortic root calcification (26% versus 54%; p = 0.008) and of atheroma in the ascending aorta (7% versus 24%; p < 0.001) are higher in aortic valve disease patients and patients coexisting coronary artery disease have more extensive arteriosclerotic changes in the thoracic aorta compared with those with aortic stenosis alone and control subjects.

The operative management of severe calcific aortic stenosis with porcelain aorta can be difficult and complex because of difficulty of clamping the ascending aorta, aortotomy, supra-annular sutures, or aortic root replacement, and the risk of calcific embolization of major branches (coronary, carotid, or other arteries), aortic dissection. Digital palpation with a lowered systemic blood pressure or epiaortic sonographic evaluation can be used to confirm that there is a softer spot in the aortic arch for cannulation intra-operatively. If there is no any healthy site on the distal ascending aorta or aortic arch for regular arterial cannulation (34%), alternative arterial cannulation should be performed through innominate (8%), axillary (24%) or femoral (34%) artery [63]. There are several alternatives to perform AVR: standard replacement, endarterectomy for calcified porcelain aorta, no touch technique under circulatory arrest (no cross-clamp, no endarterectomy, no ascending aorta replacement), total replacement of the ascending aorta replacement (with/without circulatory arrest), apico-aortic valved conduit, transcatheter AVI. I prefer standard AVR if it is possible, if not I perform David-V total ascending aortic replacement with a stentless bioprosthesis [47]. Last decade, ascending aortic replacement is the most preferred method for the treatment of porcelain aorta, but transfemoral [64] or transapical [65] AVI will replace the first choice of the treatment in this decade. These alternatives demonstrate significant advantages (especially very low incidence of neurological events, avoidance of cardiopulmonary bypass and circulatory arrest) in comparison to other conventional techniques in the setting of severe aortic calcification.

6.4. Concomitant severe coronary artery disease

Many patients with moderate or severe calcific aortic stenosis have significant coronary disease, suggesting that the degenerative changes of the aortic valve leading to aortic stenosis may be part of a similar arteriosclerotic process. Coronary lesion can be also in different coronary arteries or massif calcification involves into coronary ostia. Combined surgical treatment is the main modality, but percutaneous coronary intervention is safer in patients undergoing transcatheter AVI, or in patients with high risk (high comorbidities, reoperation, pericardial adhesion). Because hypercholesterolemia is related to increased risk of aortic valve calcification in patients with aortic stenosis, preventive treatment of hypercholesterolemia could play an important role to decrease or inhibit development of aortic valve calcification [66].

6.5. Concomitant hematologic disease

The best opportunity to improve the treatment of any hematologic disease or to prevent any complication aggravating by hematologic pathologies is avoidance from prosthetic foreign devices. Autologous tissue is the only biologic material preparing prosthetic valve, but that can be limited because of pericardial pathologies, inadequate surgical experience or technical problems. Mechanical valves have life-long durability with some possible hematologic complications such as thrombo-embolism, warfarin related hemorrhage, heparin induced thrombocytopenia, hemolysis. Prosthetic foreign material can also aggravate hematologic diseases. To decide which prosthesis can be the acceptable choice for AVR in patients with hematologic pathology is depend on patient's characteristics and patient-by-patient analysis is required. Biomaterials seem better than mechanical prostheses, and stentless aortic bioprostheses are the best alternatives because of absence of a rigid stent, biodynamic characteristics, larger EOA with lowest transvalvular obstruction, unnecessariness of anticoagulation, which might decrease hematologic complications. I prefer stentless xenografts for AVR in patients with severe hematologic pathologies [67].

Postoperative thrombocytopenia is a transient phenomenon, self–recovering after a few days without any treatment and without any observed recurrence in late follow-up. Microhemodynamic effects of the prosthesis structure or depending on the implantation technique and/or specific chemical preparations of biological prosthesis tissue could act as a trigger for the post-replacement thrombocytopenia. It seems to be possible that transient unspecific activation of platelets result in diffuse consumption and lower platelet levels. The reason for this phenomenon is unknown and the use of consistent monitoring is necessary to prevent severe falls in platelet count. It seems unrelated to the type of aortic bioprosthesis and I have not observed this phenomenon only in stentless pericardial valves, but also in different bioprostheses [68]. However, thrombocytopenia after implantation of the stentless pericardial xenografts can develop more common and becomes dangerous for the patient [69,70].

7. Surgical–technical complications

In spite of all implantation techniques of different stentless bioprostheses are demanding and require an aortic valve surgical experience, some situations can make trouble AVR intra-operatively or impair operative outcomes in the early postoperative period. Every surgeon must be aware of these troubles and keep in mind case specific technical solutions in the theater.

7.1. Severe annular calcification

To replace the diseased aortic valve in patients with calcific aortic stenosis is a serious intervention because of extensive calcification. Debridement of all calcium deposits back to soft tissue improves seating of stentless prostheses in supra-annular position and provides better performance, and may be, protects devices early calcification. I always prefer deep debridement and decalcification of all around structures. If there is no any damage on the annulus, I implant a stentless valve with the single suture technique (supra-annular implantation); if not, I prefer the classic subcoronary technique and use pledgeted sutures in subannular position to repair defects. Calcification after stentless valve implantation is complicated if a stentless bioprosthesis is implanted in young patient: faster calcification in homografts has been reported compared with xenografts [71].

7.2. Conduction disturbances

Permanent of transient conduction defects are well-known complications of aortic valve surgery [72]. Higher degree atrioventricular blocks are often reversible and disappear before discharge from the hospital. Approximately 5% of patients undergone isolated AVR require permanent pacemaker implantation. Risk factors can be patient-specific: bicuspid aorta, annular calcification, hypertension, preexisting conduction disturbances, coronary artery disease. Surgeon-specific risk factors cause mostly mechanical injury of the atrioventricular conduction pathways during aortic valve surgery: annular decalcification, deep suture placement, suturing techniques, pressure on the conduction tissue. Atrioventricular block generally results from trauma to the atrioventricular node or His bundle in the region of membranous septum and right trigone beneath the non-coronary - right coronary cusps commissure. The continuous inflow suture line is the most common cause for atrioventricular block because this suture line is placed below each commissure in a horizontal plane based on the level of the nadir of the attachments of the native aortic valve leaflets to the native aortic valve annulus. Raising the continuous inflow suture line below non-coronary - right coronary commissure prevents such conduction complication. Interrupted inflow sutures are also safer than continuous technique. The best approach is the single suture line technique which does not need any inflow suture line.

7.3. Coronary insufficiency

Coronary flow complications are uncommon after stentless AVR, in spite of calcific aortic valve stenosis appears often with coronary ostia calcification with/without coronary artery disease. Myocardial ischemia developing after AVR can develop due to several reasons. Uniform adequate myocardial preservation during operation is the main preventive strategy. Coronary artery bypass grafting should be added aortic valve surgery if any coronary artery stenosis is proved angiographically before surgery. Technical or pathologic factors must also keep in mind. Extensive calcific involvement of coronary ostia or any calcific particle embolization can block antegrade coronary blood flow postoperatively. Endarterectomy or coronary artery bypass grafting should be performed if not any coronary lesion is proved. Decalcification of the aortic root may be well without any aggressive manipulation on coronary ostia, but rupture around coronary ostia can be fatal. Implantation techniques can damage coronary blood flow due to technical errors. Besides a learning curve for these more complex procedures, other factors that could potentially contribute to excess myocardial ischemia or bleeding causing coronary ostia complications. Technical problems can occur mostly during the aortic root replacement with stentless xenografts. This type of coronary insufficiency is uncommon and more often affects the right coronary artery [73]. Coronary buttons are prepared for suturing to xenografts, but they can be damaged because of extensive cutting, dissection, or aggressive decalcification of buttons. Severe tension on the button anastomoses can cause bleeding, rupture, kinking or obstruction. Preventive maneuvers are recognition of coronary orientation, routine xenograft rotation, adequate coronary button mobilization, oversizing xenograft. The subcoronary implantation is more secure procedure than the root replacement technique and technical complication causing coronary problems can occur very seldom if running sutures bite very close to the coronary ostia.

7.4. Dehiscence

Partial or severe dehiscence of aortic prosthetic valves is a serious, but very rare complication. Complete dehiscence occurs with sudden death and it is not seen during practice life. Demand on the severity of dehiscence, the clinic scenario can be variable. Limited dehiscence can be silent and stable, more serious dehiscence shows some signs and unstable. If the aortic root replacement technique is preferred dehiscence can be very small at the proximal or distal suture line which presents bleeding, hematoma or massif hemorrhage. Dehiscence observed after the subcoronary implantation technique is associated with aortic regurgitation, but using obliterating sutures prevent usually this complication. In the aortic root inclusion technique, the dead space between native and donor aortas might be prevented adequate fusion of the walls and healing of the anastomoses, which is observed mostly in non-coronary sinus [74]. Any symptomatic dehiscence investigated by echocardiography intra- or early postoperatively should be repaired and a reoperation should be performed immediately. In the absence of valve dysfunction, progressive dehiscence, or the development of thrombus a reoperation can be not necessary and conservative management will be safe during early- and long-term follow-up [75].

7.5. Progressive sinotubular junction dilatation

This late postoperative complication is observed in some stentless xenografts when they are implanted with the subcoronary technique. Currently, little is known of the diastolic properties of stentless valves that affect stress and strain on leaflets and, hence, their durability. Despite similar systolic performances, stentless prostheses behave differently during diastole. The commissures of the stentless bioprostheses have to follow the dimensional changes of the native aortic root not only in a cyclic mode but also the increase of the aortic diameter [76]. This change pulls apart the commissures leading to reduction of coaptation area of the cusps and late aortic insufficiency develops. Aortic regurgitation is often mild or moderate depending on bioprosthesis type, especially in old generation, but re-operation rate is low. In a pressurized aortic root model, a series of in-vitro tests is conducted to determine how stentless valves behave in diastole, and how they adapt to different annulus-to-sinotubular junction (STJ) ratios [77]. Pericardial prostheses built to mimic a cylinder (ATS 3F and Sorin Solo) showed the greatest tolerance to STJ dilatation and a larger coaptation surface, but also a tendency to roll in on themselves in an italic S-shape if oversized. Valves built to mimic native aortic leaflets (porcine Prima Plus and Medtronic Freestyle) showed a reduced tolerance to STJ dilatation, resulting in regurgitation and a smaller coaptation surface, but also a reduced tendency to roll if oversized.

A significant difference of tolerance against aortic regurgitation with respect to dilatation of the sinotubular junction was found in an in vitro study: fresh porcine aortic root (higher) > fresh porcine pulmonary root > stentless porcine bioprosthesis (lower) [78]. This loss of adaptability may be related to the glutaraldehyde fixation leading stiffness and shrinkage of the bioprosthetic leaflets which leaves inadequate coaptation reserve. An increase of sinotubular junction diameter of more than 32% for the Toronto SPV and 43% for Medtronic Freestyle stentless valves results in a distinct loss of leaflet coaptation and causes aortic regurgitation.

New generation of pericardial stentless valves developed for subcoronary implantation have larger coaptation area than those old generation or porcine stentless valves, which may provide better adaptability to adverse changes in root dimensions [79]. With massif progressive stepwise dilatation at sinotubular junction level, the free edges of the leaflets are stretched wider and a triangle-shaped central coaptation defect will occur. For the 3F Aortic valve regurgitation started at approximately 156% of the labeled valve size and 145% for the Sorin Solo valve. The increased tolerance of pericardial bioprostheses may improve long-term valve performance, but durability of these valves may be affected by the redundant leaflet tissue leading increase of leaflet stress and degeneration.

To overcome this disadvantage of stentless valves, a slight oversizing of the devices may result better valve competence and hemodynamic efficiency compared to size-for-size implantation. Sizing with a supra-annular seizer is helpful to find the largest stentless valve number which is minimum equal to the sinotubular junction diameter in patients with healthy aortic root. The single suture line technique is fixed prosthetic sinuses onto the native aortic wall to prevent any leakage or stretching.

7.6. Reoperation of a stentless aortic bioprosthesis

Stentless aortic valve reoperations may become more common as these bioprostheses reach the limits of their durability, which are a challenging procedure with an increased risk of death [80].The current generation of stentless valves have been implanted since the early 1990s and are therefore starting to reach the limits of their durability. Reoperation for stentless valves is a complex procedure, especially root inclusion or full-root replacement was preferred. The risk of trauma to the coronary ostia, aortic wall, aortic annulus, anterior mitral valve, and membranous septum can all occur when severe adhesions or calcification are present around the stentless valve. Reoperation after a stentless valve is more complex than after a stented tissue or mechanical valve if root replacement techniques is used in the first operation. However, reoperation of subcoronary implanted stentless bioprosthesis is easier than any stented prosthesis because cutting only the suture line is enough to remove the degenerated bioprosthesis. Valve-in-valve replacement with transfemoral [81] or transapical [82] AVI is a more conservative alternative strategy for re-replacement of degenerated xenograft in high risk patients.

8. Clinical results

8.1. Survival

Risk of death is highest immediately after AVR in patients with severe aortic stenosis, decreased to its nadir approximately 1 year postoperatively (early hazard period), and then gradually increased (late hazard period) [83]. From approximately 2 years after operation, survival is similar to that of matched population estimates. Early outcome of patients with aortic stenosis after AVR is primarily influenced by severity of the stenosis, left ventricular hypertrophy and dysfunction at operation. Severity of aortic stenosis, severe left ventricular hypertrophy, left ventricular dysfunction, older age and patient-prosthesis mismatch worsen also long-term survival. Furthermore, stentless AVR requires longer cross-clamp and cardiopulmonary bypass times.

Several meta-analysis studies confirm that stentless AVR does not worsen the early and late outcome when compared to stented bioprostheses. Also, longer operation times do not have any adverse effect on the intra-operatively mortal complications and postoperative outcomes. Contrarily, early recovery of hemodynamic malfunctions caused by calcific stenotic native aortic valve brings better early and late outcomes.

Hospital mortality rate of stentless bioprostheses is lower than those of stented xenografts [84,85]. Early hospital or 30-day mortality is similar between stentless and stented bioprosthesis replacement in a meta-analysis (3.2% versus 2.4%; p = 0.39), and further analysis of 30-days mortality is subgroups included predominantly patients with aortic stenosis shows still no significant difference between two types of aortic bioprosthesis (3.7% versus 2.6%; p = 0.44) [86]. Only one retrospective multicenter study has shown if stentless valves are used only in selected patients (older age, female, full-root replacement) the 30-day mortality is increased when compared with stented valves (7.5% versus 3.3%; p = 0.026), but if stentless valves are used widely there is no significant difference in operative mortality between stentless and stented groups [87].Using autologous pericardium does not worse the early hospital outcome and early mortality is not seen [11].

Several studies showed an improved mid-term (< 10 years) survival after stentless AVR compared to stented valves [88,89]. A meta-analysis shows that mortality at the first year is lower after stentless aortic bioprosthesis replacement than stented bioprosthesis, but not significant: 7.5% versus 8.9%; p = 0.73 [15]. Another meta analysis also confirm no significant difference for valve-related mortality between stentless and stented xenograft replacement in the first postoperative year [86]. Lehmann and associates [89] showed in a randomized trial that 8-year survival was 78.1% ± 3.8% stentless versus 66.7% ± 4.9% stented (p = 0.03). They concluded that there was no difference in survival when compared stentless patients with an age-matched German control population.

The long-term results (≥ 10 years) with stentless valves are excellent [90]. The overall 10- and 15-year survival rates of Freestyle bioprosthesis are 60.7% and 35%, respectively [91]. The 10-year actuarial survival (44.1% ± 4.3% in subcoronary, 47.3% ± 8.15 in full-root, and 45.4% ± 13.7% in root inclusion groups; p = 0.89) and freedom from valve-related death (94.5% ± 2.9% in subcoronary, 92.9% ± 5.8% in full-root, and 87.8% ± 12.5% in root inclusion groups; p = 0.17) are similar between implants techniques with the Freestyle stentless bioprosthesis [92]. Longer follow-up (> 15 years) of stentless valves is also necessary to compare the excellent results of stented valves to establish that stentless xenografts are significantly superior than stented devices.

8.2. Durability

The rate of structural valve deterioration increases over time, especially after the initial 7 to 8 years after implantation. Structural degeneration increases long-term events and the rate of failure is < 1% at 10 years in patients older than 65 years [93]. Pericardial valves might be better than porcine valves, but all newer-generation bioprostheses are more durable. In spite of the rate of failure of any bioprosthesis decreases with the age of the patient at the time of implantation (< 10% at 10 years in patients older > 70 years), the number of implanted stentless xenografts has increased due to improved hemodynamic performance and long-term durability during last decade. Theoretically, xenogenic stentless aortic valves have better durability than stented valves. But in real life, the freedom rate from structural valve deterioration is similar in stentless and stented bioprostheses (> 90% at 10 years). CryoLife O'Brien and St Jude Toronto SPV valves have worst durability compared the other stentless valves (Medtronic Freestyle, Edwards Prima, St Jude Biocor, Sorin Pericarbon and Solo, ATS 3f).

When we focus on the implantation techniques, there are very rare papers in the literature. The overall freedom from reoperation with Freestyle stentless bioprosthesis is 91.0% and 75.0% at 10 and 15 years, whereas freedom from reoperation for structural valve deterioration was 95.9% and 82.3%, respectively. At 10 and 15 years, freedom from reoperation for structural valve deterioration is 94.0% and 62.6% for patients < 60 years of age and 96.3% and 88.4% for patients ≥ 60 years of age (p = 0.002) [90]. The actuarial freedom from reoperation (91.7% ± 3.5%

in subcoronary, 92.3% ± 6.0% in full-root, and 92.0% ± 10.7% in root inclusion groups; p = 0.82) and from structural valve deterioration (97.0% ± 2.2% in subcoronary, 96.0% ± 4.5% in full-root, and 90.9% ± 11.2% in root inclusion groups; p = 0.54) are similar between implants techniques with the Freestyle stentless valves [91].

The truly stentless autologous pericardial aortic valve may be better choice in patients who cannot or do not want to take anticoagulation, especially young population, because excellent long-term durability and easier reoperation, which is technically undemanding compared to other stentless bioprostheses. The use of autologous pericardium avoids any immune reaction between the host and the implanted valve, and minimizes tissue calcification and pannus formation, which are important causes of structural valve deterioration. The absence of a stent and sewing ring is also helpful for long-term durability with a freedom from structural valve deterioration of 100% at 7.5 years [11]. Long-term durability seems better than the other bioprostheses because it has been reported that there is no calcification, no structural dysfunction on the autologous pericardium used for aortic leaflet extension at 13 years [94]. Reoperation must be easier because there is no calcification on the aorta and pericardial aortic valve.

8.3. Echocardiographic outcomes

The advantage of stentless xenografts is providing a greater EOA index for a given valve size, which results lower transvalvular gradients compared with stented valves. These improvements have been reported in a meta analysis: lower mean aortic valve gradient (-3.57 mmHg; p < 0.01), lower peak gradient (-5.8 mmHg; p< 0.01), but higher EOA index in stentless group compared with the stented [15]. It has been shown in an experimental porcine model that the annular cross-sectional area of stentless valves is significantly larger than stented valves [23]. The EOA will increase after first postoperative year in stentless valves and significant differences in mean and/or peak pressure differences between stentless and stented valves will continue during long-term follow-up [95,96].

The Freedom SOLO stentless bioprosthesis with all size-number has a lower mean (10.6 ± 3.6 mmHg) and peak (15.9 ± 9.1 mmHg) transvalvular gradient at discharged, and below 10 mmHg in all sizes (21-27 mm) at the first postoperative year [97]. The similar results have been shown by other groups: lower mean gradient (6.7 +/- 4.1 mmHg) and a significant regression of left ventricular hypertrophy (23%) at 12 months [98].

3f aortic bioprosthesis has a satisfactory hemodynamic performance with substitutes larger than 23 mm (< 10 mmHg), but smaller valves have a significant higher mean transvalvular gradient at the 4-postoperative year (18 mmHg for 21 mm and 14 mmHg for 23 mm devices) [36]. The left ventricular mass index decreases during follow-up (showed 18% regression), but cannot reach the normal range, especially with small devices. In another study with a mean valve size 26.0 ± 1.9 mm has shown that the mean transvalvular gradient of 3f bioprostheses has increased at 5 years (15.2 ± 5.3 mmHg) [99].

The Edwards Prima Plus stentless valve bioprosthesis is a porcine aortic root cylinder and is associated with high early peak and mean transprosthetic gradients (37 ± 16 and 18 ±8 mmHg, respectively), which regress with significant improvement at 1 year (25 ±7 and 12 ±4 mmHg, respectively) and concomitant regression of left ventricular hypertrophy [100]. The Edwards Prima Plus stentless xenograft implanted with intact non-coronary sinus technique prevents the geometry of the device and has excellent long-term result (mean gradient < 10 mmHg) in all sizes (21-29 mm) [101].

There are some studies showing different results regarding transaortic gradient, which might be a result of different stentless xenografts or implantation methods. There is no any significantly difference among implantation techniques when the same stentless xeno-graft is used with different implantation techniques, but full root (4.8 mmHg) or root in-clusion technique (5.1 mmHg) has lower mean transvalvular gradient than the subcoronary technique (7.2 mmHg) [102]. Transvalvular gradient and EOA are significant-ly worse in subcoronary groups in the first postoperative period, but this difference will be insignificant due to decreasing EOA and root inclusion approach will have the worst hemodynamics at 10th postoperative year [90].

Stentless valves are the best choice in patients with small aortic annuli than large annuli, because the lower transaortic pressure difference of stentless valves has no any significant advantage over stented bioprostheses if a valve larger than 23 mm will be used [103]. The difference will be significantly when a stentless valve sized 23 mm is used (Freestyle in-clusion 11 mmHg versus Perimount 25 mmHg) [21]. The Freedom SOLO stentless bio-prosthesis seems to have better hemodynamics even in patients received a small aortic bioprosthesis with a lower mean transvalvular gradient (9 ± 2.9 mmHg for 21 mm, and 7.6 ± 5 mmHg for 23 mm) [97].

Physically active patients might benefit from stentless valves. Several studies showed that the gradient difference between different aortic stentless and stented bioprostheses of similar size with different implantation techniques increased significantly at each exercise level in favour of stentless valves [104-105106].

9. Conclusion

Aortic valve replacement means that native valve disease is replaced with prosthetic valve inadequacy affected by prosthetic valve hemodynamics, durability, and thrombogenicity. Stentless bioprostheses have better hemodynamic properties because of larger effective orifice area, better coronary flow, lower transvalvular gradient and better left ventricular mass regression than stented bioprostheses. They have also better biomechanical properties and the preserved distensibility may diminish stress considerably. Valve-related morbidity and structural valve degeneration are not worse than stented valves, but their implantation is demanding and required experience in this field. Although experienced centers give excellent results with stentless xenografts, most surgeons also prefer a stented xenograft to keep the procedure quick, safe, and simple. But, there is a trend to favor stentless valves nowadays because these valves provide larger effective orifice area, lower transvalvular gradients and excellent hemodynamics which stimulate rapid and effective reduction in left ventricular hypertrophy. It seems that the usage of stentless valves has more advantages in patients with impaired left ventricular function, small aortic, or aortic root abscess or more active patients. In future, using of stentless valves will increase with simpler implantation techniques, increased surgical experience, new design of prostheses, may be, using sutureless valves.

Author details

Kaan Kirali*

Address all correspondence to: imkbkirali@yahoo.com

Depertment of cardiovascular surgery, kosuyolu heart and research hospital, Istanbul, Turkey

References

[1] Ross DN. Homograft Replacement of the Aortic Valve. Lancet 1962;2:487.

[2] Barrat-Boyes BG. Homograft Aortic Valve Replacement in Aortic Incompetence and Stenosis. Thorax 1964;19:131-150.

[3] Binet JP, Duran CCT, Carpentier A, Langlois J. Heterologous Aortic Valve Transplantation. Lancet 1965;2:1275-1276.

[4] Sievers HH, Lange PE, Bernhard A. Implantation of a xenogenic Stentless Aortic Bioprosthesis. First Experience. Thoracic Cardiovascular Surgeon 1985;33(4):225-226.

[5] David TE, Pollick C, Bos J. Aortic Valve Replacement with Stentless Porcine Aortic Bioprosthesis. Journal of Thoracic Cardiovascular Surgery 1990;99(1):113-118.

[6] Pelletier LC, Carrier M. Bioprosthetice Heart Valves: 25 Years of Development and Clinical Experience. In: Acar J and Bodnar E (eds). Textbook of Acquired Heart Valve Disease. ICR Publishers: London; 1995. p920-956.

[7] David TE. Stentless Bioprosthetic Valves. In: Acar J and Bodnar E (eds). Textbook of Acquired Heart Valve Disease. ICR Publishers: London; 1995. p957-964.

[8] Takkenberg JJM, Klieverik LMA, Schoof PH, van Suylen R-J, van Herwerden LA, Zondervan PE, Roos-Hesselink JW, Eijkemans MJ, Yacoub MH, Bogers AJ. The Ross Procedure. A Systematic Rewiev and Meta-Analysis. Circulation. 2009;119(2): 222-228.

[9] El-Hamamsy I, Clark L, Stevens LM, Sarang Z, Melina G, Takkenberg JJ, Yacoub MH. Late Outcomes Following Freestyle versus Homograft Aortic Root Replace-

ment. Results from a Prospective Randomized Trial. Journal of American College of Cardiology 2010;55(4):368-376.

[10] Love JW. Autologous Pericardial Reconstruction of Semilunar Valves. Journal of Heart Valve Disease 1998;7(1):40–47.

[11] Chan KMJ, Rahman-Haley S, Mittal TK, Gavino JA, Dreyfus GD. Truly StentlessAutologous Pericardial Aortic Valve Replacement: An Alternative to Standard Aortic Valve Replacement. Journal of Thoracic Cardiovascular Surgery 2011;141(1):276-283.

[12] Frost MW, Funderl JA, Klaaborg KE, Wierup P, Sloth E, Nygaard H, Hasenkam JM. Leaflet Opening and Closing Dynamics of Aortic Bioprostheses. Journal of Heart Valve Disease 2010;19(4):492-498.

[13] Revanna P, Fisher J, Watterson KG. The Influence of Free Hand Sturing Technique and Zero Pressure Fixation on the Hemodynamic Function of Aortic Root and Aortic Valve Leaflets. European Journal of Cardiovascular Surgery 1997;11(2):280-286.

[14] Cohen G, Christakis GT, Joyner CD, Morgan CD, Tamariz M, Hanayama N, Mallidi H, Szalai JP, Katic M, Rao V, Fremes SE, Goldman BS. Are Stentless Valves Hemodynamically Superior to Stented Valves? A Prospective Randomized Trial. Annals of Thoracic Surgery 2002;73(3):767-775.

[15] Kunadian B, Vijayalakshmi K, Thornley AR, de Belder MA, Hunter S, Kendall S, Graham R, Stewart M, Thambyrajah J, Dunning J. Meta-analysis of Valve Hemodynamics and Left Ventricular Mass Rregression for Stentless versus Stented Aortic Valves. Annals of Thoracic Surgery 2007;84(1):73-78.

[16] Perez de Arenaza D, Lees B, Flather M, Nugara F, Huseybe T, Jasinski M, CisowskiM, KhanM, HeneinM, GaerJ, GuvendikL, BochenekA, WosS, LieM, VanNootenG, PennellD, PepperJ. Randomized comparison of Stentless versus Stented Valves for Aortic Stenosis: Effects on the Left Ventricular Mass. Circulation 2005;112(17): 2696-702.

[17] Dunning J, Graham RJ, Thambyrajah J, Stewart MJ, Kendall SW, Hunter S. Stentless vs Stented Aortic valve Bioprostheses: A Prospective Randomized Controlled Trial. European Heart Journal 2007;28(19):2369-2374.

[18] Gulbins H, Reichenspurner H. Which Patients Benefit from Stentless Aortic Valve Replacement? Annals of Thoracic Surgery 2009;88(6):2061-2068.

[19] Rabus MB, Kirali K, Kayalar N, Tuncer EY, Toker ME, Yakut C. Aortic Valve Replacement in Isolated Severe Aortic Stenosis with Left Ventricular Dysfunction: Long-term Survival and ventricular Recovery. AnatolianJournalofCardiology2009;9(1):41-46.

[20] Borger MA, Carson SM, Ivanov J, Rao V, Scully HE, Feindell CM, David TE. Stentless Aortic Valve are Hemodynamically Superior to Stented Valves During Mid-term Fol-

low-up: A Large Retrospective Study. Annals of Thoracic Surgery 2005;80(6): 2180-2185.

[21] Williams RJ, Muir DF, Pathi V, MacArthur K, Berg GA. Randomized Controlled Trial of Stented and Stentless Aortic Bioprostheses: Hemodynamic Performance at 3 Years. Seminars Thoracic Cardiovascular Surgery1999;11(4 Suppl 1):93-97.

[22] Narang S, Satsangi DK, Banerjee A, Geelani MA. Stentless Valves versus Stented Biprotheses at the Aortic Position: Midterm Results. Journal of Thoracic Cardiovascular Surgery 2008;136(4):943-947.

[23] Ali A, Halstead JC, Cafferty F, Sharples L, Rose F, Coulden R, LeeE, DunningJ, Arganov, TsuiS. Are Stentless Valves Superior to Modern Stented valves? A prospective Randomized Trial. Circulation 2006;114(1 Suppl):I535-I540.

[24] Funder JA, Ringgaard S, Frost MW, Wierup P, Klaaborg KE, Hjortdal V, NygaardH, HasenkamJM. Aortic Root Distensibility and Cross-sectional Areas in Stented and Subcoronary Stentless Bioprostheses in Pigs. Interactive Cardiovascular Thoracic Surgery 2010;10(6):976-980.

[25] Ennker JAC, Albert AA, Rosendahl UP, Ennker IC, Dalladaku F, Florath I. Ten-Year Experience With Stentless Aortic Valves: Full-Root Versus Subcoronary Implantation. Annals of Thoracic Surgery 2008;85(2):445-453.

[26] Schoof PH. Stentless Valve Dehiscence. Journal of Thoracic Cardiovascular Surgery 2008;136(1):231.

[27] Al Kindi AH, Huu AL, Shum-Tim D. Early Stenosis of Stentless Aortic Valve Prosthesis: A Word of Caution. Annals of Thoracic Surgery 2012;

[28] Tuncer A,Tuncer EY,Polat A, Mataracı İ, Keleş C, Aulasaleh S, Boyacıoğlu K, Kara İ, Kırali K. Axillary Artery Cannulation in Ascending Aortic Pathologies. Turkish Journal of Thoracic Cardiovascular Surgery 2011;19(4):539-544.

[29] Güler M, Akıncı E, Dağlar B, Kırali K, Eren E, Balkanay M, Berki T, Gürbüz A, Yakut C. Continuous Retrograde Coronary Sinus Isothermic Blood Cardioplegia with no Antegrade Combination in Aortic Valve Surgery. Turkish Journal of Thoracic Cardiovascular Surgery 1998;6(3):292-300.

[30] Kırali K, Göksedef D, Yakut C. Reverse "U" Aortotomy for Aortic Valve Replacement After Previous Coronary Artery Bypass Grafting. Journal of Cardiac Surgery 2005;20(3):269-270.

[31] Kobayashi J. Stentless Aortic Valve Replacement: An Update. Vascular Healt Risk Management 2011;7:345-351.

[32] Beholz S, Dushe S, Konertz W. Continuous Suture Technique for Freedom Stentless Valve: Reduced Crossclamp Time. Asian Cardiovascular Thoracic Annals 2006;14(2): 128-133.

[33] Song Z, lehr EJ, Wang S. An Alternative Subcoronary Implantation Technique Decreases the Risk of Complete Heart Block After Stentless Aortic Valve Replacement. Journal of Cardiovascular Disease Research 2012;3(1):46-51.

[34] Aymard T, Eckstein F, Englberger L, Stalder M, Kadner A, Carrel T. TheSorinFreedomSOLOStentlessAorticValve:TechniqueofImplantationandOperativeResultsin109Patients.Journal of Thoracic Cardiovascular Surgery 2010;139(3):775-777.

[35] Repossini A, Kotelnikov I, Bouchikhi R, Torre T, Passaretti B, Parodi O, Arena V. Single-suture Line Placement of a Pericardial Stentless Valve. JournalofThoracicCardiovascularSurgery 2005;130(5):1265-1269.

[36] Pillai R, Ratnatunga C, Soon JL, Kattach H, Khalil A, Jin XY. 3f Prosthesis Aortic Cusp Replacement: Implantation Technique and Early Results. Asian Cardiovascular Thoracic Annals 2010;18(1):13-16.

[37] D'OnofrioA, MessinaA, LorussoR, AlfieriOR, FusariM, RubinoP, RinaldiM, DiBartolomeoR, GlauberM, TroiseG, GerosaG. Sutureless Aortic Valve Replacement as an Alternative Treatment for Patients Belonging to the "Gray Zone" Between Transcatheter Aortic ValveIimplantation and Conventional Surgery: A Propensity-matched, Multicenter Analysis. JournalofThoracicCardiovascularSurgery 2012 Sep 10. pii: S0022-5223(12)00883-5. doi: 10.1016/j.jtcvs.2012.07.040. [Epub ahead of print]

[38] Shrestha M, KhaladjN, BaraC, HoefflerK, HaglC, HaverichA. A Ataged Approach Towards Interventional Aortic Valve Implantation with a Sutureless Valve: Initial Human Implants. ThoracicCardiovascularSurgeon 2008;56(7):398-400.

[39] Santarpino G, Pfeiffer S, Concistrè G, Fischlein T. ASupra-annularMalpositionofthePercevalSSuturelessAorticValve:The'χ-movement'RemovalTechniqueandSubsequentReimplantation.Interactive Cardiovascular Thoracic Surgery 2012;15(2):280-281.

[40] Folliguet TA, Laborde F, Zannis K, Ghorayeb G, haverich A, Shrestha M. Sutureless Percaval Aortic Valve Replacement: Results of Two European Centers. Annals of Thoracic Surgery 2012;93(5):1483-1488.

[41] Santarpino G, Pfeiffer S, Schmidt J, Concistrè G, Fischlein T. SuturelessAorticValveReplacement:First-yearSingle-centerExperience.Annals of Thoracic Surgery2012;94(2): 504-508.

[42] Cox JL, Ad N, Myers K, Gharib M, Quijano RC. Tubular Heart Valves: A New Tissue Prosthesis Design - Preclinical evaluation of the 3f Aortic Bioprosthesis. Journal of Thoracic Cardiovascular Surgery 2005;130(2):520-527.

[43] Risteski P, Adami C, Papadopoulos N, Sirat SA, Moritz A, Doss M. Leaflet Replacement for Aortic Stenosis Using the 3f Stentless Aortic Bioprosthesis: Midterm Results. Annals of Thoracic Surgery 2012;93(4):1134-1140.

[44] Martens S, Sadowski J, Eckstein FS, Bartus K, Kapelak B, Sievers HH, Schlensak C, Carrel T. ClinicalExperiencewiththeATS3fEnable®SuturelessBioprosthesis.European Journal of Cardiothoracic Surgery 2011;40(3):749-755.

[45] Sepehripour AH, Harling L, Athanasiou T. What Are the Current Results of Sutureless Valves In High-risk Aortic Valve Disease Patients? Interactive Cardiovascular Thoracic Surgery 2012;14(5):615-621.

[46] HolmesDRJr, MackMJ, KaulS, AgnihotriA, AlexanderKP, BaileySR, CalhoonJH, CarabelloBA, DesaiMY, EdwardsFH, FrancisGS, GardnerTJ, KappeteinAP, LinderbaumJA, MukherjeeC, MukherjeeD, OttoCM, RuizCE, SaccoRL, SmithD, ThomasJD. 2012 ACCF/AATS/SCAI/STS Expert Consensus Document on Transcatheter Aortic Valve Replacement: Developed in Collaboration with the American Heart Association, American Society of Echocardiography, European Association for Cardio-Thoracic Surgery, Heart Failure Society of America, Mended Hearts, Society of Cardiovascular Anesthesiologists, Society of Cardiovascular Computed Tomography, and Society for Cardiovascular Magnetic Resonance. AnnalsofThoracicSurgery 2012;93(4): 1340-1395.

[47] Kirali K, Mansuroğlu D, Omeroğlu SN, Erentuğ V, Mataraci I, Ipek G, Akıncı E, Işık Ö, Yakut C. Five-year Experience in Aortic Root Replacement with the Flanged Composite Graft. Annals of Thoracic Surgery 2002;73(4):1130-1137.

[48] Kirsh MEW, Ooka T, Zannis K, deux JF, Loisance DY. Bioprosthetic Replacement of The Ascending Thoracic Aorta: What Are The Options? European Journal of Cardiothoracic Surgery 2009;35(1):77-82.

[49] Urbansky PP, Hacker RW. Replacement of the Aortic Valve and Ascending Aorta with a Valved Stentless Composite Graft: Technical Considerations and Early Clinical Results. Annals of Thoracic Surgery 2000;70(1):17-20.

[50] De Paulis R, Nardi P, De Matteis GM, Polisca P, Chiariello L. Bentall Procedure with a Stentless Valve and a New Aortic Root prosthesis. Annals of Thoracic Surgery 2001;71(4):1375-1376.

[51] Kırali K, Sarıkaya S, Elibol A, Göçer S, Özer T, Altaş Ö, Ünal ÜS, Şişmanoğlu M. Aortic Root Replacement with the Reimplantation Procedure: Simplifiying the Sizing of Tubular Graft. 20th Annual Meeting for Asian Society for Cardiovascular and Thoracic Surgery, 7-11 March 2012; Bali, Indonesia.

[52] Kaya A, Heijmen RH, Kelder JC, Morshuis WJ. First 102 Patients With the Biovalsalva Conduit for Aortic Root Replacement. Annals of Thoracic Surgery 2012;94(1): 72-77.

[53] Hemmer WB, Botha CA, Böhm JO, Herrmann T, Starck C, Rein JG. replacement of the Aortic Valve and Ascending Aorta with an Extended Root Stentless Xenograft. Annals of Thoracic Surgery 2004;78(6):2150-2153.

[54] Massetti M, Veron S, Neri E, Coffin O, le Page O, Babatasi G, Buklas D, Maiza D, Gerard JL, Khayat A. Long-term Durability of Resection and End-To-End Anastomosis for Ascending Aortic Aneurysms. Journal of Thoracic Cardiovascular Surgery 2003;127(5):1381-1387.

[55] Akpınar B, Güden M, Aytekin S, Sanisoğlu I, Sagbas E, Ozbek U, Caynak B, Bayramoglu Z. The Use of Stentless Valves for Root Replacement During Repair of Ascending Aortic Aneurysms with Aortic Valve Regurgitation. Heart Surgery Forum 2002;5(1):52-56.

[56] Carrel TP, Berdat P, Englberger L, Eckstein F, Immer F, Seiler C, Kipfer B, Schmidt J. Aortic Root Replacement with a New Stentless Aortic Valve Xenograft Conduit: Preliminary Hemodynamic and Clinical Results. Journal of Heart Valve Disease 2003;12(6):752-757.

[57] Rabus MB, Kirali K, KayalarN, MataraciI, YanartasM, Ulusoy-BozbugaN, YakutC. Effects of Patient-Prosthesis Mismatch on Postoperative Early Mortality in Isolated Aortic Stenosis. Journal of Heart Valve Disease2009;18(1):18-27.

[58] Head SJ, Mokhles MM, Osnabrugge RLJ, Pibarot P, Mack MJ, Takkenberg JJM, Bogers JJCA, Kappetein AP. The Impact of Prosthesis–Patient Mismatch on Long-term Survival After Aortic Valve Replacement: A Systematic Review and Meta-Analysis of 34 Observational Studies Comprising 27 186 Patients with 133 141 Patient-years. European Heart Journal 2012;33():1518–1529.

[59] Shiono N, Watanabe Y, Kawasaki M, Yokomuro H, Fujii T, Koyama N. Evaluation of Bioprosthetic Valve for Small Aortic Root in Elderly Patients. Asian Cardiovascular Thoracic Annals 2007;15(1):102-105.

[60] Ardal H, Toker ME, Rabuş MB, Uyar İ, Antal A, Şişmanoğlu M, Mansuroğlu D, Kırali K, Yakut C. Does Aortic Root Enlargement Impair theOoutcome of Patients With Small Aortic Root? Journal of Cardiac Surgery 2006;21(5):449-453.

[61] Bical OM, Nutu O, D2eleuze P. A Technique of Aortic Annulus Enlargement with a Freestyle Stentless Bioprosthesis. Annals of Thoracic Surgery 2012;93(3):680-681.

[62] Goland S, Trento A, Czer LSC, Eshaghian S, Tolstrup K, Naqvi TZ, De Robertis MA, Mirocha J, Iida K, Siegel RJ. Thoracic Aortic Arteriosclerosis in Patients With Degenerative Aortic Stenosis With and Without Coexisting Coronary Artery Disease. Annals of Thoracic Surgery 2008;85(1):113-119.

[63] GillinovAM, LytleBW, HoangV, CosgroveDM, BanburyMK, McCarthyPM, SabikJF, PetterssonGB, SmediraNG, BlackstoneEH. The Atherosclerotic Aorta at Aortic Valve Replacement: Surgical Strategies and Results. Journal of Thoracic Cardiovascular Surgery 2000;120(5):957-963.

[64] Rode´s-Cabau J,Webb JG, Cheung A, Ye J, Dumont E, Feindel CM, Osten M, Natarajan MK, Velianou JL, Martucci G, DeVarennes B, Chisholm R, Peterson MD, Lichtenstein SV, Nietlispach F, Doyle D, DeLarochellie`re R, Teoh K, Chu V, Dancea A,

Lachapelle K, Cheema A, Latter D, Horlick E. Transcatheter Aortic Valve Implantation for theTtreatment of Severe Symptomatic Aortic Stenosis in Patients at Very High or Prohibitive Surgical Risk: Acute and Late Outcomes of the Multicenter Canadian Experience. Journal of American Collage Cardiology 2010;55(11):1080-1090.

[65] Buz S, Pasic M, Unbehaun A, Drews T, Dreysse S, kukucka M, Mladenow A, Hetzer R. Trans-apical Aortic Valve Implantation in Patients with Severe Calcification of the Ascending Aorta. European Journal of Cardiothoracic Surgery 2011;40(2):463-468.

[66] RabuşMB, KayalarN, SareyyüpoğluB, ErkinA, Kirali K, YakutC. Hypercholesterolemia Association with Aortic Stenosis of Various Etiologies. JournalofCardiacSurgery 2009;24(2):146-150.

[67] Taş S, Dönmez AA, Kırali K, Alp M, Yakut C. Aortic Valve Replacement for a Patient with Glucose-6-Phosphate Dehydrogenase Deficiency and Autoimmune Hemolytic Anemia. Jornal of Cardiac Surgery 2005;20(4):380-381.

[68] Kirali K, Aksoy E, Buyukbayrak F, Yanartas M, Elibol A, Ozer T, Boyacioglu K, Kis M, Sismanoglu M, Mataraci I. Does Thrombocytopenia Aggravate early Outcome After Aortic Valve Replacement with a Bioprosthesis. 16th World Congress on Heart Disease for Intenational Academy of Cardiology, 23-26 July 2011; Vancouver, Canada.

[69] RepossiniA, BlochD, MunerettoC, PiccoliP, BisleriG, BeholzS. Platelet Reduction After Stentless Pericardial Aortic Valve Replacement. InteractiveCardiovascularThoracicSurgery 2012;14(4):434-438.

[70] GersakB, GartnerU, AntonicM. ThrombocytopeniaFollowingImplantationoftheSstentlessBiologicalSorinFreedomSOLOValve.Journal of Heart Valve Disease 2011;20(4): 401-406.

[71] El-Hamamsy I, Zaki M, Stevens LM, ClarkLA, RubensM, MelinaG, YacoubMH. Rate of Progression and Functional Significance of Aortic Root Calcification After homograft versus Freestyle AorticRrootRreplacement. Circulation 2009;120(Suppl 1):S269-S275.

[72] Erdoğan HB, Kayalar N, Ardal H, Ömeroğlu SN, Kırali K, Güler M, Akıncı E, Yakut C. Risk Factors for Requirement of Permanent Pacemaker Implantation After Aortic Valve Replacement. Journal of Cardiac Surgery2006;21(3):211-215.

[73] Kincaid EH, Cordell R, Hammon JW, Adair SM, Kon ND. Coronary Insufficiency After Stentless Aortic Root Replacement: Risk Factors and Solutions. Annals of Thoracic Surgery 2007;83(3):964-968.

[74] Schoof P, Baur L, Kappetein A, Hazekamp M, vanRijk-Zwikker G, Huysmans H. Dehiscence of the Freestyle Stentless Bioprosthesis. Seminars in Thoracic Cardiovascular Surgery 1999;11(suppl 1):133-138.

[75] Hopkins R, Gitter H, Stave J, Bert A, Atalay M. Stable Partial Dehiscence of Aortic Homograft Inserted Freehand by Using the Subcoronary Intra-aortic Root Noncoro-

nary Sinus Ross Scallop Inclusion technique. Journal of Thoracic Cardiovascular Surgery 2008;135(1):214-216.

[76] David TE, Ivanov J, eriksson MJ, Feindel CM, Rakowski H. Dilatation of the Sinotubular Junction Causes Aortic Insufficiency After Aortic Valve Replacement with the Toronto SPV Bioprosthesis. Journal Thoracic Cardiovascular Surgery 2001;122(5): 929-934.

[77] WeltertL, NardellaS, GirolaF, ScaffaR, BellisarioA, MaselliD, DePaulisR. Diastolic Properties of the SorinSolo, ATS 3F, Edwards Prima Plus and Medtronic Freestyle Stentless Valves: An Independent in-vitro Comparison. JournalHeartValveDis-ease. 2012;21(1):99-105.

[78] Nötzold A, Scharfschwerdt M, Thiede L, Hüppe M, Sievers HH. In-vitro Study on the Relationship Between Progressive Sinotubular Junction Dilatation and Aortic Regurgitation for Several Stentless Aortic Valve Substitutes. European Journal of Cardiothoracic Surgery 2005;27(1):90-93.

[79] Scharfschwerdt M, Sievers HH, Hussein A, Kraatz EG, Misfeld M. Impact of Progressive Sinotubular Junction Dilatation on Valve Competence of the 3F Aortic and Sorin Solo Stentless Bioprosthetic Heart Valves. European Journal of Cardiothoracic Surgery 2010;37(3):631-634.

[80] Borger MA, Prasongsukarn K, Armstrong S, Feindel CM, David TE. Stentless Aortic Valve Reoperations: A Surgical Challenge. Annals of Thoracic Surgery 2007;84(3): 737-744.

[81] Finch J, Roussin I, Pepper J. Failing Stentless Aortic Valves: Redo Aortic Root Replacement or Valve in a Valve. European Journal of Cardiothoracic Surgery 2012;42():

[82] Ferrari E. Transapical Aortic 'valve-in-valve' Procedure for Degenerated Stented Bioprosthesis. European Journal of Cardiothoracic Surgery 2012;41(3):485-490.

[83] Mihaljevic T, Nowicki ER, Rajeswaran J, Blackstone EH, Lagazzi L, Thomas J, Lytle BW, Cosgrove DM. Survival After Valve Replacement For Aortic Stenosis: Implications for Decision Making. Journal of Thoracic Cardiovascular Surgery 2008;135(6): 1270-1279.

[84] Luciani GB, Casali G, Auriemma S, SantiniF, MazzuccoA. Survival After Stentless and Stented Xenograft Aortic Valve Replacement: A Concurrent, Controlled Trial. Annals of Thoracic Surgery 2002;7485):1443-1449.

[85] Dunning J, Graham RJ, Thambyrajah J, StewartMJ, KendallSW, HunterS. Stentless vs Stented Aortic Valve Bioprostheses: A Prospective Randomized Controlled Trial. European Heart Journal 2007;28(19):2369-2374.

[86] Murtaza B, Pepper JR, Jones C, Nihoyannopoulos P, Darzi A, Athanasiou T. Does Stentless Aortic Valve Implantation Increase perioperative Risk? A Critical Appraisal

of the Literature and Risk of Bias Analysis. European Journal of Cardiothoracic Surgery 2011;39(5):643-652.

[87] Westaby S, JönsonA, PayneN, SaitoS, JinXY, DelRizzoDF, GrunkemeierG. Does The Use of a Stentless Bioprosthesis Increase Surgical Risk?SeminarsThoracicCardiovascularSurgery 2001;13(4, Suppl 1):143-147.

[88] Borger MA, Carson SM, Ivanov J, RaoV, ScullyHE, FeindelCM, DavidTE. Stentless Aortic Valve Are Hemodynamically Superior to Stented valves during Mid-term follow-up: A Large Retrospective Study. Annals of Thoracic Surgery 2005;80(6): 2180-2185.

[89] Lehmann S, Walther T, Kempfert J, Leontjev A, Ardawan R, Falk V, Mohr FW. Stentless Versus Conventional Xenograft Aortic Valve Replacement: Midterm Results of a Prospectively Randomized Trial. Annals of Thoracic Surgery 2007;84(2):467-472.

[90] Bach DS, Kon ND, Dumesnil JG, Sintek CF, Ross DB. Ten-Year Outcome after Aortic Valve Replacement with the Freestyle Stentless Bioprosthesis. Annals of Thoracic Surgery 2005;80(2):480-487.

[91] Mohammadi S, Tchana-Sato V, Kalavrouziotis D, Voisine P, Doyle D, Baillot R, Sponga S, Metras J, Perron J, Dagenais F. Long-termClinicalandEchocardiographicFollow-upoftheFreestyleStentlessAorticBioprosthesis.Circulation 2012;126(11 Suppl 1):S198-S204.

[92] Bach DS, Kon ND, DumesnilJG, SintekCF, DotyDB. Ten-year Outcome After Aortic Valve Replacement With the Freestyle Stentless Bioprosthesis. AnnalsofThoracicSurgery 2005;80(2):480-486.

[93] Borger MA, Prasongsukarn K, Armstrong S, Feindel CM, David TE. Stentless Aortic Valve Reoperations: A Surgical Challenge. Annals of Thoracic Surgery 2007;84(3): 737-744.

[94] Jeong DS, Kim K-H, Ahn H. Long-term Results of the Leaflet Extension Technique in Aortic Regurgitation: Thirteen Years of Experience in a Single Centre. Annals of Thoracic Surgery 2009;88(1):83-89.

[95] Cohen G, Zagorski B, Christakis GT, Joyner CD, Vincent J, Sever J, HarbiS, Feder-ElituvR, MoussaF, GoldmanBS, FremesSE. Are Stentless Valves Hemodynamically Superior to Stented valves? Long-term Follow-up of a randomized trial Comparing Carpentier-Edwards Pericardial Valve With The Toronto Stentless porcine Valves? Journal of Thoracic Cardiovascular Surgery 2010;139(4):848-859.

[96] Chamber JB, Rimington HM, Hodson F, Rajani R, Blauth CI. The Subcoronary Toronto Stentless Versus Supra-annular Perimount Stented Replacement Aortic Valve: Early Clinical and Hemodynamic results of a Randomized Comparison in 160 Patients. Journal of Thoracic Cardiovascular Surgery 2006;131(4):878-882.

[97] Iliopoulos DC, Deveja AR, Androutsopoulou V, Filias V, Kastelanos E, Satratzemis V, Khalpey Z, Koudoumas D. Single-centerExperienceUsingtheFreedomSOLOAor-

ticBioprosthesis. Journal of Thoracic Cardiovascular Surgery 2012;(:http://dx.doi.org/
10.1016/j.jtcvs.2012.06.041)

[98] BeholzS, RepossiniA, LiviU, SchepensM, ElGabryM, MatschkeK, TrivediU, EckelL,
DapuntO, ZamoranoJL. The Freedom SOLO Valve for Aortic Valve Replacement:
Clinical and Hemodynamic Results from a Prospective Multicenter Trial. Journal-
HeartValveDisease 2010;19(1):115-123.

[99] Linneweber J, Heinbokel T, Christ T, Claus B, Kossagk C, Konertz W. Clinical Experience with the ATS 3F Stentless Aortic Bioprosthesis: Five Years' Follow Up. Journal
Heart Valve Disease 2010;19(6):772-777.

[100] TanakaK, KinoshitaT, FujinagaK, KanemitsuS, TanakaJ, SuzukiH, TokuiT. Hemody-
namicPerformanceoftheEdwardsPrimaPlusStentlessValveat1Year. GeneralThoracic-
CardiovascularSurgery2008;56(9):441-445.

[101] Luciani GB, Viscardi F, Cresce GD, Faggian G, Mazzucco A.Seven-Year Performance
of the Edwards Prima Plus Stentless Valve with the Intact Non-Coronary Sinus Tech-
nique.Journal of Cardiac Surgery 2008;23(3):221-226.

[102] Kappetein AP, Braun J, Baur LHB, Prat A, Peels K, Hazekamp MG, Schoof PH, Huysmans HA. Outcome and Follow-up of Aortic Valve Replacement with The Freestyle
Stentless Bioprosthesis. Annals of Thoracic Surgery 2001;71(2):601-607.

[103] Van Nooten G, Caes F, Francois K, Van BY, Taeymans Y. Stentless or Stented Aortic
Valve Implants in Elderly Patients? European Journal of Cardiothoracic Surgery
1999;15(1):31-36.

[104] Eriksson MJ, Rosfors S, Radegran K, Brodin LA. Effects of Exercise on Doppler-de-
rived Pressure Difference, Valve Resistance, and Effective Orifice Area in Different
Aortic Valve Prostheses of Similar Size. American Journal of Cardiology 1999;83(4):
619-622.

[105] Bleiziffer S, Eichinger WB, Wagner I, Guenzinger R, Bauernschmitt R, Lange R. The
Toronto Root Stentless Valve in the Subcoronary Position is Hemodynamically Supe-
rior to the Mosaic Stented Completely Supra-annular Bioprosthesis. Journal of Heart
Valve Disease 2005;14(6):814-821.

[106] Fries R, Wendler O, Schieffer H, Schaefers HJ. Comparative Rest and Exercise Hemodynamics of 23-mm Stentless Versus 23-mm Stented Aortic Bioprostheses. Annals of
Thoracic Surgery 2000;69(3):817-822.

Aortic Valve Replacement for Calcified Aortic Valves

Kazumasa Orihashi

Additional information is available at the end of the chapter

1. Introduction

Valve replacement has been the standard treatment for aortic stenosis until the development of transcatheter aortic valve implantation (TAVI). Although TAVI provides a treatment with fairly acceptable outcomes for patients with high surgical risk, aortic valve replacement remains essential even in the TAVI era, because surgical treatment is indicated when TAVI cannot be performed due to a small aortic annulus or inappropriate access route. In addition, surgical treatment may be necessary when complications develop during TAVI procedures. Therefore, a more meticulous procedure is required for surgeons. With an increasing number of elderly patients who need surgical treatment and are at high risk due to aging, comorbidities, or medications such as steroids or antiplatelet drugs, trivial pitfalls during surgery can lead to catastrophic results. Furthermore, many patients with hemodialysis and marked systemic calcification require aortic valve surgery in Japan [1].

Complications encountered during surgery for aortic stenosis can be associated with catastrophic events such as myocardial infarction, cerebral embolism or aortic dissection. This is because a calcified aortic valve rarely exists alone, but is often associated with marked and diffuse calcification in the aorta, coronary arteries, mitral valve or even cerebral vessels [2]. The goal of surgical treatment is to implant a prosthetic valve of adequate size in each individual patient without perivalvular leak, while avoiding undesirable complications such as stroke, cardiac events or bleeding. This chapter is devoted to the tips and pitfalls in aortic valve replacement of calcified aortic valves with a discussion of preoperative and intraoperative strategies to achieve the best possible outcomes.

2. Calcified aortic valve

2.1. Etiologies of calcification

There are three main etiologies of aortic stenosis. The location and extent of calcification in the aortic valve varies depending on its etiology (Fig. 1). In rheumatic valvular disease, there is initial thickening and fusion of the cusps with later involvement of the annulus. The fusion of cusps results in the formation of a valve orifice that looks like a fish mouth. There is also severe mitral valve calcification in patients with combined valvular disease. In arteriosclerotic aortic stenosis, calcification is most prominent in the annulus, sinus of Valsalva and ascending aorta. Calcification of the cusps and calcium deposits on them markedly limit cusp opening. In bicuspid aortic stenosis, disease on the annulus is rather mild but fusion of the commissures reduces the valve orifice area and forms a slit-like orifice. Calcification is often present in bicuspid aortic stenosis, but is rather mild compared with that in arteriosclerotic aortic stenosis.

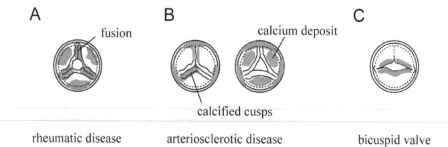

rheumatic disease   arteriosclerotic disease   bicuspid valve

Figure 1. Etiologies of aortic stenosis. A: Rheumatic disease initialy occurs on the cusps and extends toward the annulus. Fusion of the cusps causes a stenotic orifice like a fish mouth. B: Arteriosclerotic disease extends from the aorta toward the cusps. Opening of the cusps is often disturbed by rigidity of the cusps and calcium deposits on them. C: In bicuspid valve, calcification takes place mainly on the cusps.

2.2. Removal of calcium

A calcified aortic valve can be a cause of arterial embolism resulting in stroke or myocardial infarction [3-5]. A mobile mass is occasionally found attached to the calcified portion of the aortic valve. A calcified aortic valve as well as the presence of a mobile mass can be assessed by transthoracic echocardiography. Computed tomography (CT) is suitable for precisely assessing the presence and extent of calcification in the annulus and the entire aorta [6,7]. As the calcified cusps are resected, calcium in the annulus needs to be adequately removed to allow subsequent sutures for valve implantation. Calcium deposits are hard but easily crumble into pieces. They can be crushed by clamps and removed or can be fragmented by a Cavitron Ultrasound Surgical Aspirator (CUSA). Either way, loosened calcium needs to be carefully eliminated to prevent it from entering the left ventricle and causing stroke, or entering the left coronary artery and causing myocardial infarction. Digital palpation for irregularity and rigidity is helpful for evaluating the adequacy of calcium removal. To minimize the chance of perivalvular leakage following valve implantation, the inner aspect of the annulus should be smooth with the sewing cuff of the prosthetic valve sealing the small gaps between the sutures.

However, excessive removal of calcium may result in perforation of the aortic root or damage of the mitral valve [8]. Fig. 2 summarizes intraoperative transesophageal echocardiography (TEE) assessment and several measurements on the calcified aortic valve [9].

The extent of calcification should be carefully checked in the annulus and the aorta (described later). It is important to measure the dimensions of the annulus and sinotubular junction. When the latter is equal to or smaller than the former, difficult insertion of the prosthesis may be encountered. Although the valve can be narrowly inserted by distorting the bioprosthetic valve or the aorta, calcification in the aorta or sinotubular junction makes the latter difficult.

Acoustic shadow indicates the presence and extent of calcification. Fig. 3 shows three different degrees of calcification in the annulus of the noncoronary cusp. When it is transmural or continues to the anterior mitral leaflet as shown in Fig. 3C, excessive removal of calcium should be avoided and limited to a reasonable depth.

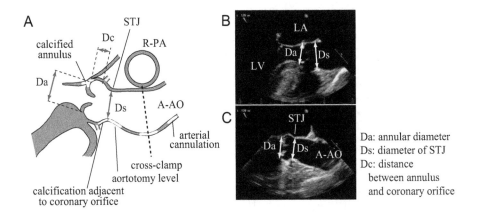

Figure 2. Intraoperative transesophageal echocardiography (TEE) assessment. A: Calcification in the annulus, sinus of Valsalva, and A-AO is assessed. Important measurements are shown. Annular diameter (Da) is usually smaller than the diameter of STJ (Ds) (B). When Ds is equal or smaller than Da (C), difficult insertion of prosthetic valve may be encountered. (modied from reference 9)

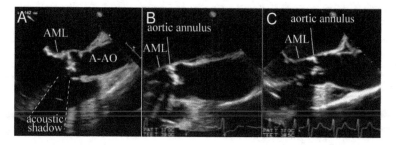

Figure 3. Calcification in the aortic annulus. A: Calcification is present on the cusps, accompanied by acoustic shadow but not in the annulus. B: Calcification in the annulus. C: Calcification extends to the AML.

2.3. Optimizing valve size

A calcified aortic valve limits the size of the prosthetic valve that can be implanted. When the aortic annulus is too small, patient-prosthesis mismatch can arise that may lead to sustained pressure overload of the left ventricle and subsequent chronic heart failure. A bioprosthetic valve is desirable for elderly patients with poor anticoagulation compliance to minimize the risk of cerebral infarction, or in patients that need antiplatelet therapy (patients with stroke or coronary stents); however, there are occasions where only a small-sized mechanical valve can be inserted due to a small aortic annulus [19]. Several solutions are illustrated in Fig. 4.

2.3.1. Annular dilatation

To enlarge the annulus, the aortotomy incision line is extended proximally toward the commissure between the left and non-coronary cusps or toward the noncoronary sinus of Valsalva (Fig. 4A) [11]. However, a markedly calcified annulus and/or sinus of Valsalva makes this procedure difficult or even increases the risk of uncontrollable bleeding at the suture line. Preoperative CT assessment or intraoperative TEE is helpful for making a decision.

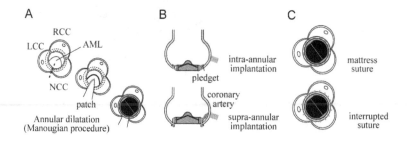

Figure 4. Solutions for small aortic annulus. A: Annular dilation by Manougian procedure. The commissure between LCC and NCC is incised and a patch is placed. B: Supra-annular implant. Care should be taken to avoid an obstruction of coronary artery. C: Interrupted suture. Cutting of annular tissue while tying is a pitfall.

2.3.2. Supra-annular implantation

This allows implantation of a prosthetic valve that is one size larger and is commonly used in many institutes (Fig. 4B). A non-everting suture is placed along the annulus. However, this generates a risk of occlusion of the coronary ostium when it is located at an unusually low level. It can be evaluated by CT, but may be missed by coronary angiography. Intraoperative TEE is helpful for making a decision (Fig. 2A).

2.3.3. Interrupted suture

Although mattress sutures slightly reduce the circumference of the aortic annulus, interrupted sutures allow insertion of a prosthetic valve with the same size as the annulus (Fig. 4C). This slightly increases the number of sutures required. Since appropriate seating of the sewing ring on the annulus cannot be confirmed by the pledget adjacent to the sewing cuff, it needs to be inspected through the valve by manually opening the leaflet. When the annulus is severely calcified, it is important to prevent a gap between the annulus and sewing ring. Furthermore, cutting of annular tissue should be avoided while the suture is tied. Two other solutions are stentless aortic valve implant [12,13] and apicoaortic conduit [14-16]. The reader should consult the literature for further details on these two methods.

3. Calcified aorta

Calcification in the aorta occasionally necessitates modification of the surgical strategy because of the safety of arterial cannulation, aortic cross-clamping, insertion of a root cannula, aortotomy and suture closure of the aorta. Calcification can be precisely assessed by preoperative CT. The principal strategy can be selected based on the CT findings. Intraoperative TEE and/or epiaortic echo may be used to identify the precise location and extent of calcification and atheromatous plaque in the surgical field. Echo-guided marking of calcification on the aorta can be helpful for subsequent surgical procedures. Three-dimensional (3D) TEE is capable of visualizing the entire ascending aorta (Fig. 5). The xPlane mode allows serial sections of the aorta to be scanned from the aortic valve to the aortic arch. The diseased portion of the aorta can be located by digital compression of the aorta during visualization by TEE.

Fig. 6 demonstrates several TEE images of calcified aortas. Fig. 6A shows a calcified aortic wall just distal to the sinotubular junction, accompanied by acoustic shadow. The aortotomy line needs to be shifted distally. Calcification can take place at the level of the aortic cross-clamp, where the right pulmonary artery crosses behind the ascending aorta (Fig. 6B). Fig. 6C shows calcification at the level of arterial cannulation. The use of epiaortic echo is desirable to accurately locate the site of calcification. Fig. 6D is a TEE image of rather mild calcification. In this case, the aorta could be clamped without cerebral complications. Fig. 6E shows atheromatous plaque on the anterior wall of the ascending aorta at the level of cross-clamping and insertion of the root cannula. Since enhanced CT is not often employed for preoperative assessment before aortic valve replacement, care should be taken to avoid missing such findings. Palpation of the aorta cannot detect the presence of atheroma. TEE or epiaortic echo is needed to avoid an embolic event.

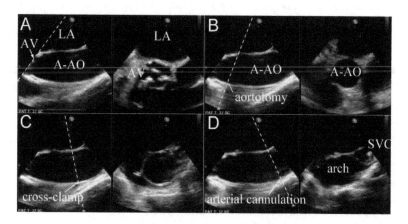

Figure 5. Scanning the entire A-AO using xPlane mode. In the midesophageal A-AO long-axis view, the scanning plane orthogonal to the reference plane is tilted from the AV up to the arch level. Short-axis view of A-AO can be visualized.

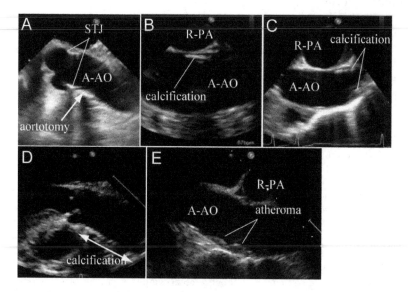

Figure 6. Examples of TEE images of calcified A-AO. A: Calcification of anterior wall just distal to STJ. B: Calcification at the level of cross-clamping (R-PA level). C: Calcification at the arterial cannulation level. D: Mild calcification of A-AO. E: Atheromatous plaque in the A-AO.

3.1. Arterial cannulation and insertion of a root cannula

Calcification often involves the distal portion of the ascending aorta and makes arterial cannulation difficult (Fig. 6C). Since an adequate space for aortotomy needs to be spared for procedures on the aortic valve, the cannulation site should not be too proximal. Arterial cannulation of a calcified aorta might cause aortic dissection at the time of cannulation and/or difficult hemostasis following decannulation. When aortic cannulation is not desirable, the axillary or femoral artery can be used as an alternative perfusion route. However, in patients with a calcified aorta, there can also be stenosis or atheromatous lesions in the innominate or iliac artery; thus, it is mandatory to check for these lesions before surgery. The insertion site of the root cannula should be carefully determined. Epiaortic echo is helpful for examining the presence and location of calcification and atheroma. A safe placement of the root cannula requires a certain length of nearly normal wall, which allows secure closure of the puncture site. When an adequate area is not available, an elastic needle may be used instead.

3.2. Aortic cross-clamp

In cases with severe and diffuse calcification of the aorta (porcelain aorta), concomitant replacement of the ascending aorta should be considered [17-19]. However, in the majority of calcified aortic valve cases, calcification is present but not severe; it is often scattered without apparent atheromatous plaque on the intima. It is important to determine the safety of aorta cross-clamp in all cases, since cross-clamp of a calcified aorta potentially causes fracture of the calcified layer that can lead to aortic dissection or embolism of fragmented calcium.

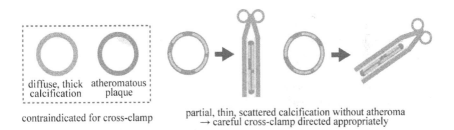

diffuse, thick   atheromatous
calcification   plaque

contraindicated for cross-clamp

partial, thin, scattered calcification without atheroma
→ careful cross-clamp directed appropriately

Figure 7. Strategies for clamping in cases of calcified aorta. When calcification is diffuse and thick or atheromathous plaque is present, cross-clamp is avoided. If calcification is partial and thin without atheroma, the aorta can be clamped according to the distribution of calcified portion.

Fig. 7 shows the strategy of the author. When calcification is diffuse and thick or atheromatous plaque is present, aortic cross-clamp is avoided. If the calcified layer is partial and not thick, the aorta may be clamped with some fracture of the calcified portion, but without incompetent clamp or the development of dissection. The clamp may be applied as parallel to the calcified wall as possible to minimize fracture of the calcified section and the shear force on the intima. Initially, the ratchet is locked slowly and less deeply. The blood flow in the proximal aorta is checked with TEE before antegrade cardioplegia is given. When there is some leak through the clamp site, the ratchet is advanced. If full clamp is not effective, another straight clamp is added adjacent to the first clamp or conversion to aortic repair is considered, depending on the risk of aortic repair in each individual case. It should be kept in mind that a clamp on the calcified aorta flattens the proximal aorta and narrows the surgical field following aortotomy. In the case shown in Fig. 6D, the aorta was carefully clamped and valve replacement was performed without neurologic sequelae. For porcelain aorta, endovascular clamping may be another option [20].

3.3. Aortotomy

An incision line is determined based on the distribution of calcification. It may be modified from the standard J-shaped incision line to a rather transectional or more oblique and distal incision. In the case shown in Fig. 6A, aortotomy at a more distal level or meticulous removal of calcification is needed. If there is an insufficient margin for suture closure of the aortotomy (at least 1 cm in width), the surgeon should be prepared for difficult suturing. When the calcified portion of the aorta is to be incised and sutured, calcium needs to be carefully removed following aortotomy, but before implanting a prosthetic valve. The use of CUSA is helpful for reducing the amount of calcium, enabling an adequate attachment of the aortic walls during suture closure. A new device for this purpose may be helpful [21].

4. Coronary arteries

Myocardial protection is one of the most important issues in aortic valve replacement. Left ventricular hypertrophy and/or coronary artery disease is often associated with aortic stenosis. In addition, surgical procedures may potentially cause new myocardial ischemia. Therefore, careful observation of coronary perfusion is essential. Fig. 8 shows visualization of the coronary arteries with TEE. The coronary arteries can be visualized bilaterally in the majority of cases and coronary artery assessment is done routinely in our institute. The ostia of the right and left coronary arteries are depicted in the short-axis view at the level of sinus of Valsalva (Fig. 8 A,B). The right coronary artery travels in the groove between the right atrium and right ventricle, whereas the left coronary artery crosses behind the pulmonary artery. The left main truncus divides into the left anterior descending and left circumflex arteries. The right coronary ostium can also be depicted in the midesophageal aortic valve long-axis view, giving an idea of its distance from the annulus (Fig. 8C).

To further visualize the distal portion of the left coronary artery, the scanning plane is rotated counterclockwise from the midesophageal aortic valve long-axis view (Fig. 8D). The left coronary sinus takes the place of the noncoronary sinus, and the short-axis view of left main truncus appears. The left anterior descending artery courses toward the 6 to 7 o'clock direction. The distal portion of the left circumflex artery is visualized in the atrioventricular groove. With the 3D en face view, the height of coronary take-off can be observed (Fig. 8E). The author meticulously uses TEE for intraoperative assessment of coronary perfusion, because it is the most important factor that affects the outcomes of aortic valve replacement, especially for calcified aortic valves. Several pitfalls related to myocardial ischemia are shown in Fig. 9.

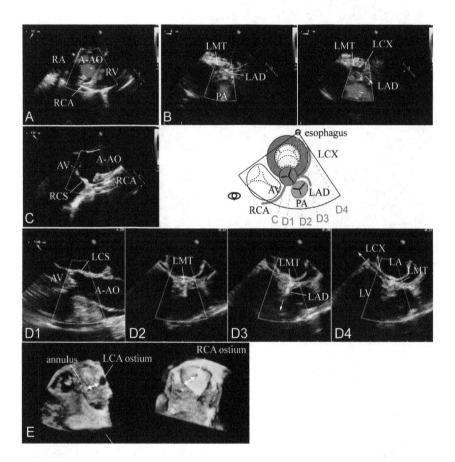

Figure 8. Visualization of coronary arteries with TEE. A: In short-axis view at the level of sinus of Valsalva, RCA arises from RCS at 6 o'clock position directed to the groove between RA and RV. B: The LCA takes off from LCS at 3 o'clock position. LMT courses behind PA and divides to LAD and LCX. C: In midesophageal AV long-axis view, RCA arises from RCS (C). D: As the probe is rotated counterclockwise, LCA arises from LCS and LMT divides to LAD and LCX. LAD is directed toward the LV apex and LCX courses posteriorly along the atrioventicular groove between LA and LV. E: In 3D en-face view, distance from AV annulus to the ostia is recognized.

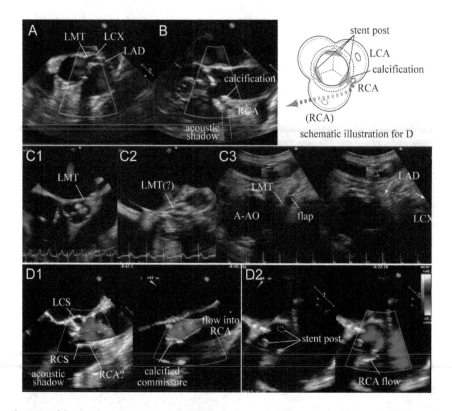

Figure 9. Pitfalls related to coronary artery in aortic valve replacement. A: Short LMT divides to LAD and LCX near the ostium. B: Calcification adjacent to RCA ostium. C: New dissection in the LMT. LMT was intact before bypass (C1), but no flow was detectable during wearing from bypass (C2) associated with akinetic LV. Epicardial echo following coronary bypass to the LAD shows a flap obstructing the LMT and blood flow from LAD toward LCX (C3). D: Anomalous origin of RCA. RCA was not found in the RCS, but at the commissure between RCC and LCC (D1). Following valve replacement, RCA was seen originating from the commissure in front of the stent post (D2). Schematic illustration of D is shown.

4.1. Short left main truncus

The left main truncus is occasionally found to be short (Fig. 9A). As the cannula is forcefully thrust into the ostium, the cannula tip may enter either the left anterior descending or left circumflex artery. Any unperfused region of the left ventricle may be poorly protected during the procedure.

4.2. Calcified ostium

The coronary ostium as well as the surrounding wall of the coronary sinus of Valsalva may be rigid or irregular, occasionally making it difficult to selectively infuse cardioplegic solution into the coronary artery, because the cannula tip does not fit properly and there is significant leakage. When calcification accompanied by acoustic shadow is present adjacent to the coronary ostium (Fig. 9B), this pitfall may occur. A highly echogenic projection accompanied by acoustic shadow, usually on the side of the sinotubular junction, is a typical TEE finding. Calcification in the aortic root also makes it difficult to locate the right coronary ostium, especially when the sinus wall of Valsalva is rigid and cannot be folded back. Unsuccessful infusion of cardioplegic solution potentially leads to right heart failure, since the right coronary region cannot be adequately perfused via the retrograde approach. Although a large-bore cannula tip does not adequately fit the calcified ostium, a small-caliper cannula causes little leakage but the velocity of jet stream ejected out of the cannula can exceed 2 m/sec, potentially causing intimal damage or dissection. Fig. 9C shows the TEE findings of dissection that occurred in the left coronary artery following cardiopulmonary bypass in a case of difficult coronary perfusion. Although the left coronary artery was intact before bypass, no blood flow was detected during weaning from bypass in the area that was thought to contain the left main truncus. Since the anterior and posterior walls of the left ventricle were akinetic, immediate coronary bypass grafting to the left anterior descending artery was performed. Subsequent epicardial echo revealed a flap in the left main truncus and retrograde blood flow in the left anterior descending artery from the coronary bypass graft that perfused the left circumflex artery.

4.3. Anomalous origin of the right coronary artery

Anomalous origin of the right coronary artery is rather rare (Fig. 9D), but is difficult to diagnose based on preoperative coronary angiography. In a case of aortic stenosis with an intact right coronary artery in preoperative coronary angiography, the right coronary ostium could not be found in the right coronary sinus of Valsalva. Selective perfusion of the left coronary artery caused backflow from the right coronary ostium, which was identified at the commissure between the right and left coronary cusps. Calcified protrusion was continuous from the commissure to the ostium. The right coronary artery was successfully perfused, and the calcium at the orifice was left unresected. However, when calcium is exposed without being covered by the sewing ring, there is the potential for thrombus formation adjacent to the right coronary ostium. Following aortic valve replacement, TEE demonstrated that the stent post was located in front of the right coronary ostium, because the stent posts were oriented so that the left coronary ostium was not covered by the stent post. The right coronary artery coursed along the right coronary sinus and could have been inadvertently injured by the surgical procedures.

4.4. Myocardial perfusion during cardioplegia

Retrograde cardioplegia is a solution for difficult antegrade coronary perfusion. However, the region perfused by the right coronary artery is poorly protected because the cardioplegic solution predominantly enters the coronary veins along the left coronary artery (great cardiac vein) but not the middle or small cardiac veins. Although the latter may be perfused via collaterals between the veins, this is not certain. Also, in cases where it is difficult to fit the coronary perfusion cannula and there is considerable leakage, perfusion of the myocardium is a concern. A myocardial thermometer was conventionally used, but may not be useful in warm heart surgery. Real-time assessment of myocardial perfusion is desired, especially in cases with deteriorated cardiac function. Here, a novel method for noninvasively assessing myocardial perfusion is demonstrated (Fig. 10). The transgastric basal or midventricular short-axis view is visualized. In pulsed-wave Doppler mode, the sample volume is placed on the myocardium. When this portion of myocardium is perfused, a flow signal is detected. Under selective perfusion of the left coronary artery, blood flow is detected in the anterior wall but not in the inferior wall. As coronary perfusion is discontinued, the flow signal instantaneously disappears. The perfused region is identified by mapping the myocardium. This can be helpful for examining the extent of retrograde delivery of cardioplegic solution.

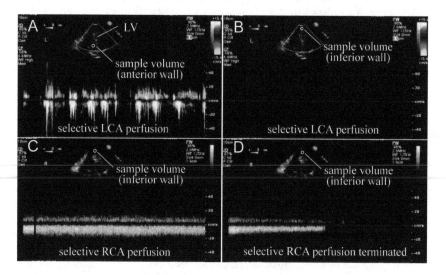

Figure 10. TEE assessment of myocardial blood flow during cardioplegia. Under selective perfusion to LCA, blood flow is detectable in the anterior wall (A) but not in the inferior wall (B). As selective RCA perfusion is terminated, blood flow detected in the inferior wall (c) instantaneously disappears (D)

5. Assessment following implantation

After the aortotomy is closed, several pitfalls need to be checked (Fig. 11,12). If an unexpected event is detected, a prompt decision for additional intervention should be made.

5.1. Perivalvular or transvalvular leakage

During weaning from bypass, the surgeon should check for perivalvular leakage. A calcified aortic valve can result in inadequate contact between the annulus and the suture ring of the prosthetic valve. It is readily examined by TEE in the midesophageal long-axis view (Fig. 11A). A minor leak that originates inside of the ring and deviates inwards is transvalvular leak and is not significant (Fig. 11B). When significant leakage is detected in the left ventricular outflow tract that originates outside of the suture ring, perivalvular leakage is probable (Fig. 11C). The assessment of leakage is difficult in cases with concomitant mitral valve replacement. The ring of the prosthetic valve implanted in the mitral position casts an acoustic shadow on the left ventricular outflow tract (Fig. 11D). In such an instance, leakage is assessed in the deep transgastric long-axis view via the left ventricular apex (Fig. 11E).

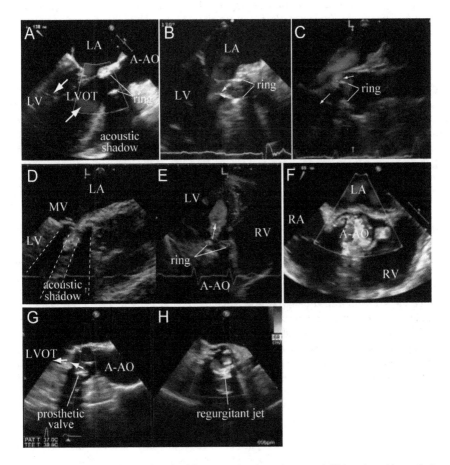

Figure 11. TEE assessment of prosthetic valve following aortic valve replacement. A: Midesophageal long-axis view without abnormal leak from the prosthetic valve. B: Minor transvalvular leak. C: Significant perivalvular leak around the valve. D: Leakage is suspected but visualization is disturbed by the valve in mitral position. E: Deep transgastric view shows mild transvalvular leak F: Blood flow in the entire area of ascending aorta just distal to the prosthetic valve indicates good opening of discs. G,H: Massive transvalvular leak from the bioprosthesis due to everted leaflet.

Valve dysfunction should be checked during weaning from bypass. Dysfunction of a mechanical valve includes an immobilized disc at the open or closed positions. Since the disc itself is hardly depicted by TEE, dysfunction is examined in the color Doppler mode. In the short-axis view of the ascending aorta at the level just above the valve, opening of both discs can be confirmed by the flow signal, which fills the entire area of the aorta (Fig. 11F). Incompetence of the valve is caused by an immobilized disc of a mechanical valve at the open position probably due to debris or calcium between the disc and ring or by jammed leaflets of a bioprosthetic valve. It can be recognized by massive aortic regurgitation, demonstrated by a regurgitant jet in the left ventricular outflow tract originating from inside of the ring in midesophageal or deep transgastric view (Fig. 11G,H). In this case, exploration revealed that there was unintended eversion of a leaflet on the noncoronary side without jamming or leaflet damage. The leaflet was returned to the normal position and the aortotomy was closed [22].

5.2. Coronary ostium and ventricular contraction

Obstruction of coronary ostium is checked during weaning from bypass to minimize myocardial damage under warm ischemia. This event is important especially for the valve implanted in the supra-annular position. In the early timing following aortic declamping, patency and blood flow in both coronary arteries is checked. Both ostia can be visualized in the short-axis view just above the valve (Fig. 12A). In the midesophageal aortic valve long-axis view, the right coronary ostium is seen above the sewing ring (Fig. 12B). The presence of flow and distance from the ring of the prosthetic valve is checked.

Blood flow in the left coronary artery is examined proximal to its bifurcation into the LAD and LCX as shown in Fig. 8. Fig. 12D shows TEE views in a case of a low origin of the LMT. Before cardiopulmonary bypass, the midesophageal long-axis view showed a short distance between the aortic annulus and left main truncus. Following valve replacement at the intra-annular position, knots were found to be in front of the left coronary ostium and accelerated flow was seen. In the midesophageal long-axis view, the left coronary ostium was just above the ring. Surprisingly, the left main truncus was just behind the annulus. A deep suture could have injured the left main truncus. Fig. 12E and F demonstrate a case with a normal origin of the main left coronary artery. Before cardiopulmonary bypass, the coronary orifice was approximately 1 cm above the aortic annulus (Fig. 12E1,2). The 3D en face view clearly demonstrated an adequate distance (Fig. 12 E3). After replacement, TEE showed that there was no obstacle in front of the left main truncus in the short-axis view (Fig. 12F1). In the long-axis view, there was adequate distance between the ring and left main truncus (Fig. 12F2). 3D TEE also clearly showed safe implant of the prosthetic valve (Fig. 12F3). As ventricular contraction recovers, regional wall motion abnormalities can be assessed in the midesophageal, 2-chamber and 4-chamber views, or the transgastric basal or mid-short-axis views.

If coronary obstruction is suspected as in Fig. 9, early coronary revascularization is to be considered for minimizing myocardial damage. Ischemia can develop not only by obstruction of coronary ostium but by poor myocardial protection or embolism of dislodged calcium or even intracardiac air. Sustained circulatory support may be advantageous or retrograde cardioplegia may potentially help to displace any calcium or air embolus toward the coronary ostium.

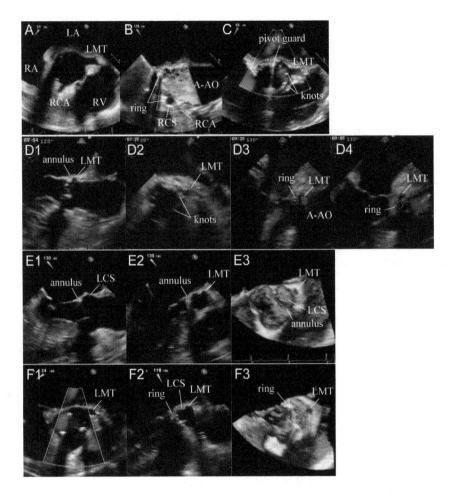

Figure 12. TEE assessment of coronary arteries in aortic valve replacement. A; Short-axis view at the level of the sinus of Valsalva that shows patent ostia of the RCA and LMT. B: RCA flow in midesophageal AV long-axis view. Distance from the ring to RCA ostium is checked. C: LMT flow in short-axis view of sinus of Valsalva. Knots are seen without obstruction. D: Low take-off of LMT (D1). Following valve replacement, the knots are in front of LMT ostium. A mild acceleration of blood flow is seen (D2). In midesophageal long-axis view, the LMT orifice is just above the ring (D3). LMT was found to course very close to the suture (D4). E: Normal take-off of LMT. LMT originates from the LCS at approximately 1 cm above the aortic annulus (E1 to E2). 3D en face view clearly demonstrates the distance of LMT from the annulus (E3). F: TEE views following valve replacement. There is no obstruction in front of the LMT (F1). There is adequate distance from the ring to the LMT orifice, depicted in midesophageal long-axis view (F2) and 3D en face view (F3)

5.3. New mitral regurgitation

Mitral regurgitation may appear following aortic valve replacement. One reason is perforation of the mitral annulus caused by excessive decalcification of the aortic annulus. Another mechanism is systolic anterior motion of the mitral leaflet, which is caused by reduced left ventricular dimensions and/or a sigmoid septum due to left ventricular hypertrophy. When several measures are not effective, emergent mitral valve replacement should be considered.

5.4. Aortic dissection

Following aortic declamping, the aorta distal to the clamp site should be checked for new dissection. It may potentially develop due to detachment of the calcified aortic wall, and inner or outer layer. Dissection can also originate from the arterial cannulation site, root cannula site or aortotomy site.

In conclusion, it is essential to watch for pitfalls in aortic valve replacement for calcified aortic valve, because it is commonly associated with various pathologies that can affect the surgical outcomes. Meticulous monitoring and intraoperative diagnostic imaging are helpful for achieving the best possible results in cases with increased risk factors.

Abbreviations for figures

A-AO ascending aorta

AML anterior mitral leaflet

AV aortic valve

LA left atrium

LAD left anterior descending artery

LCA left coronary artery

LCC left coronary cusp

LCS left coronary sinus

LMT left main truncus

LVOT left ventricular outflow tract

MV mitral valve

NCC noncoronary cusp

PA pulmonary artery

RA right atrium

RCA right coronary artery

RCC right coronary cusp

RCS right coronary sinus

R-PA right pulmonary artery

RV right ventricle

STJ sinotubular junction

SVC superior vena cava

Author details

Kazumasa Orihashi

Department of Cardiovascular Surgery, Kochi Medical School, Kochi, Japan

References

[1] Tanaka, K, Tajima, K, Takami, Y, et al. Early and late outcomes of aortic valve re-placement in dialysis patients. Ann Thorac Surg (2010). , 89, 65-70.

[2] Kaden, J. J, Eckert, J. P, Poerner, T, et al. Prevalence of atherosclerosis of the coronary and extracranial cerebral arteries in patients undergoing aortic valve replacement for calcified stenosis. J Heart Valve Dis (2006). , 15, 165-8.

[3] Staico, R, Armaganijan, L, & Lopes, R. D. Coronary embolism and calcified aortic valve: is there a correlation? J Thromb Thrombolysis (2012). , 34, 425-7.

[4] Mannino, G, Romano, M, Calanchini, M, Mannino, C, & Cascone, N. C. Branch reti-nal artery embolization due to calcific aortic valve stenosis. Eur J Ophthalmol (2010). , 20, 625-8.

[5] Mahajan, N, Khetarpal, V, & Afonso, L. Stroke secondary to calcific bicuspid aortic valve: case report and literature review. J Cardiol (2009). , 54, 158-61.

[6] Rivard, A. L, Bartel, T, Bianco, R. W, et al. Evaluation of aortic root and valve calcifi-cations by multi-detector computed tomography. J Heart Valve Dis (2009). , 18, 662-70.

[7] Aviram, G, Sharony, R, Kramer, A, et al. Modification of surgical planning based on cardiac multidetector computed tomography in reoperative heart surgery. Ann Thor-ac Surg (2005). , 79, 589-95.

[8] Islamoglu, F, Apaydin, A. Z, Degirmenciler, K, et al. Detachment of the mitral valve anterior leaflet as a complication of aortic valve replacement. Tex Heart Inst J (2006). , 33, 54-6.

[9] Orihashi, K. Intraoperative imaging in aortic valve surgery as a safety net (Chapter 1). IN: Motomura N, ed. Aortic Valve Surgery. InTech Co., Croatia, (2011). , 3-18.

[10] Taniguchi, S, Noguchi, M, Onohara, D, et al. Aortic valve replacement with 17-mm St. Jude Medical Regent prosthetic valves for a small calcified aortic annulus in elderly patients. Gen Thorac Cardiovasc Surg (2010). , 58, 506-10.

[11] Coutinho, G. F, Correia, P. M, Paupério, G, et al. Aortic root enlargement does not increase the surgical risk and short-term patient outcome? Eur J Cardiothorac Surg (2011). , 40, 441-7.

[12] Karimov, J. H, Cerillo, A. G, Solinas, M, et al. Stentless aortic valve implantation in heavily calcified aorta. J Cardiovasc Med (Hagerstown) (2009). , 10, 813-4.

[13] Di Matteo G Masala N, Swanevelder J, et al. Clinical outcome of a simplified technique for aortic valve replacement with stentless bioprostheses. J Heart Valve Dis (2009). , 18, 111-8.

[14] Shin, H, Mori, M, Suzuki, R, et al. Apicoaortic valved conduit with an apical connector for aortic stenosis with a calcified aorta. Gen Thorac Cardiovasc Surg (2009). , 57, 467-70.

[15] Chahine, J. H, Rassi, I, & Jebara, V. Apico-aortic valved conduit as an alternative for aortic valve re-replacement in severe prosthesis-patient mismatch. Interact Cardiovasc Thorac Surg (2009). , 9, 680-2.

[16] Crestanello, J. A, Zehr, K. J, Daly, R. C, et al. Is there a role for the left ventricle apical-aortic conduit for acquired aortic stenosis? J Heart Valve Dis (2004). , 13, 57-62.

[17] Chung, S, Park, P. W, Choi, M. S, et al. Surgical experience of ascending aorta and aortic valve replacement in patient with calcified aorta. Korean J Thorac Cardiovasc Surg (2012). , 45, 24-9.

[18] Iliopoulos, D. C, Deveja, A. R, Satratzemis, V, et al. Deep hypothermic arrest for aortic valve replacement in case of porcelain aorta. Asian Cardiovasc Thorac Ann (2009). , 17, 415-6.

[19] Okamoto, H, Fujimoto, K, Tamenishi, A, et al. Aortic valve replacement in a heavily calcified "porcelain" aorta. Jpn J Thorac Cardiovasc Surg (2001). , 49, 453-6.

[20] Ooi, A, Iyengar, S, Langley, S. M, et al. Endovascular clamping of porcelain aorta in aortic valve surgery using Foley Catheter. Heart Lung Circ (2006). , 15, 194-6.

[21] Kudo, M, Misumi, T, & Koizumi, K. Aortotomy and endarterectomy of the ascending aorta for aortic valve replacement in a patient with porcelain aorta. Surg Today (2005). , 35, 1000-3.

[22] Orihashi, K, Kurosaki, T, & Sueda, T. Everted leaflet of a bovine pericardial aortic valve. Interact Cardiovasc Thorac Surg (2010). , 10, 1059-60.

Chapter 8

Indications for Transcatheter Aortic Valve Implantation

Ibrahim Akin, Stephan Kische, Henrik Schneider,
Tim C. Rehders, Christoph A. Nienaber and
Hüseyin Ince

Additional information is available at the end of the chapter

1. Introduction

Rising life expectancy results in an increase of degenerative and neoplastic diseases. Popula-tion-based observational studies report that 1% to 2% of patients older than 65 years have moderate-to-severe aortic stenosis (AS) [1]. Surgical aortic valve replacement (AVR) dates back to 1960 and is currently the only treatment option for severe AS that has been shown to improve survival, regardless of age [2]. In the ideal candidate, surgical AVR has an estimat-ed operative mortality of 4% [2]. Unfortunately, up to one-third of patients with severe AS are ineligible for corrective valve surgery, either because of advanced age or the presence of multiple comorbidities [3]. Current treatment options for those patients not offered surgery include medical treatment or percutaneous balloon aortic valvuloplasty, although neither has been shown to reduce mortality. Medically treated patients with symptomatic AS have 1- and 5-year survival of 60% and 32%, respectively [4,5]. With the introduction of percuta-neous aortic valve implantation in 2002, there seems to be an alternative for these patients.

2. Selection of patient

Due to the existence of tried and tested surgical AVR with good long-term results, the selec-tion of patients for transcatheter aortic valve implantation (TAVI), which should done in a multidisciplinary consultation between cardiologists, surgeons, imaging specialists, and an-esthesiologists, involves several critical steps [6]. Candidates considered for TAVI must have severe symptomatic AS in addition to a formal contraindication to surgery or other charac-teristics that would limit their surgical candidacy because of excessive mortality or morbidity (Figure 2). The procedure should be offered to patients who have a potential for functional improvement after valve replacement. It is not recommended for patients who simply refuse surgery on the basis of personal preference.

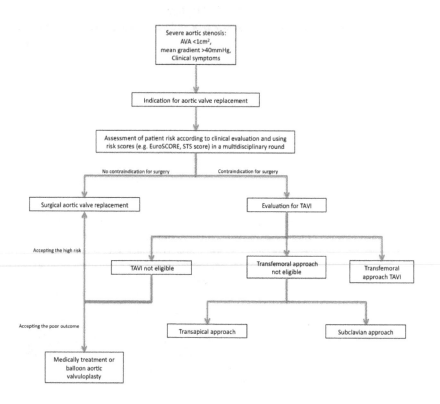

Figure 1. Algorithm to determine the treatment options of patients with severe AS (AVA: aortic valve area; TAVI: transcatheter aortic valve implantation)

3. Confirming the severity of aortic stenosis

Actually, TAVI is indicated only for patients with calcified pure or predominant symptomatic AS. The different imaging modalities can assist in the selection process by providing important information on the aortic valve, coronary arteries, and vascular structures. First, the severity of AS should be assessed. Both transthoracic (TTE) and transesophageal (TEE) Doppler echocardiography are the preferred tools (Figure 2).

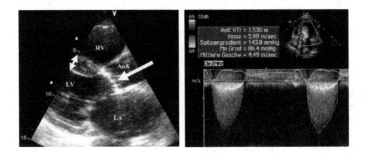

Figure 2. TTE in the assessment of severe AS

In addition, the exact anatomy of the aortic valve should be assessed. Echocardiography, multislice CT (MSCT), and magnetic resonance imaging (MRI) can all help to distinguish between a bicuspid and a tricuspid aortic valve. It is important to point out that implantation of available percutaneous prostheses is contraindicated in the case of a bicuspid aortic valve, because of the risk of incomplete deployment, significant paravalvular regurgitation, and displacement of the prosthesis [6,7] (Figure 3).

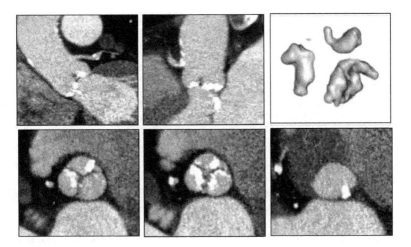

Figure 3. ECG-gated CT-scan in a patient with severe aortic valve stenosis (the upper right panel shows the isolated calcification of the tricuspid aortic valve)

A severely calcified aortic valve may result in the inability to cross the native valve with the catheter. Bulky leaflets and calcifications on the free edge of the leaflets may increase the risk of occlusion of the coronary ostia during aortic valve implantation. Therefore, the extent and exact location of calcifications should be carefully assessed before the implantation procedure. Assessing coronary anatomy is also important in the selection process. Conventional coronary angiography, which remains the "gold standard", should be done to exclude the presence of significant coronary artery disease (Figure 4).

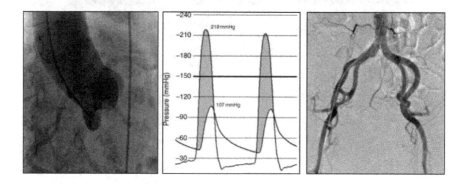

Figure 4. Invasive diagnostic prior TAVI, including aortography and access vessels as well as transvalvular gradient

4. Analysis of surgical risk and evaluation of life expectancy and quality of life

The precise evaluation of surgical risk in a specific patient is not easy and involves an attempt at individualization based on statistical data from databases containing a large number of procedures. The most accepted and validated algorithms that are widely available today are the EuroSCORE, the STS (Society of Thoracic Score) score,and the Parsonnet score. These algorithms predict the surgical risk by assigning weight to various factors that affect the clinical result, but it is clear that they can underestimate or overestimate the risk in certain groups of patients who are not represented satisfactorily in the population used to generate the algorithm [8]. There is some evidence in the literature of the incorrect prediction of aortic AVR outcome using the EuroSCORE model [9]. The key element for establishing whether patients are at high risk for surgery is multidisciplinary clinical judgment, which should be used in association with a more quantitative assessment, based on the combination of several scores (for example, expected mortality >20% with the EuroSCORE and >10% with STS score). This approach allows the team to take into account risk factors that are not covered in scores but often seen in practice, such as chest radiation, previous aortocoronary bypass with patent grafts, porcelain aorta, liver cirrhosis.

5. Assessment of feasibility and exclusion of contraindications for TAVI

After criteria of severe symptomatic aortic valve stenosis and high surgical risk are evaluated, the technical evaluation of the patient's suitability for the percutaneous implantation technique begins (Table 1).

Indication for Transcatheter aortic valve implantation
Severe aortic stenosis (AVA: <1cm², mean gradient "/>40mmHg, severe symptoms)
Contraindication for surgical valve replacement
Contraindication for Transcatheter aortic valve implantation
Mild to moderate aortic stenosis
Asymptomatic patients
Life expectancy <1 year
Surgical aortic valve replacement possible, but patient refused
Aortic anulus <18 or "/>25mm (balloon-expandable) and <20 or "/>27mm (self-expandable)
Bicuspid aortic valve
Asymetric heavy valvular calcification
Aortic root "/>45mm at the aortotubular junction
Presence of left ventricular apical thrombus
Contraindication for transfemoral approach
Severe calcification, tortuosity, small diameter of the iliac arteries
Previous aortofemoral bypass
Severe angulation, severe atheroma of the aorta
Coarctation of the aorta
Aneurysm of the aorta with protruding mural thrombus
Contraindication for transapical approach
Previous surgery of the left ventricle using a patch
Calcified pericardium
Severe respiratory insufficiency
Non-reachable left ventricular apex

Table 1. Actually proposed indications and contraindications for TAVI

The two most basic parameters are the suitability of the peripheral arteries and the size of the aortic valve annulus. Contrast angiography is needed to assess the former, while the latter requires an initial assessment of the diameter of the aortic annulus on a TTE. In general terms, a large artery with dominant elastic elements should have a diameter up to 1 mm smaller than the external diameter of the sheath that has to be introduced for the valve implantation. Thus, current systems with an external sheath diameter of 28 F (SAPIEN 26 mm, Edwards Lifescience LLC, Irvine, CA), 25 F (SAPIEN 23 mm, Edwards) and 22 F (CoreValve, Medtronic, Inc., Minneapolis, MN) require minimum diameters of 8, 7, and 6 mm, respectively. Apart from the minimum diameter, the existence of significant vessel tortuosity (>90°), especially when combined with wall calcifications, makes advancing the large sheath problematic, with a high risk of vascular complications that could potentially affect the final outcome. In addition, the existence of extensive circumferential calcifications limits the elastic dilation of the artery; thus, the minimum diameters referred to above are underestimated. Patients who do not meet the criteria of suitable peripheral arterial access may still be candidates for transapical implantation. For the assessment of aortic annulus diameter, we should keep in mind that TTE underestimates its size by a mean of 1.4 mm compared with TEE [6,10], while the latter method also underestimates the size by 1.2 mm compared with intraoperative measurement [10]. Therefore, in order to avoid undesirable and often catastrophic displacement of the prosthesis, there should be a margin of at least 1-2 mm between the diameter of the valve and the size of the aortic annulus estimated using TEE, so that the former may be successfully and safely anchored within the latter. Computed tomography scan aortography and angiography of the ascending aorta are the most appropriate examinations for investigating these aspects. Those examinations will also be used for the measurement of the dimensions of the ascending aorta and the aortic arch, which are essential for checking eligibility for the CoreValve (the most important being the diameter of the ascending aorta, which should be <4.3 cm) (Figure 5).

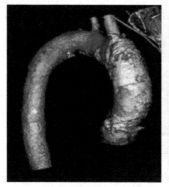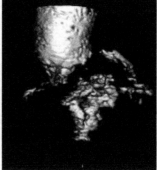

Figure 5. ECG-gated CT-scan of a patient with severe aortic valve stenosis and porcelain aorta after radiation exposure

The anatomy of the thoracic aorta (any chance of porcelain aorta) and the abdominal aorta should be studied by some imaging method for the existence of extensive atheromatosis, mural thrombi and aneurysm (Figure 6).

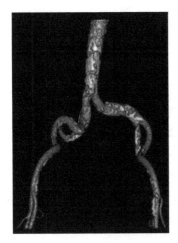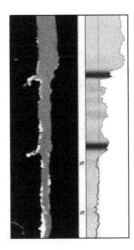

Figure 6. Three-dimensional reconstruction of contrast-enhanced CT angiography to assess morphology of femoral arteries (left) and centerline stretched view (right)

6. Different transcatheter aortic valves

On the basis of first results from clinical trials, CoreValve Revalving System and Edwards Lifescience SAPIEN obtained CE mark approval in 2007 with the specification that these valves are intended for patients with a high or prohibitive risk for surgical valve replacement or who cannot undergo AVR. The first generation balloon-expandable valve was entitled Cribier-Edwards valve (Edwards Lifesciences), whereas at present the Edwards SAPIEN valve (Edwards) is commercially available (Figure 7). The Edwards Lifesciences SAPIEN THV device is a balloon-expandable valve. It consists of bovine pericardium that is firmly mounted within a tubular, slotted, stainless steel balloon-expandable stent. Two valve sizes have been developed (23mm and 26mm). At present, available prosthesis sizes are 23 and 26 mm for aortic annulus diameters between 18–22 mm and 21–25 mm, respectively. The CoreValve Revalving device is a self-expanding frame-valve prosthesis (Figure 7). It consists of a porcine pericardial tissue valve that is mounted and sutured in a multilevel self-expanding nitinol frame. It is available in 26, 29 and 31 mm sizes. The device has a broader upper segment (outflow aspect), which yields proper orientation to the blood flow. The first-generation valve used bovine pericardial tissue and was constrained within a 25 French (F) delivery catheter. The second-generation valve was built with porcine pericardial tissue within a 21 F catheter to allow access through smaller-diameter vascular beds. The third-generation of the device features a catheter with a valve delivery sheath size of 18 F and a follow-on shaft of 12 F.

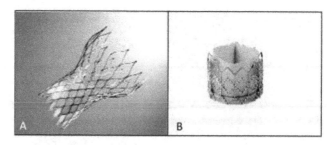

Figure 7. Profile of the CoreValve Revaving System (A) and Edwards SAPIEN Transcatheter Heart Valve (B)

Newer devices that have first-in-man application include Paniagua (Endoluminal Technology Research, Miami, FL), Enable (ATS, Minneapolis, MN), AoTx (Hansen Medical, Mountain View, CA), Perceval (Sorin Group, Arvada, CO), Jena (JenaValve Technology, Wilmington, DE), Lotus Valve (Sadra Medical, Campbell, CA), and Direct Flow percutaneous aortic valve (Direct Flow Medical, Inc., Santa Rosa, CA). TAVI represents a unique challenge for anesthesiologists. As with other invasive procedures, a careful preoperative assessment, appropriate intraoperative monitoring and imaging, meticulous management of hemodynamics, and early treatment of expected side effects and complications is of utmost importance. An unexpected decrease or increase in systemic vascular resistance resulting in decreased coronary perfusion pressure or acute heart failure by elevated left ventricular end-diastolic pressure should be avoided by maintaining a normotensive blood pressure and heart rate between 60 bpm and 100 bpm. The choice of anesthetic technique, either local anesthesia with mild sedation promoting spontaneous respiration, deep intravenous sedation with insertion of a laryngeal mask, or general anesthesia, varies among centers and is probably not associated with a significant difference in outcome. Post valvuloplasty and implantation, which were done under rapid right ventricular pacing due to reduce left ventricular ejection and cardiac motion, may require some additional inotropic support. Tracheal extubation can usually be done at the end of the procedure. Close postoperative monitoring is necessary, and admission to an intensive care unit is required. However, at present a retrograde approach through the femoral artery is used. During the procedure, a balloon valvuloplasty is first done to facilitate passage of the native aortic valve. During rapid right ventricular pacing, the prosthesis is positioned and deployed under fluoroscopy and echocardiographic guidance. Alternatively, in patients with difficult vascular access because of extensive calcifications or tortuosity of the femoral artery or aorta, a transapical approach can be used. After a partial thoracotomy, direct puncture of the apical portion of the left ventricular free wall is done to gain catheter access to the left ventricle and aortic valve. The prosthesis is subsequently positioned and deployed, similar to the antegrade approach.

7. Implantation approaches

With regard to the delivery systems and their introduction into ascending aorta, two specific pathways have been explored so far: the antegrade pathway, which uses direct transapical access, and the retrograde pathway, which uses either transfemoral or trans-subclavian or trans-axillary access [11].

7.1. The transapical approach

The main advantages of using transapical procedures are: [1] the feasibility does not rely on the absence of a concomitant peripheral vascular disease or previous aortic surgery; [2] the delivery system seems to be more "steady" and the procedure itself more "straightforward"; and [3] this access potentially reduces the risk of calcium dislodgement due to the passage of a stiff transfemoral device into a diseased aortic arch. A transapical approach can be used in the operating room, in a hybrid room, or in a catheterization laboratory with a patient under general anesthesia. Regardless of where the transapical approach is done, it is a prerequisite that high-quality fluoroscopic imaging must be guaranteed. Apical bleeding is very rare, mostly related to patient tissue fragility or to the team learning curve, and represents the most dangerous complication related to transapical access itself. In transapical TAVI, the cardiac apex is prepared through a small left anterolateral mini-thoracotomy using a purse-string or a crossing suture reinforced by pledgets and, after the procedure, a chest tube is routinely inserted into the left pleura with pain releasers injected in the intercostal tissue (Figure 8).

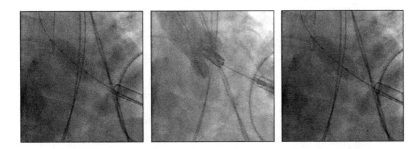

Figure 8. TAVI using the transapical approach

7.2. The transfemoral approach

The transfemoral approach is used mostly in cardiac catheterization laboratory or a hybrid room. One of the main advantages of this technique is that it allows fully percutaneous implantation in conscious patients, as long as the peripheral vessels are of an adequate caliber (more than 6mm diameter), there are no very tortuous vessels, and vascular closure devices are available (Figure 9). Alternatively, the standard technique requires surgical preparation of the common femoral artery under local or general anesthesia. Major and minor postoperative vascular complications have been reported quite often in recent series [12,13] and some critical events (vessel dissections, ruptures or avulsions) might be catastrophic when not promptly and adequately treated.

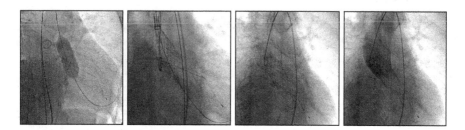

Figure 9. TAVI using the transfemoral approach

7.3. The trans-subclavian approach

Trans-subclavian access is an alternative retrograde pathway that has been recently explored. It requires a surgical exposure of the left subclavian artery and an adequate minimal vessel inner diameter for 18F delivery systems (Figure 10). There are some advantages in using this approach: firstly, the distance between the site of introduction and the aortic valve is short, compared with the transfemoral option, and it results in a steadier pathway. Secondly, as long as the subclavian artery is intact, the trans-subclavian procedure can be done in case of a concomitant vascular disease involving the abdominal aorta or the legs, and it does not require a thoracotomy. Unfortunately, the presence of a patent internal mammary artery, such as a diseased subclavian artery, in redo coronary surgery contraindicates this approach. However, at this moment, this interesting approach remains "off-label" and is not yet formally recommended by the industry.

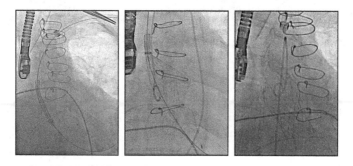

Figure 10. TAVI using the subclavian approach

7.4. The trans-aortic approach

In case of severe vascular disease and a concomitant contraindication to transapical proce-dures, an alternative, interesting, retrograde approach has been proposed: through an upper "J-shape" mini-sternotomy, the guidewire and the delivery system are inserted, retrograde-ly, into the ascending aorta and are secured with a double-string suture. TAVI is then done as a transfemoral procedure. The presence of "porcelain" aorta and the risk of postoperative massive bleeding limit this approach to selected patients.

8. Results from the literature

8.1. Cribrier-Edwards valve

Cribier *et al.* did the first human implantation in 2002 [14]. The Edwards SAPIEN valve was approved for use in the European Union in November 2007 (for the transfemoral approach) and in January 2008 (for transapical delivery). In the Initial Registry of EndoVascular Im-plantation of Valves in Europe (I-REVIVE) trial, followed by the Registry of Endovascular Critical Aortic Stenosis Treatment (RECAST) trial, a total of 36 patients (mean (SD) Euro-SCORE 12 (2)) were included [15]. Twenty-seven patients underwent successful percutane-ous aortic valve implantation (23 antegrade, 4 retrograde). The 30-day mortality was 22% (6 of 27 patients), and the mean AVA increased from $0.60 \pm 0.11cm2$ to $1.70 \pm 0.10cm2$ (p<0.001). Importantly, this improvement in AVA was maintained up to 24 months follow-up [16]. Since these first trials, the Cribrier-Edwards prosthesis and the Edwards SAPIEN prosthesis have been used in numerous studies. Overall, acute procedural success is ach-ieved in 75–100% of the procedures, and 30-day mortality ranges between 8–50% in the pub-lished studies. Using the transapical technique and the Sapien valve, Walther et al. [17] has reported their initial multicenter results of 59 consecutive patients, which is the largest feasi-bility study published thus far. Procedural success using the transapical technique was ach-ieved in 53 patients. Thirty-day mortality was 13.6% and none of these were thought to be valve related as there was good valve function at autopsy. The overall procedural success of 1038 SAPIEN implants from 32 centers within the European SOURCE registry was 93.8%. The 30-day survival within SOURCE was 93.7% (transfemoral) and 89.7% (transapical) [18]. The 1-year survival of the cohort was 81.1% (transfemoral) and 72.1% (transapical), respec-tively. In cohort B of the PARTNER randomized trial, 179 patients receiving transfemoral SAPIEN aortic valve with 179 patients receiving standard medical therapy (including bal-loon aortic valvuloplasty), confirmed the superiority of transfemoral TAVI with regard to overall survival and cardiac functional status [19]. The Kaplan-Meier 1-year mortality from any cause was 30.7% (TAVI) versus 50.7% (standard medical therapy), corresponding to a 0.55 hazard ratio with TAVI (p<0.001). The fraction of surviving patients at 1-year, in New York Heart Association functional class III-IV, was lower in the TAVI group (25.2% versus 58%; p<0.001). Nevertheless, the TAVI group had a higher 30-day incidence of major stroke (5.0% versus 1.1%; p=0.06) and major vascular complications (16.2% versus 1.1%; p<0.001). Early and 1-year outcomes from the REVIVAL trial, which consisted of 55 patients with a

mean AVA of 0.57±0.14cm2 and a mean logistic EuroSCORE of 33.5±17%, have been reported [20]. TAVI was successful in 87%. Mean echocardiographic AVA improved from 0.56±14
to 1.6±0.48cm2 after the procedure (p<0.0001). Thirty-day all-cause mortality and major adverse cardiac events (MACE) were 7.3% and 20%, respectively. These rates increased to
23.6% and 32.7%, respectively, at 1 year, with most late events related to underlying comorbidities. The mean NYHA functional class improved from 3.22±0.66 at baseline to 1.50±0.85
at 1-year follow-up (p<0.001).

8.2. CoreValve ReValving

Since the first implantation of the CoreValve prosthesis in a patient in 2005 [12], a large
number of patients have been treated with this device. The feasibility and safety of this
valve was studied in a prospective, multicenter trial [12]. A total of 25 symptomatic patients
with an AVA < 1cm^2 were enrolled in the study. The device was successfully implanted using the retrograde technique in 22 of 25 patients. Procedural success and aortic mean pressure gradients were markedly improved immediately following implantations with pre-
procedure gradients 44.24 ± 10.79 mmHg to 12.38 ± 3.03 mmHg post-procedure, and were
about the same at 30-day follow-up (11.82 ± 3.42 mm Hg). NYHA functional class improved
by 1 to 2 grades in all patients. MACE, defined as death from any cause, major arrhythmia,
myocardial infarction, cardiac tamponade, stroke, urgent or emergent conversion to surgery
or balloon valvuloplasty, emergent percutaneous coronary intervention, cardiogenic shock,
endocarditis, or aortic dissection, occurred in 8 of the 25 hospitalized patients. Recently,
Grube et al. [21] reported the results with the three different generations of the CoreValve
Revalving system in a non-randomized, prospective study of 136 patients. Ten patients were
treated with first-generation devices, 24 patients with second-generation, and 102 patients
with third-generation devices. At baseline, mean AVA was 0.67cm^2 and mean logistic Euro-
SCORE was 23.1% in the overall study population. With the new-generation devices, the
overall procedural success rate significantly increased from 70.0% and 70.8% to 91.2% for
the first-, second-, and third-generation prostheses, respectively (p = 0.003). Interestingly, using newer devices, periprocedural mortality decreased from 10% (first-generation) to 8.3%
(second-generation) to 0% (third-generation). Overall 30-day mortality for the three generations was 40%, 8.3% and 10.8%, respectively. Pooled data demonstrated a significant improvement in mean NYHA functional class (from 3.3 to 1.7, p<0.001), without a difference
between the three generations. Importantly, NYHA functional class and mean pressure gradient remained stable up to 12 months follow-up in all three generations. In addition, the
results of a multicenter registry with the third-generation CoreValve Revalving system have
recently been reported [22]. A total of 646 patients from 51 centers were included in the registry. It was a high-risk elderly population (mean age: 81 years) with a poor functional class
(85% of the patients in NYHA class III or IV), and a high logistic EuroSCORE (mean: 23.1%).
Procedural success was achieved in 628 of the 646 patients (97.2%). All-cause 30-day mortality was 8%, and the combined end point of procedural related death, stroke, or myocardial
infarction was reached in 60 patients (9.3%). After successful implantation, mean pressure
gradient decreased from 49 mmHg to 3 mmHg [22]. The FRANCE real-world registry of 244
consecutive high-risk patients with symptomatic severe AS, enrolled from 16 centers over a

period of 5 months in 2009, reported 98.3% procedural success for both Edwars SAPIEN and Medtronic CoreValve (66% transfemoral, 5% subclavian, and 29% transapical) prostheses [13]. The 30-day mortality was 12.7%, and, at 1 month, 88% of patients were in NYHA class I-II. Buellesfeld *et al.* [23] reported on a 2-year follow-up of 126 patients who underwent TA-VI. Thirty-day all-cause mortality was 15.2%. At 2-years, all-cause mortality was 38.1%, with a significant difference between the moderate-risk group and the combined high-risk groups (27.8% versus 45.8%; p=0.04). This difference was attributable to an increased risk of noncardiac mortality in high-risk groups. Hemodynamic results remained unchanged during follow-up (mean gradient: 8.5±2.5mmHg at 30 days and 9.0±3.5mmHg at 2 years) without any incidence of structural valve deterioration.

The larger CoreValve prostheses (26, 29 and 31 mm) were the only device for annulus between 26 and 29 mm, before the currently available 29-mm SAPIEN XT valve for transapical implantation. The CoreValve prosthesis had previously been the only device suitable for transarterial implant in patients with limited iliofemoral artery access, but this has changed with the SAPIEN NovaFlex delivery system. The growing experience with the subclavian artery approach, however, allows the CoreValve prosthesis to be implanted in patients with unusable iliofemoral arteries. Because of these results, the indications for TAVI expanded (e.g. in patients with porcelain aorta, with previous cardiac surgery, etc.) [24] (Figure 11,12).

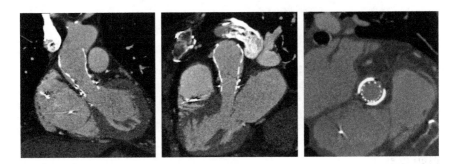

Figure 11. TAVI in a patient with a history of AVR

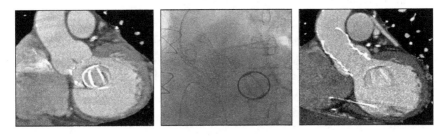

Figure 12. TAVI in a patient with a history of mitral valve replacement

9. Conclusion

Transcatheter aortic valve implantation was developed to provide an alternative and less invasive method of treating aortic valve stenosis. Actually, it has been proved that the method is feasible, with results that have been reproduced by many physicians in many centers (approximately 10,000 implantations to date). Today there are at least 10 new transcatheter aortic valves that have had their first implantation in humans, many more that have reached the level of animal experiments, and even more that are still in the initial design stage. As a new treatment tool, it has to be evaluated in randomized controlled trials with long-term follow-up in order to assess safety and efficacy. Therefore, TAVI should be restricted to a limited number of high-volume centers, that have both cardiology and cardiac surgery departments as well as expertise in structural heart disease intervention and high-risk valvular surgery. Because of excellent results with surgical valve replacement, patient selection, which should be done in multidisciplinary conferences, is of utmost importance. Like other interventional procedures, there is a learning curve with significant improvements in the success rate and the clinical results after the first 25 procedures, which implies that the TAVI procedure should initially be done by and thereafter supervised by a special team [25,26]. In addition to patient selection and intervention of TAVI, a close follow-up with assessment of clinical and objective parameters is mandatory for defining the indications of this technique.

Author details

Ibrahim Akin, Stephan Kische, Henrik Schneider, Tim C. Rehders,
Christoph A. Nienaber and Hüseyin Ince

University of Rostock, Germany

References

[1] Nkomo VT, Gardin JM, Skelton TN, et al. Burden of valvular heart disease: a population-based study. Lancet 2006;368(9540): 1005-11.

[2] Kvidal P, Bergstrom R, Horte LG, et al. Observed and relative survival after aortic valve replacement. J Am Coll Cardiol 2000;35(3): 747-56.

[3] Iung B, Cachier A, Baron G, et al. Decision-making in elderly patients with severe aortic stenosis: why are so many denied surgery. Eur Heart J 2005;26(24): 2714-20.

[4] Varadarajan P, Kapoor N, Bansal RC, et al. Clinical profile and natural history of 453 nonsurgical managed patients with severe aortic stenosis. Ann Thorac Surg 2006;82(6): 2111-5.

[5] Ross J Jr, Braunwald E. Aortic stenosis. Circulation 1965;38(2): V61-7.

[6] Vahanian A, Alfieri O, Al-Attar N, et al. Transcatheter valve implantation for pa-
     tients with aortic stenosis: a position statement from the European Association of
     Cardio-Thoracic Surgery (EACTS) and the European Society of Cardiology (ESC), in
     collaboration with the European Association of Percutaneous Cardiovascular Inter-
     ventions (EAPCI). Eur Heart J 2008;29(11): 1463-70.

[7] Zegdi R, Ciobotaru V, Noghin M, et al. Is it reasonable to treat all calcified stenotic
     aortic valves with a valved stent? Results from a human anatomic study in adults. J
     Am Coll Cardiol 2008;51(5): 579-84.

[8] Roques F, Nashef SA, Michel P, et al. Risk factors for early mortality after valve sur-
     gery in Europe in the 1990's: lesson from the EuroSCORE pilot program. J Heart
     Valve Dis 2001;10(5): 572-8.

[9] Grossi EA, Schwartz CF, Yu PJ, et al. High-risk aortic valve replacement: are the out-
     comes as bad as predicted. Ann Thorac Surg 2008; 85(1): 102-6.

[10] Babaliaros VC, Liff D, Chen EP, et al. Can balloon aortic valvuloplasty help deter-
     mine appropriate transcatheter aortic valve size. JACC Intv 2008;1(5): 580-6.

[11] De Robertis F, Asgar A, Davies S, et al. The left exillary arter-a new approach for
     transcatheter aortic valve implantation. Eur J Cardiothorac Surg 2009;36(5):807-12.

[12] Grube E, Laborde JC, Gerckens U, et al. Percutaneous implantation of the CoreValve
     self-expanding valve prosthesis in high-risk patients with aortic valve disease: Sieg-
     burg first-in-man study, Circulation 2006;114(15): 1616-24.

[13] Eltchaninoff H, Prat A, Gilard M, et al. Transcatheter aortic valve implantation: early
     results of the France (French Aortic National CoreValve and Edwards) registry. Eur
     Heart J 2011; 32(2): 191-7.

[14] Cribrier A, Eltchaninoff H, Bash A, et al. Percutaneous transcatheter implantation of
     an aortic valve prosthesis for calcific aortic stenosis: first human case description.
     Circulation 2002;106(24): 3006-8.

[15] Cribrier A, Elchaninoff H, Tron C, et al. Early experience with percutaneous trans-
     catheter implantation of heart valve prosthesis for the treatment of end-stage inoper-
     able patients with calcific aortic stenosis. J Am Coll Cardiol 2004;43(4): 698-703.

[16] Cribrier A, Elchaninoff H, Tron C, et al. Treatment of calcific aortic stenosis with the
     percutaneous heart valve: mid-term follow-up from the initial feasibility studies: the
     French experience. J Am Coll Cardiol 2006;47(6): 1214-23.

[17] Walther T, Simon P, Dewey T, et al. Transapical minimally invasive aortic valve im-
     plantation: multicenter experience. Circulation 2007;116(Suppl 11): I240-5.

[18] Thomas M, Schymik G, Walther T, et al. Thirty-day results of the SAPIEN aortic Bio-
     prosthesis Outcomes (SOURCE) Registry: A European registry of transcatheter aortic
     valve implantation using the Edwards SAPIEN valve. Circulation 2010;122(1): 62-9.

[19] Leon MB, Smith CR, Mack M, et al. Transcatheter aortic-valve implantation for aortic stenosis in patients who cannot undergo surgery. N Engl J Med 2010;363(17): 1597-607.

[20] Kodali SK, O'Neill WW, Moses JW, et al. Early and late (one year) outcomes follow-ing transcatheter aortic valve implantation in patients with severe aortic stenosis (from the United States REVIVAL Trial). Am J Cardiol 2011;107(7): 1058-64.

[21] Grube E, Buellesfeld L, Mueller R, et al. Progress and current status of percutaneous aortic valve replacement: results of three device generation of the CoreValve Revalv-ing system. Circ Cardiovasc Intervent 2008;1(3): 167-75.

[22] Piazza N, Grube E, Gerckens U, et al. Procedural and 30-day outcomes following transcatheter aortic valve implantation using the third generation (18 Fr) CoreValve revalving system: results from the multicentre, expanded evaluation registry 1-year following CE mark approval. EuroIntervention 2008;4(2): 242-9.

[23] Buellesfeld L, Gerckens U, Schuler G, et al. 2-year follow-up of patients undergoing transcatheter aortic valve implantation using a self-expanding valve prosthesis. J Am Coll Cardiol 2011;57(16): 1650-7.

[24] Wenaweser P, Buellesfeld L, Gerckens U, Grube E. Percutaneous aortic valve replace-ment for sévère aortic régurgitation in degenerated bioprosthesis : the first valve in valve procédure using Corevlave Revalving system. Catheter Cardiovasc Interv 2007 ;70(5) :760-4.

[25] Walther T, Dewey T, Borger MA, et al. Transapical aortic valve implantation: step by step. Ann Thorac Surg 2009;87(1): 276-83.

[26] Webb JG, Pasupati S, Humphries K, et al. Percutaneous transarterial aortic valve re-placement in selected high-risk patients with aortic stenosis. Circulation 2007 ;116(7): 755-63.

Chapter 9

Congenital Aortic Stenosis in Children

Hirofumi Saiki and Hideaki Senzaki

Additional information is available at the end of the chapter

1. Introduction

Congenital aortic stenosis (AS) is caused by abnormal morphological development of the aortic valve. [1, 2] Valvular abnormalities may be accompanied by supra- or sub-valvular stenosis. The embryogenic process that forms aortic valves begins approximately 31–32 days of gestation. Cavity formation in the basal portion of the truncus arteriosus is a key process in the development of the leaflet and sinus of Valsalva, which are important components of the aortic valve. Therefore, incomplete formation of the cavity causes various morphological abnormalities of the aortic valve, including bicuspid valve with or without commissural fusion, tricuspid valve with commissural fusion, monocuspid valve, and myxomatoid leaflet valve (dysplastic valve). The most frequent type of congenital AS is a bicuspid aortic valve, [3] accounting for approximately 90% of AS cases.

Although the morphological features of the aortic valve are closely associated with the AS severity, the pathophysiology and resultant clinical manifestation of AS are fundamentally determined by the severity of the stenosis (effective orifice area). In this sense, congenital AS in children is classified into 2 major types: severe AS that becomes symptomatic and necessitates interventions during the neonatal period or early infancy and a milder form of AS with signs and/or symptoms that develop later in childhood.

In this chapter, we will outline the pathophysiology, clinical characteristics, and management of congenital AS observed in children (from fetus to adolescence) for each type of AS mentioned above. We will also briefly discuss the differences in ventricular adaptation, which are strongly linked to the clinical manifestation of AS, to the increased afterload caused by AS between children and adults.

2. Pathophysiology of congenital AS

The mechanism underlying the increase in severity of AS in children is similar to that seen in adults. The orifice size can decrease because of increased thickness and rigidity of the valve leaflets, independent of the morphological anomalies of the aortic valve, although native abnormal morphological features have greater impact on the progression of stenosis in children than in adults. The mechanisms underlying the exacerbation of stenosis also need to be determined. Valvular fibrosis, lipid accumulation, [4,5] inflammatory changes, [6] and acquired fibrotic fusion of commissures, which increase cusp thickness/stiffness, [5,7] could also be associated with the development of valvular stenosis, even in childhood AS. Metabolic syndrome is an emerging issue even in children and may be associated with these exacerbating mechanisms, [8] resulting in calcification, which reduces the possibility of valvular plastic surgery. In addition, bicuspid aortic valves possibly develop aortic calcification earlier than tricuspid aortic valves. [9,10] In this section, we will discuss the hemodynamic aspects of aortic stenosis in fetuses, neonates, and children.

2.1. AS with signs and symptoms that develop during the fetal or neonatal period

The fundamental underlying pathophysiology of AS involves an increase in afterload to the left ventricle (LV). The mechanism by which the LV copes with this increase in afterload is an increase of myocardial mass (hypertrophy) to generate a higher force to confront the increased afterload. If the aortic valve stenosis is too severe to allow the LV to become adaptive, LV contractility is depressed and the LV becomes markedly dilated. In this critical condition, the fetal circulation can maintain, to some extent, the systemic output using the right ventricle (RV), because there are interatrial communication (foramen ovale) and ductus arteriosus in the fetal ciculation. The ascending aortic flow and sometimes even the coronary arterial flow rely on retrograde blood flow from the ductus arteriosus. However, an LV exposed to massive afterload with relatively reduced coronary blood flow supply is at high risk of progressive ventricular failure, and is associated with an increased risk of sudden cardiac death. If the patient can survive this condition for a certain period, a marked increase in LV end-diastolic pressure (EDP) hinders the blood flow from the left atrium entering into the LV, leading to a gradual reduction of LV cavity volume. This process is postulated as one mechanism of evolving hypoplastic left heart syndrome (HLHS). Degeneration of the endocardium may accompany this process, representing a condition known as endocardial fibroelastosis. [11]

In other cases, an increase in LV afterload may allow the LV to exert its adaptive mechanism of hypertrophy, which also inhibits LV inflow due to increased LV stiffness and resultant EDP rise. [12] This is another form of evolving HLHS physiology (Figure 1A).

Of course, the above pathophysiological mechanisms should be understood as a continuum, [13, 14] and some patients may be born with a markedly dilated LV and depressed contractility, known as critical AS (Figure 1B). Such patients suffer from severe circulatory failure and pulmonary congestion, which is often life threatening and requires emergency intervention, either by catheters or surgery, as discussed below.

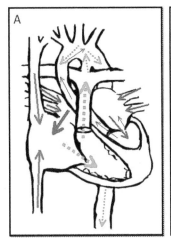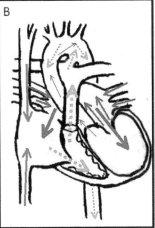

Figure 1. A schema of hypoplastic left heart syndrome (A) and that of critical aortic stenosis (B).

2.2. AS with signs and/or symptoms that develop during late infancy and school age

When the severity of AS is mild such that the LV can cope with the increased afterload, patients present with clinical symptoms during late infancy or school age. Although their LV exhibits hypertrophy, AS may be mild enough in patients such that they will be asymptomatic. There are also a group of patients who had no signs and symptoms other than heart murmur. In general, the aortic valves of this group of patients can supply the systemic blood flow during the neonatal period. This is verified by the fact that the ductus flow during the neonatal period shows left-to-right shunting. The timing of the onset of AS symptoms in this group is dependent on the severity of stenosis that is associated with the LV's capability to exert its adaptive mechanism to increased afterload. Of note, unlike adult onset AS, the severity of AS in children is also influenced by somatic growth, which induces a relative increase in the blood flow through the aortic valve and thereby causes augmentation of LV afterload. In addition, it was reported that an increased pressure gradient across the aortic valve is related to earlier progression of stenosis and a higher frequency of complicating aortic regurgitation. [15, 16] Therefore, the pathophysiology of AS in this age group may be dependent on preload change due to aortic regurgitation as well as the increasing afterload. In the clinical setting, it is important to follow-up with these patients periodically to detect such changes and to determine the appropriate timing and method of treatment. Therefore, we will discuss methods for monitoring the dynamic changes in AS in this particular group of patients in the following section.

2.2.1. Monitoring methods for AS

Clinical symptom evaluation, physical examination, electrocardiogram (ECG), and echocardiography are essential sources for obtaining comprehensive information for appropriate management of AS in this patient group. If fainting, convulsion, or resuscitated cardiac arrest are observed, relieving AS is indicated for preventing further adverse events. [17, 18] Although angina and syncope are reported to be observed only in <10% of patients whose peak-to-peak pressure gradient is greater than 80 mmHg, chest pain is an important clinical sign indicating the need for intervention, as adverse events are likely to occur within a few years after the complaint of initial chest pain.

ECG examinations are informative if ST-segment changes are observed. Usually, severe AS shows a 0–90°QRS-axis with high voltages in the left precordial leads. However, it is important to note that the above ECG findings of LV hypertrophy do not necessarily reflect the severity of the stenosis. Wagner et al. reported that one-third of AS patients with peak-to-peak pressure gradients greater than 80 mmHg do not exhibit the above LV hypertrophic findings on ECG. [17] In contrast, the ST strain pattern in the left precordial leads is thought to be more specific to LV hypertrophy and reflects the severity of AS (Figure 2).

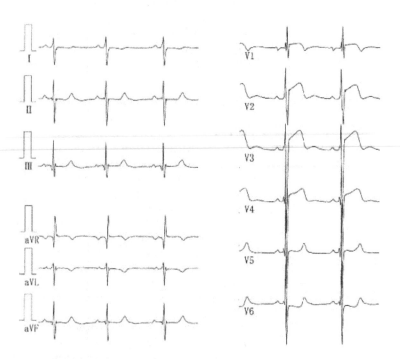

Figure 2. Electrocardiogram of severe aortic stenosis. This is an electrocardiogram (ECG) of a patient with severe aortic stenosis with an estimated pressure gradient of 140mmHg. Surprisingly, ECG shows no prominent finding of left ventricular hypertrophy other than changes in ST-T segment.

Holter ECG is also useful for predicting sudden deaths, even in asymptomatic AS patients. Wolfe et al. reported that multiform ventricular premature contraction, couplet, and ventricular tachycardia are serious arrhythmias that are associated with sudden cardiac death. [19]

Exercise testing may provide more accurate information about the risk of cardiac events than other examinations. Lewis et al. demonstrated the usefulness of exercise testing to identify subclinical ischemia in patients with severe AS. [26] Thus, exercise testing and Holter ECG may play a key role in clinician decision making for the management of AS patients.

Echocardiography is a direct method for evaluating the anatomical features and severity of AS. Valvular anatomy can be assessed for leaflet number, balance, thickening, or doming. The annulus diameter is also important, particularly when intervention is indicated. M-mode study in short-axis view provides information regarding LV pressure calculated by Glanz's equation: LV systolic pressure=225*LVPWs/LVIDs, where LVPWs and LVIDs represent LV systolic posterior wall thickness and LV systolic diameter, respectively. [20] This equation is clinically useful, because the peak-to-peak pressure gradient can be evaluated when coupled with the arterial pressure measurement. The LV dimension and wall thickness values provide information regarding the risk of cardiac events and ischemia. In addition, combining an echocardiography study with exercise testing may be useful for predicting a higher risk of cardiac events, even in asymptomatic patients. [21] Velocity measurement by spectral pulse wave and continuous wave Doppler reflects the severity of AS if cardiac function is not impaired. The pressure gradient calculated by applying the Bernoulli equation in the outflow tract is one of the guides for determining the need for intervention, although it has some limitations. [22, 23] Spectral pulse wave Doppler could also be a powerful tool for confirming the localization of obstruction and estimating the valvular area.

The indication for the catheter examination is limited, but this modality provides accurate information regarding coronary arteries and severity of AS. Because the LV outflow tract is truncated, the severity of AS tends to be over-estimated by velocity-derived pressure gradient. In contrast, a precise PIPG as well as a peak-to-peak gradient can be evaluated by the catheter examination (Figure 3). The aortic valve area is also calculated by Gorlin's method. [24]

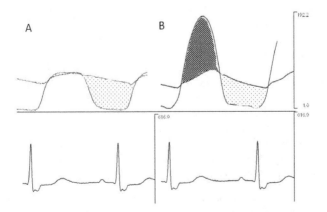

Figure 3. Simultaneous measurements of ascending aortic pressure and left ventricular pressure by the catheter examination. Both instantaneous and peak to peak pressure gradient can be clearly monitored. A; normal, B; aortic stenosis

3. Treatment of AS

3.1. Fetal and neonatal AS

If the patients have an established HLHS circulation with an underdeveloped LV, all the treatment options are directed to the future completion of the Fontan circulation, a final goal for patients with single ventricular circulation. However, if the LV size and components are to be sufficient to generate systemic output when the excessive afterload due to AS is relieved, interventions for the aortic valve per se are indicated, including either catheters or surgery. [25] The most attractive merit of catheter intervention (percutaneous transluminal aortic valvuloplasty [PTAV]) is that it is less invasive. In this procedure, cardiopulmonary bypass, which is a prerequisite for surgical procedures, can be avoided. PTAV is known to accelerate annular growth even in small sized aortic valve [26] if mitral valve stenosis is not complicated [27] .In performing PTAV, the carotid artery is generally used for blood access because lower body hypoperfusion makes it difficult to achieve access from the femoral artery and has a high risk of arterial obstruction with a prolonged sheath insertion, and because the curvature of aortic arch makes it difficult to manipulate the catheter and successfully pass it through the tiny aortic orifice (Figure 4). Therefore, central nervous system damage can be a potential adverse event associated with PTAV. More importantly, PTAV is a procedure used to enlarge the aortic orifice area by tearing the weak portions of the valve, not necessarily in the anatomically proper portion (commissures). Therefore, PTAV cannot be applied to valves with pre-existing aortic regurgitation because the procedure generally worsens this condition, which could be fatal. It was reported that 15% of 113 patients younger than 60 days old who had undergone PTAV developed significant aortic regurgitation. [26] Surgical interventions in this patient group include aortic valve plasty (AVP) and aortic valve replacement (AVR) with the autologous pulmonary artery valve (Ross procedure). The advantage of open AVP is that surgeons can perform the procedure on the basis of a detailed examination of the valve anatomy, which may reduce the risk of aortic regurgitation. Bhabra et al. [28] reported that if the aortic valve is tricuspid, the rate of freedom from reintervention after open AVP was 92% and that of AVR was 100% at a 10-year follow-up. These rates for bicuspid valves were only 33% and 57%, respectively. This report emphasizes the importance of valve morphology as a determinant of outcome following AVP. The other surgical option is the Ross procedure, which is particularly useful when sub/suprastenosis coexists with valvular stenosis (Ross-Konno procedure). The survival rate for the Ross procedure was 77% and rate of freedom from reintervention was 50%, comparable to the results of the Norwood procedure. [29-31] To apply the Ross procedure, autologous graft (pulmonary valve) function is important. Concha et al. reported that the rate of freedom from autograft failure at a 5-year follow-up was 95%, demonstrating a low incidence of autograft failure. [32] However, future pulmonary insufficiency remains as a matter of concern in long-term follow-ups.

We often encounter intermediate cases between established HLHS with underdeveloped LV and potentially normal-sized LV under excessive afterload. In such situations, accurate diagnosis about whether the LV has the potential to generate systemic output after relieving afterload is of primary importance. If the LV is judged to be incapable of generating systemic output, then the systemic circulation should rely on the RV. In such a case, the Fontan procedure becomes a goal of treatment. Multicenter studies have elucidated that the outcome of biventricular repair with a small LV is much worse than that of the Fontan procedure [13, 14], although the survival rate of Fontan completion for patients with a small LV or severely reduced LV function is only approximately 50-70%, even in the recent reports. [33-35]

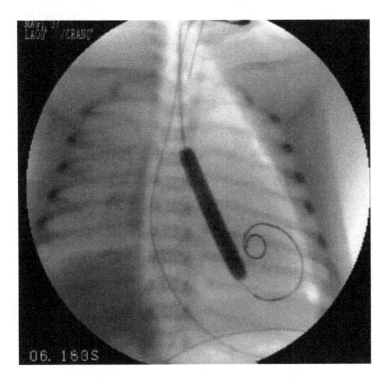

Figure 4. Percutaneous transluminal aortic valvuloplasty performed for a patient with critical aortic stenosis

Based on the pathophysiology of evolving HLHS as previously discussed and the poor survival rate of HLHS patients, fetal intervention has been attempted, aimed at relieving AS at earlier stages before the LV cavity is reduced. For the first time, Maxwell et al. reported their experience of intrauterine balloon dilatation of the fetal aortic valve in 1991. [36] Thereafter, a case series of 12 fetuses that underwent balloon valvuloplasty in the third trimester were reported, with no improvement was observed in their LV growth. [37] Tworetzky et al. also reported the results of fetal intervention for 24 AS patients (ranging from 21 to 29 weeks of gestation) who were thought to have a high probability of developing HLHS. [38] Technical success was achieved in 14 patients, but only 3 patients were able to undergo two-ventricular repair. Therefore, fetal intervention should be regarded as experimental at present, as many issues remain to be solved.

3.2. AS with signs and symptoms that develop during late infancy and school age

The treatment strategy for AS in which signs and/or symptoms develop later in childhood is different from that for neonatal AS. The American College of Cardiology/American Heart Association Guidelines for the management of AS of this group [31] recommended that patients with a peak instantaneous pressure gradient (PIPG) measured by Doppler echocardiography ≥70 mmHg be considered for cardiac catheterization and treatment in asymptomatic children and young adults. If the patients desire to participate in competitive sports or become pregnant, a PIPG of 50–70 mmHg is an indication for further evaluation and interventions. If patients have symptoms (angina, syncope, or dyspnea on exertion), a PIPG ≥50 mmHg is the indication for treatment. If the PIPG is less than 50 mmHg and a symptom is present, another origin of the symptom should be investigated.

There are several treatment options for cases in which intervention is indicated, including PTAV, open AVP, the Ross procedure, and AVR. Procedure selection is primarily dependent upon whether the patient's somatic size (aortic annular size) is large enough to use a prosthetic valve, because AVR is considered as the first-line procedure at present. If the prosthetic valve is not available, procedures other than AVR are selected so that patients can live with their own valve until they can use a prosthetic aortic valve. In such situations, the most important concept for treatment is that the procedure should be regarded as a bridge to AVR. Therefore, the aim of any intervention should be to reduce the afterload without any significant aortic regurgitation so that patients can grow uneventfully until AVR can be performed. In this sense, if these patients do not have heart failure but have exertion-induced ischemic signs, restriction of exercise without invasive intervention may be selected to achieve a better outcome. Application of PTAV in this age group is relatively limited because AVP is thought to be better than PTAV in terms of preserving aortic valve function, [39, 40] and because aortic insufficiency caused by valvuloplasty is known to be progressive in nature. [15, 16] However, some patients may still benefit from PTAV to achieve the therapeutic goal in this AS group. The Ross procedure is also not regarded as a definitive repair surgery, because neoaortic regurgitation and pulmonary insufficiency are frequently observed postoperative complications, which require further interventions in the future. [40, 41] Therefore, the Ross procedure indication is limited to patients who cannot grow due to severe aortic insufficiency.

4. The hemodynamic effects of AS on ventricular function in children

In this last section, we briefly comment on the differences in LV geometric and functional changes between adult- and child-onset of AS. The natural history of LV geometric and functional changes in adult-onset AS is characterized by LV concentric hypertrophy in the early stage, followed by diastolic dysfunction, systolic dysfunction with eccentric hypertrophy, and heart failure at the end-stage. [42] Most of the patients who are candidates for surgical intervention are ranked in the state between diastolic and systolic ventricular dysfunction. Delayed relaxation characterizes early-stage ventricular diastolic dysfunction, and thus is observed in almost all AS patients, [43] while increased diastolic stiffness is observed in more advanced stages in which LV hypertrophy and fibrosis may coexist. The degree of diastolic dysfunction is important for predicting prognosis because it takes years to achieve reverse remodeling of diastolic function after normalization of afterload. [44]

In contrast to the relatively uniform geometric and functional LV changes observed in adult-onset AS, such changes in children's AS are diverse and somewhat different from those of adults. The difference primarily stems from the diversity of the initial impact of afterload on the LV. Because adult onset of AS is largely due to a bicuspid valve or atherosclerotic change with aging, AS gradually increases LV afterload. This allows the LV to confront the increased afterload by inducing hypertrophic changes. However, the severity of AS that initially imposes afterload on the LV is diverse in children, as previously discussed, thus excessive afterload may not allow the LV to become hypertrophic, resulting in LV dilation and systolic dysfunction as observed in critical AS. With increasing age, the LV geometry and function gradually resembles those of adult AS: a hypertrophic LV with diastolic dysfunction. However, it is rare in children to observe a marked increase in LV diastolic stiffness, even in cases of hypertrophic LV (Figure 5). In addition, it is interesting that LV relaxation appears to be relatively preserved in children with AS and hypertrophic LV. These differences in LV functional responses between children and adults may have a clue to a better management of patients with AS.

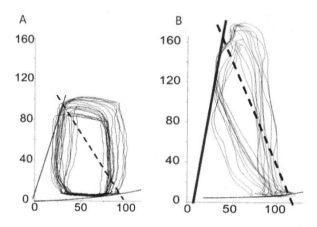

Figure 5. Examples of left ventricular pressure-volume relationships in a control patient (A) and a patient with aortic stenosis (B). The steep slope of the end-systolic pressure-volume relationship (solid line) and arterial elastance (dashed line) indicate increased ventricular contractility and afterload. Note that the slope of the end-diastolic pressure-volume relationship in aortic stenosis is comparable to that of control.

5. Conclusions

In adults, AS generally develops slowly, with the progression of valve calcification or leaflet degeneration being independent of the existence of substrates for congenital abnormalities.

This allows the LV to adapt to the increased afterload by becoming concentrically hypertrophied. Therefore, it takes a long time before LV systolic function is severely impaired and critical events occur.[45] Because valvular calcification is a commonly observed morphological change and because a prosthetic valve is generally available for adults, aortic valve replacement is selected as a first-line treatment and plastic surgery is seldom chosen for this population. Thus, the treatment strategy is rather straightforward.

In contrast, as discussed in this chapter, a wide range of clinical phenotypes is seen in pediatric AS. Depending on the severity of the native aortic valve abnormality and associated hemodynamic features, AS could be one of the most severe forms of congenital heart defects in children, leading to a critical condition in neonates or even during fetal life. In the milder form of pediatric AS, no clinical symptoms are seen throughout the patient's life. Therefore, the complexity of the treatment approach depends upon the patient's age, body size, and associated cardiac anomalies. In particular, because of the limited availability of prosthetic aortic valves for small children, the native valve morphological features constitute an extremely important determinant of treatment strategy. A detailed assessment of LV function as well as accurate anatomical diagnosis, including analysis of the potential utility of the native aortic valve, is essential for achieving a better outcome for patients. The use of specific medications [46] and prevention of metabolic syndrome from childhood may help improve outcomes.

Accumulation of information regarding the outcomes of underdeveloped valves, detailed mechanisms underlying disease progression, surgical outcomes, and improvements in surgical techniques should lead to considerably improved outcomes in the pediatric population.

Author details

Hirofumi Saiki and Hideaki Senzaki*

Department of Pediatric Cardiology, Saitama Medical Center, Saitama Medical University, Saitama, Japan

References

[1] Falcone, M. W, Roberts, W. C, & Morrow, A. G. Perloff JK: Congenital aortic stenosis resulting from a unicommisssural valve. Clinical and anatomic features in twenty-one adult patients. *Circulation* (1971).

[2] Aortic StenosisIn Moss's Heart disease in infants, Children, and adolescents, Baltimore The Lippincott Wiliams and Wilkins Co. (2001).

[3] Michelena, H. I, Desjardins, V. A, & Avierinos, J. F. Natural history of asymptomatic patients with normally functioning or minimally dysfunctional bicuspid aortic valve in the community. *Circulation* (2008).

[4]   Palta, S, Pai, A. M, & Gill, K. S. Pai RG: New insights into the progression of aortic stenosis: implications for secondary prevention. *Circulation* (2000).

[5]   Pohle, K, Maffert, R, & Ropers, D. Progression of aortic valve calcification: association with coronary atherosclerosis and cardiovascular risk factors. *Circulation* (2001).

[6]   Olsson, M, Dalsgaard, C. J, Haegerstrand, A, Rosenqvist, M, & Ryden, L. Nilsson J: Accumulation of T lymphocytes and expression of interleukin-2 receptors in nonrheumatic stenotic aortic valves. *J Am Coll Cardiol* (1994).

[7]   Parolari, A, Loardi, C, & Mussoni, L. Nonrheumatic calcific aortic stenosis: an overview from basic science to pharmacological prevention. *Eur J Cardiothorac Surg* (2009).

[8]   Capoulade, R, Clavel, M. A, & Dumesnil, J. G. Impact of metabolic syndrome on progression of aortic stenosis: influence of age and statin therapy. *J Am Coll Cardiol* (2012).

[9]   Pomerance A: Pathogenesis of aortic stenosis and its relation to age. (1972). *Br Heart J.*

[10] Hope, M. D, Urbania, T. H, Yu, J. P, & Chitsaz, S. Tseng E: Incidental aortic valve calcification on CT scans: significance for bicuspid and tricuspid valve disease. *Academic radiology* (2012).

[11] Mcelhinney, D. B, Vogel, M, & Benson, C. B. Assessment of left ventricular endocardial fibroelastosis in fetuses with aortic stenosis and evolving hypoplastic left heart syndrome. *Am J Cardiol* (2010).

[12] Mcelhinney, D. B, Marshall, A. C, & Wilkins-haug, L. E. Predictors of technical success and postnatal biventricular outcome after in utero aortic valvuloplasty for aortic stenosis with evolving hypoplastic left heart syndrome. *Circulation* (2009).

[13] Lofland, G. K, Mccrindle, B. W, & Williams, W. G. Critical aortic stenosis in the neonate: a multi-institutional study of management, outcomes, and risk factors. Congenital Heart Surgeons Society. *J Thorac Cardiovasc Surg* (2001).

[14] Jacobs, J. P, Mavroudis, C, & Jacobs, M. L. Lessons learned from the data analysis of the second harvest ((1998). of the Society of Thoracic Surgeons (STS) Congenital Heart Surgery Database. *Eur J Cardiothorac Surg* 2004, 26(1):18-37.

[15] Eroglu, A. G, Babaoglu, K, & Saltik, L. Echocardiographic follow-up of congenital aortic valvular stenosis. *Pediatr Cardiol* (2006).

[16] Davis, C. K, Cummings, M. W, & Gurka, M. J. Gutgesell HP: Frequency and degree of change of peak transvalvular pressure gradient determined by two Doppler echocardiographic examinations in newborns and children with valvular congenital aortic stenosis. *Am J Cardiol* (2008).

[17] Wagner, H. R, Weidman, W. H, & Ellison, R. C. Miettinen OS: Indirect assessment of severity in aortic stenosis. *Circulation* (1977). Suppl):I, 20-3.

[18]   Wagner, H. R, Ellison, R. C, Keane, J. F, & Humphries, O. J. Nadas AS: Clinical course
       in aortic stenosis. *Circulation* (1977). Suppl):I, 47-56.

[19]   Wolfe, R. R, Driscoll, D. J, & Gersony, W. M. Arrhythmias in patients with valvar aortic
       stenosis, valvar pulmonary stenosis, and ventricular septal defect. Results of hour ECG
       monitoring. *Circulation* (1993). Suppl):I89-101., 24.

[20]   Glanz, S, Hellenbrand, W. E, & Berman, M. A. Talner NS: Echocardiographic assess-
       ment of the severity of aortic stenosis in children and adolescents. *Am J Cardiol* (1976).

[21]   Lancellotti, P, Lebois, F, Simon, M, Tombeux, C, & Chauvel, C. Pierard LA: Prognostic
       importance of quantitative exercise Doppler echocardiography in asymptomatic
       valvular aortic stenosis. *Circulation* (2005). Suppl):I, 377-82.

[22]   Little, S. H, & Chan, K. L. Burwash IG: Impact of blood pressure on the Doppler
       echocardiographic assessment of severity of aortic stenosis. *Heart* (2007).

[23]   Giardini, A. Tacy TA: Pressure recovery explains doppler overestimation of invasive
       pressure gradient across segmental vascular stenosis. *Echocardiography* (2010).

[24]   Gorlin, R. Gorlin SG: Hydraulic formula for calculation of the area of the stenotic mitral
       valve, other cardiac valves, and central circulatory shunts. I. *Am Heart J* (1951).

[25]   Mccrindle, B. W, Blackstone, E. H, & Williams, W. G. Are outcomes of surgical versus
       transcatheter balloon valvotomy equivalent in neonatal critical aortic stenosis?
       Circulation (2001). Suppl 1):I, 152-8.

[26]   Mcelhinney, D. B, Lock, J. E, Keane, J. F, & Moran, A. M. Colan SD: Left heart growth,
       function, and reintervention after balloon aortic valvuloplasty for neonatal aortic
       stenosis. *Circulation* (2005).

[27]   Han, R. K, Gurofsky, R. C, & Lee, K. J. Outcome and growth potential of left heart
       structures after neonatal intervention for aortic valve stenosis. *J Am Coll Cardiol* (2007).

[28]   Bhabra, M. S, Dhillon, R, & Bhudia, S. Surgical aortic valvotomy in infancy: impact of
       leaflet morphology on long-term outcomes. *Ann Thorac Surg* (2003).

[29]   Shinkawa, T, Bove, E. L, Hirsch, J. C, & Devaney, E. J. Ohye RG: Intermediate-term
       results of the Ross procedure in neonates and infants. *Ann Thorac Surg* (2010). discussion
       32.

[30]   Hansen, J. H, Petko, C, Bauer, G, Voges, I, & Kramer, H. H. Scheewe J: Fifteen-year
       single-center experience with the Norwood operation for complex lesions with single-
       ventricle physiology compared with hypoplastic left heart syndrome. *J Thorac Cardio-
       vasc Surg* (2012).

[31]   Feinstein, J. A, Benson, D. W, & Dubin, A. M. Hypoplastic left heart syndrome: current
       considerations and expectations. *J Am Coll Cardiol* (2012). Suppl):S, 1-42.

[32]   Concha, M, Aranda, P. J, & Casares, J. The Ross procedure. *Journal of cardiac surgery*
       (2004).

[33] Feinstein, J. A, Benson, D. W, & Dubin, A. M. Hypoplastic left heart syndrome: current considerations and expectations. *J Am Coll Cardiol,* 59(1 Suppl):S, 1-42.

[34] Graham, E. M, Zyblewski, S. C, & Phillips, J. W. Comparison of Norwood shunt types: do the outcomes differ 6 years later? *Ann Thorac Surg,* , 90(1), 31-5.

[35] Photiadis, J, Sinzobahamvya, N, & Hraska, V. Asfour B: Does bilateral pulmonary banding in comparison to norwood procedure improve outcome in neonates with hypoplastic left heart syndrome beyond second-stage palliation? A review of the current literature. *Thorac Cardiovasc Surg,* , 60(3), 181-8.

[36] Maxwell, D, & Allan, L. Tynan MJ: Balloon dilatation of the aortic valve in the fetus: a report of two cases. *Br Heart J* (1991).

[37] Kohl, T, Sharland, G, & Allan, L. D. World experience of percutaneous ultrasound-guided balloon valvuloplasty in human fetuses with severe aortic valve obstruction. *Am J Cardiol* (2000).

[38] Tworetzky, W, Wilkins-haug, L, & Jennings, R. W. Balloon dilation of severe aortic stenosis in the fetus: potential for prevention of hypoplastic left heart syndrome: candidate selection, technique, and results of successful intervention. *Circulation* (2004).

[39] Rehnstrom, P, Malm, T, & Jogi, P. Outcome of surgical commissurotomy for aortic valve stenosis in early infancy. *Ann Thorac Surg* (2007).

[40] Miyamoto, T, Sinzobahamvya, N, & Wetter, J. Twenty years experience of surgical aortic valvotomy for critical aortic stenosis in early infancy. *Eur J Cardiothorac Surg* (2006).

[41] Williams, I. A, Quaegebeur, J. M, & Hsu, D. T. Ross procedure in infants and toddlers followed into childhood. *Circulation* (2005). Suppl):I, 390-5.

[42] Lund, O, Flo, C, & Jensen, F. T. Left ventricular systolic and diastolic function in aortic stenosis. Prognostic value after valve replacement and underlying mechanisms. *Eur Heart J* (1997).

[43] Murakami, T, Hess, O. M, Gage, J. E, & Grimm, J. Krayenbuehl HP: Diastolic filling dynamics in patients with aortic stenosis. *Circulation* (1986).

[44] Villari, B, Vassalli, G, Monrad, E. S, Chiariello, M, & Turina, M. Hess OM: Normalization of diastolic dysfunction in aortic stenosis late after valve replacement. *Circulation* (1995).

[45] Rosenhek, R, Binder, T, & Porenta, G. Predictors of outcome in severe, asymptomatic aortic stenosis. *N Engl J Med* (2000).

[46] Leskela, H. V, Vuolteenaho, O, & Koivula, M. K. Tezosentan inhibits uptake of proinflammatory endothelin-1 in stenotic aortic valves. *J Heart Valve Dis* (2012).

Permissions

The contributors of this book come from diverse backgrounds, making this book a truly international effort. This book will bring forth new frontiers with its revolutionizing research information and detailed analysis of the nascent developments around the world.

We would like to thank Elena Aikawa, MD, PhD, for lending her expertise to make the book truly unique. She has played a crucial role in the development of this book. Without her invaluable contribution this book wouldn't have been possible. She has made vital efforts to compile up to date information on the varied aspects of this subject to make this book a valuable addition to the collection of many professionals and students.

This book was conceptualized with the vision of imparting up-to-date information and advanced data in this field. To ensure the same, a matchless editorial board was set up. Every individual on the board went through rigorous rounds of assessment to prove their worth. After which they invested a large part of their time researching and compiling the most relevant data for our readers. Conferences and sessions were held from time to time between the editorial board and the contributing authors to present the data in the most comprehensible form. The editorial team has worked tirelessly to provide valuable and valid information to help people across the globe.

Every chapter published in this book has been scrutinized by our experts. Their significance has been extensively debated. The topics covered herein carry significant findings which will fuel the growth of the discipline. They may even be implemented as practical applications or may be referred to as a beginning point for another development. Chapters in this book were first published by InTech; hereby published with permission under the Creative Commons Attribution License or equivalent.

The editorial board has been involved in producing this book since its inception. They have spent rigorous hours researching and exploring the diverse topics which have resulted in the successful publishing of this book. They have passed on their knowledge of decades through this book. To expedite this challenging task, the publisher supported the team at every step. A small team of assistant editors was also appointed to further simplify the editing procedure and attain best results for the readers.

Our editorial team has been hand-picked from every corner of the world. Their multi-ethnicity adds dynamic inputs to the discussions which result in innovative outcomes. These outcomes are then further discussed with the researchers and contributors who give their valuable feedback and opinion regarding the same. The feedback is then collaborated with the researches and they are edited in a comprehensive manner to aid the understanding of the subject.

Apart from the editorial board, the designing team has also invested a significant amount of their time in understanding the subject and creating the most relevant covers. They scrutinized every image to scout for the most suitable representation of the subject and create an appropriate cover for the book.

The publishing team has been involved in this book since its early stages. They were actively engaged in every process, be it collecting the data, connecting with the contributors or procuring relevant information. The team has been an ardent support to the editorial, designing and production team. Their endless efforts to recruit the best for this project, has resulted in the accomplishment of this book. They are a veteran in the field of academics and their pool of knowledge is as vast as their experience in printing. Their expertise and guidance has proved useful at every step. Their uncompromising quality standards have made this book an exceptional effort. Their encouragement from time to time has been an inspiration for everyone.

The publisher and the editorial board hope that this book will prove to be a valuable piece of knowledge for researchers, students, practitioners and scholars across the globe.

List of Contributors

Mehmet Demir
Bursa Yüksek İhtisas Education and Research Hospital, Cardiology Department, Bursa, Turkey

George Tokmaji, Dave R. Koolbergen and Bas A.J.M. de Mol
Department of Cardiothoracic Surgery, Academic Medical Center, Amsterdam, The Netherlands

Berto J. Bouma
Department of Cardiology, Academic Medical Center, Amsterdam, The Netherlands

Dave R. Koolbergen
Department of Cardiothoracic Surgery, Leiden University Medical Center, Leiden, The Netherlands

Fahrettin Oz and Huseyin Oflaz
Istanbul University, Istanbul School of Medicine, Department of Cardiology, Turkey

Fatih Tufan
Istanbul University, Istanbul School of Medicine, Department of Internal Medicine, Division of Geriatrics, Turkey

Ahmet Ekmekci
Istanbul University, Istanbul School of Medicine, Department of Internal Medicine, Turkey

Omer A. Sayın
Istanbul University, Istanbul School of Medicine, Department of Cardiovascular Surgery, Turkey

Stamenko Šušak, Lazar Velicki and Dušan Popović
Institute of Cardiovascular Diseases Vojvodina, Sremska Kamenica, Serbia

Ivana Burazor
Clinical Centers, Nis, Serbia

Omer Leal and Juan Bustamante
Department of Cardiovascular Surgery, Hospital Universitario La Princesa, Madrid, Spain

Sergio Cánovas
Department of Cardiac Surgery, Hospital General Universitario de Valencia, Valencia, Spain

Ángel G. Pinto
Department of Cardiac Surgery, Hospital Universitario Gragorio Marañon, Madrid, Spain

Kaan Kirali
Depertment of cardiovascular surgery, kosuyolu heart and research hospital, Istanbul, Turkey

Kazumasa Orihashi
Department of Cardiovascular Surgery, Kochi Medical School, Kochi, Japan

Ibrahim Akin, Stephan Kische, Henrik Schneider, Tim C. Rehders, Christoph A. Nienaber and Hüseyin Ince
University of Rostock, Germany

Hirofumi Saiki and Hideaki Senzaki
Department of Pediatric Cardiology, Saitama Medical Center, Saitama Medical University, Saitama, Japan

Printed in the USA
CPSIA information can be obtained
at www.ICGtesting.com
JSHW011421221024
72173JS00004B/616

9 781632 410252